Contents

Communication Difficulties in Childhood

A practical guide

Edited by
James Law and Alison Parkinson
with Rashmin Tamhne

Foreword by
David Hall
Professor of Community Paediatrics
University of Sheffield

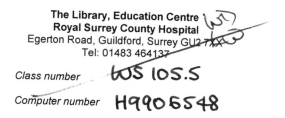

Radcliffe Medical Press

Radcliffe Medical Press Ltd
18 Marcham Road, Abingdon, Oxon OX14 1AA

British Library Cataloguing in Publication Data

A catalogue record for this book is available from the British Library.

ISBN 1 85775 098 5

Typeset by Acorn Bookwork, Salisbury, Wiltshire
Printed and bound by TJ International Ltd, Padstow, Cornwall

Foreword

Bees, whales and chimpanzees have some remarkable communication techniques, but Homo sapiens is unique in the extent of his ability to manipulate and share ideas and information. It is all the more surprising then that the study of how children acquire this skill in all its richness and variety, and why it goes wrong, has been a respectable area of clinical and scientific enquiry for barely half a century.

In the sixties and seventies, clinical approaches to children with speech and language problems were, in retrospect, somewhat naïve and were rarely subjected to dispassionate investigation. But now the whole field is expanding fast and is benefiting from the recent emphasis on evidence-based medicine. Better understanding of the range and limits of normality, more careful classification of clinical disorders and ingenious experimental design characterise the material available to authors. Perhaps the most exciting opportunities are those arising from collaborative work between language experts and other disciplines, notably genetics and neuro-imaging.

Application of basic epidemiological principles to concepts like screening has resulted in a re-examination of previous assumptions about which children need intervention and how they can be identified. In turn, the need for robust studies on whether, when and how intervention works has become increasingly evident. Primary prevention, by applying recent insights into language acquisition, seems unlikely to eliminate the problem of severe 'specific' language impairment, which may well have a biological basis, but it does offer the possibility of raising the overall level of language functioning. Instead of asking whether a child has or has not got a language problem, we could apply the Geoffrey Rose principle and ask – how much of it has he got? This approach might lead us into a classic public health opportunity to raise the general level of language function and usage, particularly for children whose exposure to quality language learning experiences is limited.

The authors have assembled an impressive array of material and experts in this book. A glance at the contents page shows the breadth of the subject matter. There is something here for everyone interested in the problems of children who do not develop language at the usual rate or whose language structure and use are atypical.

David Hall
July 1999

Preface

Speech, language, and indeed all manifestations of communication, play a central role in the psychological well being of the child and the family. A child who experiences difficulties in developing communication skills is vulnerable because such difficulties have the potential to interfere with that well being. Consequently it is the responsibility of both health and educational services to identify children with such difficulties and provide intervention in the most appropriate manner. Children with communication difficulties of one sort or another are relatively common, but the conditions that they experience have a rather uncertain natural history in the first few years. If they persist thereafter they can result in long-term problems for the individuals concerned. Although communication difficulties are experienced by people from all walks of life, many of those affected come from families with histories of learning difficulties and by definition may not be able to find a voice for themselves in a way that many other clinical groups have done. Likewise the inability to communicate can effectively put a barrier up between the individual and what society can offer. This places the onus fairly and squarely on the professionals with whom children with communication difficulties come into contact to identify their needs and to respond appropriately. But the paradox is that many professionals have found it hard to know what they are looking for and equally challenging to judge what weight to attach to observed symptoms. When is it best to assess speech and language and which speech and language skills best predict future development? What is the best sort of advice to give to parents?

This book is intended for people in regular contact with children, especially those who may be in a position to identify children who stand to gain from clinical support. It is targeted at medical personnel, general practitioners and at those involved in primary care groups, at rehabilitation co-ordinators and at those with special responsibility for commissioning services for children. It will also be useful for psychologists, speech and language therapists, teachers and others involved in the provision of special education. It is particularly intended for those working with young children.

Communication is made up of a range of identifiable components (vocabulary, syntax, the ability to understand spoken language, the ability to interact effectively) and no observation is complete without consideration of all of these. It is not simply a matter of assessing a child on a single occasion. Each one of these components has its own developmental progression and to make matters more complicated they interact differently across time. Vocabulary may be a useful marker at two years of age but by four years must be taken in the context of the child's use of syntax and the ability to retell stories. Any assessment or intervention must also include careful analysis of the child's communication environment. Each child develops his or her communication skills in the context of the home, the school and, as they get older, their peer group, together with all the other shared activities with which the child becomes involved. While it is possible that, in extreme cases, those activities may contribute to the problem, the assumption made here is that for most children there is a major organic component to their communication difficulty. But, as in other aspects of genetic research, the interesting question is not what percentage is predetermined and what is left for the environment to impact upon, but what features of the environment can be altered to help the child maximise his or her potential and what risk and protective factors need to be taken into consideration. It is, after all, this fusion of the individual child and the context in which he or she is raised that creates the person in the longer term.

Whereas it was once thought that apparent difficulties in the early years resolved spontaneously, a different picture is now emerging. It is true that a sizeable number of children who are slow to start speaking may go on to cope perfectly well in school, but equally it is now clear that many children will be struggling to cope with their difficulty into adulthood. It may affect their literacy skills and thus their access to all curriculum subjects. It may well affect their capacity to interact with peers. Equally, of course, such difficulties may impact on those with whom they come into contact, their family, their friends and their peers in school. But what does a developmental speech and language difficulty look like in adulthood? Although many would recognise their own early history of reading and writing problems impacting on their current performance, it is less easy to ascertain what impact these difficulties would have on relationships, on employment or on lifestyle. In the modern, highly competitive, labour market, which prizes articulate presentation and flexible reasoning, there may be little in the way of opportunities for the young adult with communication difficulties. Communication difficulties may prove to be an antecedent of social exclusion for many and as such of considerable social importance in modern society.

But it is not enough to identify that a child is experiencing difficulties. Appropriate and useful intervention is what parents are searching for. Intervention is then the application of appropriate techniques to both the child and the family at an appropriate time in the development of the condition. Too early and it may lack relevance to the child or the family and may serve to label a child prematurely. Too late and there is a risk of not optimising the child's potential, resulting in a raft of secondary conditions, such as behaviour problems and reluctance to socialise with peers. In such circumstances early communication difficulties may reasonably be seen as a pre-symptomatic stage. It is important to stress that interventions may focus on the child, but it is as likely that they will focus on modifying the environment for that child. So rather than aiming to remove an impairment, to cure a child of his or her communication difficulty, the intervention may aim to improve the communication skills of those around the child by helping them to provide an optimum communica-

tive environment for the child. Throughout the book there is also a recognition that
there is a need for evidence-based practice, the use of the best available evidence to
inform clinical and policy decision making. As in much of medicine it is often easier
to speak of evidence-based practice than it is to find the definitive sort of evidence
that would enable such decisions to be made. But the practice related to communication difficulties is now beginning to move in this direction, although there is still
much work to be done in the identification of the most appropriate outcomes.

Although this book is not concerned with a description of services as such, it is
noteworthy that services for communication-impaired children may be arranged
differently from those available for other client groups. For example, provision relies
heavily on the interaction between different agencies, of which the health services
are only one part. The independent sector plays an important role in this area both
in providing services and in supporting and representing parents. Similarly education services necessarily play an integral role in supporting families and children as
the children go into preschool and then school. Indeed the provision of services to
these children is characterised by the need for multi-agency collaboration at all
stages.

The book is divided into two sections. Part one provides the backbone of the text.
Chapter 1 gives an overview of the key areas subsumed under the rather amorphous
term 'communication' and highlights the need to recognise that the most apparent
aspects of a difficulty, those that the listener hears, such as speech itself, are not
necessarily the most clinically important. Chapter 2 deals with prevalence, summar-
ising many of the findings. It concludes that the application of a single figure for the
prevalence of communication difficulties gives a misleading impression of homoge-
neity for a group of conditions which manifests itself in different degrees of severity
and in formulations. Chapter 3 tackles the process of identification and screening and
emphasises the role that the primary health clinician plays in making good use of
parental judgement. Chapter 4 focuses on the medical assessment and the main areas
which need to be tackled by medical personnel wishing to examine possible aetiologies and to search for treatable antecedents. Chapter 5 describes the assessment from
the perspective of a speech and language therapist, providing a clear picture of what
needs to be assessed within the communication system. Chapter 6 extends this assessment process, looking at assessment and treatment in a multicultural society and
helps resolve some of the complex issues of whether a communication difficulty is
present independent of a bilingual upbringing. As it stands, bilingual children are
often the last to be referred for speech and language therapy or other support because
it is wrongly assumed that the bilingualism accounts for all their difficulties. Chapter
7 looks at the available literature on intervention for speech and language difficulties
and Chapter 8 reports the findings of a study of the long-term implications of speech
and language impairments.

Part two provides a series of short pieces on the speech and language difficulties
associated with a number of different conditions. Each one follows the same pattern,
describing the condition with some illustrations, outlining treatment, and providing

some helpful literature. Each of these is written by a recognised practitioner/researcher in the field and presents good practical advice to the clinician.

There has been much discussion in recent years about the different labels that are used to describe the possible problems of children with communication difficulties. The use of the term 'difficulty' rather than 'impairment', 'delay' or 'disorder' is used because it describes what others see. It makes no assumptions about underlying pathology and avoids making use of what has come to be recognised as a rather artificial distinction between delay and disorder. The term 'communication' is sometimes associated with more complex developmental conditions in which speech and language are only one component and hints at a difficulty in conveying messages in any modality. Communication encompasses speech and language but incorporates all the other aspects of behaviour which refer to the interaction between individuals. For example, while there are children whose speech and language is obviously affected either because they are unintelligible or because they are unable to formulate sentences as well as other children of their age, for others the difficulty may lie in less obviously verbal aspects of communication. Many of these children exhibit behavioural symptoms (Chapter 12) which are as important to those around them as, for example, their receptive language difficulties. Similarly the selectively mute child (Chapter 21) may not have a speech problem as such but clearly the withdrawal from communication represents a communication difficulty. The book is principally concerned with communication difficulties which are primary in nature, that is those that cannot readily be associated with other developmental conditions. However, a glance at Part two will reveal that a number of conditions have been included which might account for the communication difficulties experienced by the child, such as autism (Chapter 11), cerebral palsy (Chapter 14), hearing loss (Chapter 17) or learning disability (Chapter 19). These have been incorporated because the communication difficulties are frequently a distinctive feature of the condition. To make the text accessible, chapters are not, for the most part, heavily referenced.

Many people have been involved in the production of this book. In particular our thanks go Rashmin Tamhne, paediatrician, who had the original idea for the book, and Frances Glascoe from the department of Pediatrics of Vanderbilt University in Nashville for her considerable contribution and for providing the contact with the many US authors, the majority of whom are from Vanderbilt University in Tennessee.

We would also like to thank the following: Kathryn Mann, speech and language pathologist, for her contributions to the writing on expressive language disorder; Deborah Plummer, speech and language therapist, for her contribution to the discussion on stammering and for her helpful suggestions on Chapters 1 and 5; Dr Miriam Ish-Horowicz, paediatrician, for her comments on Chapter 1; Dr Gabrielle Laing, paediatrician, for her discussion of prevalence in the context of Chapter 2; Lindsay Thomason, speech and language therapist for her contribution to Chapter 15; Ros Herman, speech and language therapist, for her comments on Chapter 17; Dr Sue Roulstone, speech and language therapist, and Christine Cassell, senior educational psychologist, for their comments regarding the current educational context.

Finally thanks go to Gillian Nineham and Kathryn Shellswell from Radcliffe Medical Press for their support and advice throughout the project.

James Law
Alison Parkinson
July 1999

List of contributors

Linda Ashford
Assistant Professor
Division of Child Development
Vanderbilt University School of Medicine
Nashville, USA

Anna Baumgaertel
Assistant Professor
Division of Child Development
Vanderbilt University School of Medicine
Nashville, USA

Helen Cockerill
Newcomen Centre
Guy's Hospital
London, UK

Steven R Couch
Assistant Professor
Division of Child Development
Vanderbilt University School of Medicine
Nashville, USA

Frances Page Glascoe
Associate Professor
Division of Child Development
Vanderbilt University School of Medicine
Nashville, USA

James W Hall III
Associate Professor
Department of Hearing and Speech
   Sciences
Vanderbilt University School of Medicine
Nashville, USA

Corinne Haynes
Speech and Language Therapist
Nottingham, UK

Susie Hoddell
Speech and Language Therapist
West Park Hospital
Surrey, UK

James Law
Senior Lecturer
Department of Clinical Communication
   Studies
City University, London, UK

Janet Lees
Honorary Research Fellow
Neurosciences Unit
Institute of Child Health
Wolfson Centre, London, UK

Deirdre Martin
Senior Lecturer
School of Education
University of Birmingham, UK

Tim Milward
Consultant in Plastic, Aesthetic and Hand
   Surgery
BUPA Hospital
Leicester, UK

Anthony Narula
Consultant ENT Surgeon
Department of Otolaryngology
The Leicester Royal Infirmary, UK

Opal Y Ousley
Developmental Psychologist
Department of Psychology and Human
    Development
Vanderbilt University School of Medicine
Nashville, USA

Alison Parkinson
Speech and Language Therapist
Leicestershire and Rutland Healthcare
    Trust
Leicester, UK

Suzanne Pate
Speech-Language Pathologist
Division of Child Development
Vanderbilt University School of Medicine
Nashville, USA

Theodora Phea Pinnock
Assistant Professor
Division of Child Development
Vanderbilt University School of Medicine
Nashville, USA

Maureen Sanger
Assistant Professor
Division of Community Pediatrics
Vanderbilt University School of Medicine
Nashville, USA

Alice Sluckin
Honorary Visiting Fellow
Department of Psychology
University of Leicester
Leicester, UK

Wendy L Stone
Associate Professor
Division of Child Development
Vanderbilt University School of Medicine
Nashville, USA

Ray Sturner
Associate Professor of Pediatrics
Johns Hopkins University
Baltimore, USA

Rashmin Tamhne
Consultant Paediatrician
Leicestershire and Rutland Healthcare
    Trust
Leicester, UK

Geoff Thorley
Clinical Psychologist
Child and Family Psychiatric Services
Leicestershire and Rutland Healthcare
    Trust
Leicester, UK

Mark L Wolraich
Professor of Pediatrics
Division of Child Development
Vanderbilt University School of Medicine
Nashville, USA

Doris J Wossum
Neuropsychologist
Division of Child Development
Vanderbilt University School of Medicine
Nashville, USA

PART ONE

CHAPTER 1

Children's communication: development and difficulties

James Law

Mum: *What do you want me to do?*
Child (aged 2;2):   *Put back hat on.*

Anyone who has listened to the speech of small children knows that it is full of simple and often rather endearing errors of this type. But are they really errors? They may be wrong if we compare them to the adult model but they are common in the speech of children of this age. Children's communication skills must always be seen in the context of what would be expected for the child's age. This is obvious when we are listening to two-year-olds but it is also relevant when we are considering the older child relative to his or her peers. The type of error illustrated above is to be expected in the language of a child of that age but would be inappropriate in that of a monolingual seven-year-old. Care has to be taken to distinguish between *speech* and *language*. The term 'speech' should be confined to the speech sounds themselves. As a generic term it is helpful to use the term 'communication' and see it as made up of a web of intersecting skills of which speech is one. Separating out communication skills in this way helps to identify the child's strengths and weaknesses across a range of skills and this is important for the purposes of both diagnosis and treatment.

This chapter begins by outlining a highly inclusive model of communication development. This model is compared to the structure of a tree in Box 1.1. The chapter goes on to discuss the normal course of speech and language development, focusing particularly on the very early years because it is here that the roots of language first develop. Likely presenting features of speech and language difficulties will be described.

A model of communication

Communication is a dynamic process. On the one hand it represents an interaction between the individual and the environment. On the other there is also an interplay between the component parts of the communication system.

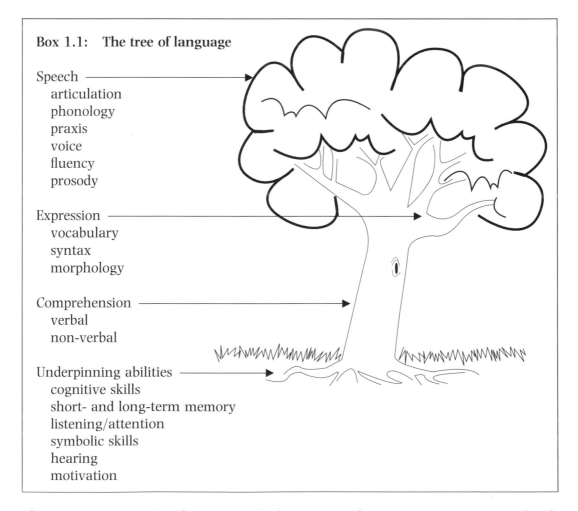

Box 1.1:   The tree of language

Speech
   articulation
   phonology
   praxis
   voice
   fluency
   prosody

Expression
   vocabulary
   syntax
   morphology

Comprehension
   verbal
   non-verbal

Underpinning abilities
   cognitive skills
   short- and long-term memory
   listening/attention
   symbolic skills
   hearing
   motivation

The roots of the tree can be seen as the factors contributing to communicative development. *Motivation* is an obvious example. Without motivation it is unlikely that the child's communication system will develop adequately. There are also structural concerns, such as the development of the necessary cerebral and anatomical structures. Hearing clearly comes into this category, although we should be careful not to see it as a prerequisite for communication. Children who are deaf can learn to communicate perfectly adequately. Children who are not deaf but have mild-to-moderate conductive hearing losses associated with otitis media with effusion often present a more complex picture. The child must have the necessary underpinning *cognitive skills* in order to process and retain incoming information and to formulate the appropriate response. In particular the child must have sufficient short-term and long-term memory. It is the child's short-term auditory memory coupled with the capacity to discriminate auditory phenomena which are critical here. Clearly it is difficult to separate out the roles played by memory and language since memory relies so heavily on linguistic monitoring of input. One way that researchers have attempted to do this is with the use of non-word repetition tasks where a child repeats back a word which has the structure of the native language in terms of the sounds used but has no meaning which the child can use to facilitate recall. Also closely linked is the need for adequate *attention* and *listening skills* such that the child can discriminate appropriate from inappropriate information. At the early stages it is important to identify the child's ability to attend to the object or person to which reference is being made or to direct others to a given object. As the child comes to the end of the preschool years and moves into school the principal issue is whether he or she can control his or her attention, shifting it between competing stimuli – the parent and a toy, the teacher and another child.

Finally the child must learn to understand the symbolic nature of the linguistic world, that is to recognise that one phenomenon can stand for another, connected by means of an ostensibly arbitrary association – a word. Without this skill he or she will find the manipulation of linguistic symbols difficult and language acquisition may well be restricted to a rote learning task. Of particular interest here in the young child is the ability to transform objects in symbolic play, for example by pretending that a banana is a telephone. Interestingly this skill develops in most children at the same time as the child moves from the single-word vocabulary stage in their development to the use of syntax. Different explanations for the exact nature of the relationship between play and language have been suggested.

The trunk of the tree represents the child's *verbal comprehension*, often overlooked by clinicians involved in primary care as they respond to the parent's concerns about speech. It is now widely recognised as a critical area to be covered in the diagnostic process.[1] For example, children with expressive language problems frequently have delayed comprehension skills which would in themselves explain or, at the very least, contribute to their expressive difficulties. Equally, delayed comprehension is often related to delayed cognitive skills and to difficulties associated with behaviour. In the first instance poor comprehension is associated with a poor understanding of vocabulary items and for any child the acquisition of word meaning can remain an obstacle to linguistic progress. Subsequently it can be seen in an inability to extract the relevant meaning from sentences. For many children the main difficulty is that posed by decoding the message 'on line', i.e. at the speed that they hear it. It is important to distinguish between verbal comprehension and *non-verbal comprehension*. The former can be context-free, the latter is usually context-dependent. At its most sophisticated, non-verbal comprehension may refer to alternative methods of communication such as augmentative, manual or 'signed' systems. But it may also refer to the interpretation of noises used in a conventional manner, such as the symbolic noise of a car favoured by many children or the use of sighs, laughter, etc., which may have meaning at an affective rather than a symbolic level. Children often become very skilled in extracting sufficient meaning from the context to determine the gist of a given request without actually understanding what has been said. For example, a child may function at an acceptable level in nursery by watching others and picking out key words used by the teacher. Being able to do this is obviously an adaptive skill but it is important that parents and professionals recognise when it is happening.

The branches of the tree comprise the child's expressive language skills. In particular we are referring here to *vocabulary development* and to the *development of syntax*. For most children, formulating sentences quickly becomes an automatic skill, but for some the complex relationships between subjects and verbs, the construction of conjoined sentences (connected *with*, *and*, *but*, etc.) and the embedding of sentences within one another (this ball's like the one *that I have at home*) is too complex a task. A number of children who have particular difficulty with the manipulation of syntax often have specific difficulties with the small changes to words that affect meaning. These are known as *morphological changes* and comprise the skills necessary to change verb endings (-ing, -es, etc.) and mark plurals (*inflectional morphology*) or to derive one word from another (*discussion* from *discuss*) which is known as *derivational morphology*. Children start marking morphological changes at 18–24 months, but as with all other aspects of language development in this early stage many continue to make errors well into primary school years.

Expression is obviously about the formal aspects of language but it is also about the *semantics*, the child's intended meaning. Initially the child has a very limited range of such meanings. Perhaps he or she points, meaning 'it's over there' and raises his or her arms, meaning 'pick me up' or 'help me', but gradually a range of linguistic functions develops which expands dramatically once they are supported by syntax. The important point here is that the same words may often be used for different functions and establishing the level of a child's vocabulary may not be an adequate way of revealing what he or she is doing with the words that he or she does have. From the parent's perspective the child who has a wide range of semantic functions is generally perceived to be more communicative and probably receives more verbal responses than the child with a much more restricted range of intended meanings even if the two children have the same tested vocabulary level. Expression characteristically refers to *narrative skills* in the older child. Sentence structure is obviously important, but as the child goes into school it is the capacity to report on actions and retell stories which characterises his or her communication skills. Indeed there is some suggestion that it is these skills in particular which best discriminate children with poor language skills when assessed at four years of age.[2]

The leaves on the tree signify the more external aspects of communication development, the sounds which go to make up language. The production of sound can be divided into three categories. Those functions associated with the structure and function of the oral space are referred to as *articulation*. These include the tongue, lips, palate and the connections between the oral, nasal and pharyngeal cavities. Any child will have his or her own set of sounds which will approximate to a greater or lesser extent to the adult norm. Those functions are associated with the pattern in which the individual learns to differentiate one sound from another, patterns which are distinct for different languages. This is known as *phonological development*. There is also the interaction between articulation and phonology, the capacity of the child to control the rapid motor sequences necessary to produce target phonological output. These sequences are built up into automatic sequences such that not every sound is articulated in isolation. The repetition which is commonly associated with very early language development probably goes a long way to facilitate this co-ordination. It is unclear whether this calls for a separate term but it may be helpful to think of it as *praxis*, and it can reasonably be construed as the link between the formulation of the sound string that goes to make up the word and its execution.

When we listen to a speaker the focus of the attention is on the message. If that message is unintelligible because the articulation or phonological system is impaired this will affect our interpretation of the message. But our interpretation is also affected by other, less tangible, aspects of speech. For example, we may be influenced by a person's *voice* quality, whether they sound hoarse or strained, and by their *fluency*, how much they hesitate, whether they appear able to get the words out easily. In most cases the process is so effortless that we pay little attention to it. We become aware of these characteristics of speech when the child has severe difficulties, for example when they stammer. Finally there is the intonation or *prosody*, which carries the message, emphasises salient words and adds nuance to meaning. It might be considered that difficulties in this area are of a different nature to speech or language difficulties. This is probably true but again the central role of prosody is brought home when a speaker is unable to modulate an utterance. It is often difficult to decode the intended meaning and can lead to conversational mismatches.

While morphological, syntactic and phonological features are clearly integral to the process of communication it is important to recognise that communication takes place between individuals not solely within the language centres in the temporal lobe. The process reflects the way people interact and share meaning with one another. This is the very stuff of communication and, without pushing the analogy too far, may be seen as the water flowing through the roots, trunk and branches of the tree. The term sometimes used for this aspect of communication is *pragmatics* and it refers to the skills necessary to interact effectively, to interpret what the speaker is meaning to say, to read between the lines of the more obvious structural aspects of communication. It is clear from the child who brings the biscuit tin to his mother with an appealing look on his face that there is more to communication than the formal properties of language. This is an important distinction which remains a part of an interchange once language develops. For example in the following exchange ...

Mum:	*Will you put your boots on?*
Child (aged 4;2)	*I'm not going on the bike.*

we have a mismatch between the question and the response. A very ordinary request receives an apparently bizarre response which can only be interpreted by an unfamiliar observer when provided with additional knowledge of the context. In this case the child has produced a seemingly anomalous utterance in the context of what the mother has said. In many other instances speakers imply more than is actually said. For young children this can often prove problematic because they are not able to make the link between the implicit and the explicit information and the literal interpretation can be very unrewarding in such instances. The issue becomes more sophisticated as the child has to learn to decode metaphor, sarcasm, etc.

This organic 'tree' analogy is helpful because it relates the various subcomponents one with another in an active sense. Nothing about communication is static either in terms of the interaction between individuals or in terms of the developmental sequence of the individual skills. Furthermore none of these skills develops completely independently of one another.

Developing communication skills across childhood

The first year of life

The development of intention

There is now considerable evidence that children are expressing needs from birth and indeed even *in utero*.[3] Of course, it is impossible to describe these early interactions as far as the child is concerned. Initially he or she is responding to the immediate physical environment, simply reacting to internal imperatives, rather than deliberately conveying a message. But parents often interpret such involuntary movements as communicative and respond accordingly. For example, they may comment on the personality of the baby in the womb and speak to him or her accordingly. Similarly, as soon as he or she is born, parents often speak to the child as if he or she knew what was going on around him or her. It is something of a moot point as to whether the child conditions the parent in this process or vice versa, but the two are clearly collaborating on the task of communication from the word go. Communication in its broadest sense is not something that the infant acquires as an individual but something that he or she shares with those around him or her. Furthermore it starts very early on in life and not when the child starts to speak, a common misconception of which all professionals working with small children need to be aware.

Listening and attention

One of the earliest skills that the child needs to acquire is the capacity to attend and to listen. He or she must learn to recognise the human voice and determine which ones are the most important to listen to. Likewise he or she must learn to discriminate human faces and to recognise which are the most important. It seems that there are some evolutionary adaptations which have the specific effect of facilitating this process. Infants very quickly learn to discriminate the face and voice of their primary care giver and there is some suggestion that the higher frequency ranges found in the female voice may receive preferential treatment as far as the child is concerned. The child quickly learns to listen to words and to break up the sentences that the adults around him or her are saying. Long before he or she is able to use any of the words, he or she is able to distinguish a wide range of familiar words and there is even some evidence that the child is able to discriminate between nouns and verbs well before his or her first birthday. In essence the brain is using the environment to lay down a template over which later experience can be laid.

The increasing control over speech output

Initially, as we have noted, the sounds that the child uses are involuntary. Gradually these come under the child's volitional control and by the age of perhaps six months the child has begun to babble or play with sounds in a consistent manner. Initially we hear the cooing often associated with contentment and consonant/vowel sounds [*ma ma ma*] or [*ba ba ba*] when in a more heightened state. Gradually these sounds come to be assembled into strings of similar sounds or *reduplicated babbling* at perhaps nine or ten months. At this point we often hear parents attributing the child with their first words. Sometimes disappointed mothers will say that the child said [*dada*] and enquire why [*mama*] did not come first. It would be wrong to see the child as necessarily choosing what to say at this stage. The parent has simply extrapolated from what the child has said to the adult model. In fact it is the context in which the words are said which provides the meaning, not the explicit intention of the child. But by this stage it is becoming very difficult to distinguish between the two.

For some years there has been an argument as to whether the sounds used in babbling are continuous with those in the first words that a child uses. In fact there is some evidence that children use a very wide range of sounds in their babbling, but they seem to start again when they begin to use words. It is as if the two skills, babbling and speaking, fulfil different functions. The former is primarily a motor function with a broad communicative intent 'I'm here!'. It also starts the child practising the motor sequences which make up the building blocks of speech development. Clearly children do not articulate every sound in every word. Rather they acquire automatic sequences which allow them to speak at speed and this process starts with the endless repetition which begins so early on in the communicative process. The latter, by contrast, seems more clearly linked into language. In effect, babbling is superseded by early speech and no longer becomes functionally very useful. It is interesting that some children seem to return to using strings of undifferentiated speech or *jargon* later on, particularly when they are under emotional pressure, for example at the birth of a younger sibling.

The development of play

It is now widely recognised that there is a symbiotic relationship between play and language in the early years and nowhere is this more apparent than in the child's development of symbolic representations. As indicated above, these correspond to the understanding that one thing can stand for something else in the way that a word can stand for an object or referent and that this relationship is communicable. Children do not usually develop a working understanding of this relationship until the second year of life but that understanding itself is based on underpinning manipulation skills and social skills which develop in the first year. Of particular interest here is the development of the child's understanding of social routines and what amount to simple jokes. For example, it is common to see a child taking an active role in setting up social routines, such as smiling coupled with putting his or her head on one side. The game is developed with one parent, extended into the family and then tried on others. Similarly children learn to manipulate an object in their environment thereby acquiring an understanding of its physical properties. It is no coincidence that it is these familiar objects which are often the first to be named.

Motor control and the development of referencing

There is one other prelinguistic behaviour that needs to be highlighted at the end of the first year. As the babbling increases so does the child's motor co-ordination. Walking follows quickly on from this but we also need to note what the child is doing with his or her hands. By ten months children have started pointing in a qualitatively different way. They have shifted from what is known as the 'proto-imperative' point in which the child points, implying 'I know it's there and I want it!' to the 'proto-declarative' point in which the child points, looks at the object and then looks to his or her parent and back to the object and so on. The message is qualitatively different because it suggests the child sharing his or her meaning with the parent. He or she is saying 'I know that you know what I am referring to'. In effect, he or she is beginning to communicate in a symbolic way, indicating an understanding of shared meaning. Initially these points may be accompanied by an undifferentiated noise, but parents usually map a word on to this context and this becomes the slot into which the child starts to insert his or her first words. Interestingly, for most children once words start to fill these slots the purpose of this type of referencing becomes redundant and is discarded. If children continue to use this referential pointing beyond 18 months it is usually a sign that spoken language is not yet functional for them.

The first year is characterised by the understanding of the role of the listener in conversation and the development of intentional communication. In addition we see the early development of attention and listening skills and the laying down of early motor patterns which subsequently become associated with speech. Above all it is the child's motivation to communicate that develops in this period and it is this that sets the child up for participation in the more obviously 'linguistic' aspects of communication which start to come on-stream in the second year of life. None of the skills is lost. All are adapted to different functions. It is important to recognise that difficulties in acquiring any of these early, prelinguistic skills may result in subsequent difficulties acquiring language. As we shall see below there are a great many conditions that affect a child's capacity to listen in the first year. Equally there are conditions with a pronounced motor component, which will affect the child's capacity to produce sounds. Finally any of these difficulties may affect the level of interaction between parent and child. Difficulties on the part of the child or inappropriate expectations on the part of the parent may lead to a disruption in the timing of the interaction between parent and child – the dance – as it is sometimes called.[4] The level at which the difficulty occurs inevitably determines where we need to intervene.

The shift to words

Parents and professionals often collude in the emphasis they place on the first few words that a child uses. In fact, as work on the MacArthur Communicative Development Inventories has shown, the variability between individual children is such that it is relatively difficult to interpret the data clinically (*see* Figure 1.1).[5] Nonetheless it is clear that although the actual words that children acquire may differ, the uses to which they are put probably do not. Initially, words may not have a specific syntactic role. 'Drink' may be used for a noun – the cup or the liquid – or for the verb – the process of drinking. But gradually the child's need to differentiate the message forces him or her to make the meaning clearer for the listener. Initially, he or she may do this with accompanying gesture but this will soon be replaced by other words, e.g. 'more drink' or 'there drink'. The important point to reiterate here is the role of the listener in providing the contexts for the child's language to develop. Some authors have spoken of the adult providing the 'scaffolding' giving the structure and allowing the child to make use of the communicative opportunities.[6] Typically, parent and child will create routines – bath or feeding time for example – and will go through the same rituals both reinforcing each other. Later the games will lose their potency and be re-enacted only as a memory of their former importance. But in the early

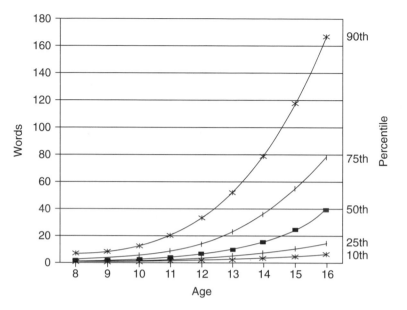

Figure 1.1 The development of vocabulary production. From the MacArthur Communicative Development Inventories.[5]

stages of communicative development one must not underestimate the importance of these games.

The acquisition of the first few words is often quite an effortful process for the young child. He or she struggles to differentiate speakers' words from the speech stream that he or she hears. But once the child has understood the idea that the word can be mapped directly on to the context this seems to trigger an extraordinary hunger to extend this process to the labelling of the world around him or her. Once this is in action the child starts to carry out a process which is sometimes referred to as 'fast mapping' – mapping the word heard to the context at speed.[7] This increase in speed then allows him or her to become involved in processing conversation rather than single words. The child is then on his or her way to becoming a linguistic rather

Table 1.1 Early relational meanings

Category	Example
Existence, nomination or notice	*hi spoon, that book*
Non-existence or disappearance	*all gone*
Reoccurrence	*more read*
Action	*go home*
Location	*where doggie gone*
Possession	*mine*
Attribution	*big truck*

than an intuitive communicator. As young children come to understand and observe more about their world, their vocabulary begins to reflect new insights and knowledge. At the same time they come to learn that there are rules governing the way words are used. For example, they may learn the word 'dada' and apply it in a number of contexts before homing in on the conventional application.

As vocabulary expands children begin to express a range of different semantic relational meanings (*see* Table 1.1).[8] Although many of these are clearly word combinations there are some authors who make the point that this early combinatorial stage does not really reflect early syntactic development as such.[9]

Non-verbal behaviour

It is all too easy to assume that once the child starts to communicate verbally, speech and language is the only method of communication worth considering. In fact there are a great many clues to be found in observing the child's behaviour above and beyond the level of verbal response. There is a constant stream of visual and auditory information available during an interaction and participants ignore this information at their peril. In fact the greater part of meaning in a communicative interaction may be made up of this type of information. For example, the way someone sits or stands and the clothes they wear may be just as important in determining whether the hearer believes what they are saying as the content of what they say, their accent or their vocal pitch. It seems likely that the use of such information is highly dependent on the age, class, gender and culture of the participants. Children start to learn how to make sense of this type of information very early on in their communicative careers. They often scrutinise faces and copy gestures recognising that this is a way into the social world of those around them. Of course, at a more formal level non-verbal behaviour may have a specific communicative intent in the form of specific gestures. These are often at an iconic level in that the relationship between the action and the intended communication is transparent, e.g. lifting a hand to the mouth for drinking. They can reach a symbolic level in the case of the signing systems used by the deaf community or those with learning disabilities.

The relative role of genetics and the environment

Critically important to our understanding of both the way speech and language develop and the potential for modifying its course, is the role played by the environment. Intervention to remediate communication difficulties depends on the extent to which its course in the individual is or is not predetermined and the malleability of the individual. At one level it is self-evident that the environment plays a considerable role. Children learn the language to which they are exposed and they pick up many of the turns of phrase of their parents. But does the way in which the parents speak to the child, effectively train the child to speak and can a given style accelerate that development? The parental style which has been most often studied is referred to as

---

Box 1.2:   Child-directed speech

Accentuated pitch
Increased repetition
Exaggeration of prominent words
Simplification of syntax
Speech style slow and deliberate
Exaggerated bodily and facial expression

'motherese' or more recently 'child directed speech' (*see* Box 1.2).[10] The terms relate to the way in which more experienced communicators use language when interacting with the child before they can keep up with the conversation.

Whether this recognisable style actually teaches children to speak or accelerates that development remains unclear. Of all the aspects that have been studied, the only specific relationship that has been identified is the relationship between the adult's use of question forms and the child's acquisition of auxiliary verbs (have, do, are, etc.). Given that these come at the beginning of a question this is probably not surprising. That there are not more obvious grammatical links is perhaps more surprising. In fact children do not learn to imitate the motherese style when they start to speak. Furthermore, while there is now considerable evidence that this style is not common to all cultures, there is no evidence that children from cultures which do not embrace this style necessarily have greater difficulty learning language. Rather it seems that the style draws the child's attention to language in a meaningful way. It makes the spoken word especially interesting, but having done this engages the child's own language-processing skills. The essence of the function of these behaviours seems to be the development of *semantic contingency* – the highlighting of relevant aspects of the context to encourage the child to process the links between what is said and what is referred to.[11]

The discussion related to child-directed speech has had considerable implications for the way in which we have come to understand language development. As with all behaviour there is a commonly recognised interplay between nature and nurture, between the way in which the environment and the organism interact. In many cases this is probably rather a sterile argument. It is obvious that both are involved and it is rather invidious to attribute percentages one way or another. In the case of language development it is necessary to consider whether children could reasonably acquire language simply from the language they hear in their environment. Some have indeed suggested that the environment is paramount. Indeed the earlier emphasis on the role of the parent as communicative partner would rather support this argument. However, it remains highly improbable, given the low level of active tuition that most parents give their children, that they would be able to develop the most complex cognitive function known to man within such a short period of time.

Most authors nowadays would accept that the human child is preprogrammed or 'hard wired' to make sense of and acquire language.[12] They speak of rather abstract concepts such as a 'language acquisition device' or 'linguistic canalisation'. Some speak of specific constraints that the child brings to bear on the incoming information in order to make sense of it. Unfortunately little is known about the neurological nature of this black box, the language processor, and much is left to hypothesis and speculation on the basis of the external behaviour of the child. Some progress has been made in recent years in establishing the genetic origins of speech and language development. For a long time it has been known that communication difficulties run in families and there is emerging evidence that heritability is stronger among those with the poorest language skills.[13] Increasingly there is a suggestion of genotypes related to specific language impairment (SLI).[14,15]

Even accepting the rationale for such a processor it is still necessary to look for an explanation of how it interacts with its environment. It is fairly clear now that the organism probably provides the lower threshold but the environment provides the upper threshold. The input the child receives can help accelerate the development of skills but, except in extreme cases of neglect or neurological insult, probably does not actively interfere with the process of language acquisition in a clinical sense. As Pinnock and Wolraich indicate in Chapter 22, while there is an overall socioeconomic effect on language development, performance cannot necessarily be predicted from the environment in which the child is raised.

Difficulties arising at the early verbal stage

One of the most common concerns expressed to family doctors relates to slow language development. If this is expressed before the child is two and a half years this is most likely to be a concern about the development of vocabulary. Often it comes from direct comparison made with other children of the same age or siblings when they were at the age in question. These worries may be expressed as a result of the parent seeking out the professional concerned and/or they may arise out of routine surveillance or screening (*see* Chapter 3).

It is important to take parental concerns seriously. The evidence suggests that parents who express such concerns are usually right about their child having a difficulty.[16] The aetiology of the condition may not be so readily available and parental expression of concern about vocabulary development may also be a request for help about other aspects of health or development, both recognised and unacknowledged. The central point is that these concerns are likely to reflect real clinical problems. Although it is true that some of these are likely to resolve spontaneously, it is unlikely that the differential diagnosis can be made with any certainty. The vocabulary level can usefully be seen as a litmus paper, a marker, for a range of other conditions or may be the problem in its own right.

It is also important to monitor other *paralinguistic* features, those which are not linguistic as such but underpin the linguistic system, such as attention and listening skills on the one hand and social skills on the other. By the end of the first year and throughout the second we should also be looking for children who are not able to focus their attention on people or objects. Poor attention to objects and sound is likely to preface difficulties with both receptive and expressive language. If the child is not able to focus his or her attention to the environment, extracting the appropriate information about labels or about the way in which language is used, he or she may be at risk of slow language development. Again it is likely that hearing and general learning abilities may be a contributory problem but this may not be the case. A child who passes a hearing test at ten months may still experience difficulties attending to spoken language.

Problems related to the development of social skills are likely to prove difficult to disentangle from the normal range of social skills in very young children. However, by 18 months it may be possible to distinguish the child who actively resists social engagement or shows indifference to people. Recent attempts at screening for early symptoms of autism in children at this age have had some success.[17]

The second year and the period when vocabulary appears in most children at such a rate is one in which it is notoriously difficult to identify clinical problems with great accuracy. The noise of normal development seems to swamp the signal that clinicians are looking for. Nonetheless there are clearly problem areas which can be monitored if parents or professionals are concerned. Poor vocabulary development accompanied by poor attention skills and a lack of interest in social interaction characterise one end of the spectrum. At the other end are the children who seem to have intact underlying skills and clearly want to communicate but for whom the whole process of expression is problematic. The important point about these very early attempts at identifying and classifying communication problems is that, for the most part, the children are being identified on the basis of their communication skills. The differential diagnosis of what it is that is happening to the individual, and thereby the establishment of the likely outcome of such difficulties, is often some way in the future.

Moving to syntax

The first phenomenon that the parent usually notices once the first ten or so words have been acquired is the speed at which the child's expressive vocabulary proceeds to develop. By 18 months nearly half of all children are using more than 100 words.[5] By 30 months 70% of children are using 500 or more words. But it is not as if they simply go on adding new words. By 18 months 68% of girls and 49% of boys are combining words. Most researchers would now argue that the rapidly expanding range of needs that the child is wishing to express is driving the acquisition of new structures. The child wants to comment on the world but also to control it. He or she wants to use others to get what he or she wants and wants to stop them from doing things. It is often assumed that the child knows what he or she is intending to say but that those around the child miss the point. A common illustration is the use of what are sometimes known as 'pivot phrases', such as 'mummy sock', which combine two words but which still need to be heavily interpreted by the listener according to the context. Does the child mean 'that's mummy's sock' or 'mummy put on/take off my sock'?

From the child's point of view real progress is made when he or she begins to make sense of and use verbs effectively. Once he or she is able to 'map' verbs in the way that he or she can map nouns on to context, a whole new vista of possibilities opens up. Verbs are generally much more difficult for a child to acquire because they carry with them all sorts of additional information. Who does what and to whom? When was it carried out – the past, present or future? Each form requires a knowledge of how to 'mark' the verb. Again the variability across children in their acquisition of syntactic forms can be considerable, as the distribution for the acquisition of phrases illustrated Figure 1.2 suggests, and this can make it difficult to determine where the low range of average merges with 'problem' levels of syntactic development.

Morphology

The child at this stage makes great strides in their use of morphology. For example he or she learns that the third person singular carries an 's', that the past tense carries an 'ed' ending. Of course there is also the issue of the irregular verbs, which are much more common in English than they are in most other languages. It is an interesting, commonly observed, phenomenon that children often start by imitating constructions

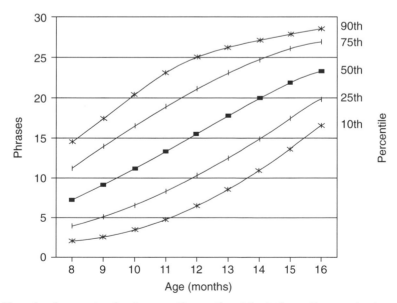

Figure 1.2 The development of phrases. From the MacArthur Communicative Development Inventory.[5]

they hear and get them correct but then as they begin to use the construction for themselves rather than just in direct imitation of the adult model they start to make mistakes again. For example an 18-month-old might say 'we went to the shops' but then three months later say 'we goed to the shops' or even 'we wented to the shops'. Some children seem particularly proficient in acquiring morphology, others continue to make errors of this kind up until four or five years of age.

Social skills

The skills already identified as relating to communication development in the first year of life then mesh into these linguistic skills. As the child becomes more aware not only of other communicative partners but of their different roles and status he or she begins to mark this accordingly. He or she learns more about turn-taking and by two years of age may be able to hold a conversation. However, we need to remember that children at this stage remain very self-orientated and the responsibility often rests on the conversational partner to keep the conversation going and repair mistakes when they occur.

Speech

The child's articulation and phonological system are also developing apace. By his or her second birthday most of the *plosive consonants* [p,b,t,d,k,g] and *vowels* have been added to the child's phonetic inventory. Yet the child still simplifies words which are unfamiliar or too long. In particular the *fricative consonants* [th,f,v,s,z,sh], the sounds which require careful control of the airstream, still prove very difficult for most children. Parents often bring this lack of clarity to the attention of primary care workers but, except in the most extreme cases, where feeding and oro-motor difficulties are involved it is very difficult to predict whether lack of phonological precision is really a problem at 18 months or two years.

Box 1.3:   Normal sequence of speech sound acquisition

Age at which 90% of children have acquired the sound
3 years   m b p h w   plus vowels
4 years   k g t d n ng f
5 years   s z l v y th sh ch
6 years   r j

Intelligibility to strangers
2 years   25%
2.5 years   60%
3 years   75%
4 years   90%

Difficulties emerging as the child starts to acquire syntax

As the language of the majority of children takes its course, children who are struggling begin to stand out more. Vocabulary is still a clear marker of weakness in this area and poor vocabulary is often assumed to have a direct link to syntactic development.[9] It seems quite plausible that there is a critical mass of vocabulary items that must be acquired before the child's syntactic development can progress. At a simple level this is obvious. To produce meaningful syntactic utterances the child must be in a position to draw upon a pool of vocabulary items which is both deep enough, in the sense that there are sufficient nouns to represent the labels needed in his or her immediate environment, and wide enough, in the sense that there is a sufficient range of items, nouns, verbs, prepositions and adjectives to allow meaningful sentences to be constructed.

Not surprisingly children with poor early vocabularies are generally slow to construct sentences. When they do, their sentences are marked by the limited range and simple nature of the verbs used, by the telegraphic nature of the utterances and by the lack of adjectives to colour the sentence. So at one level these children have difficulties which can be characterised by limited output and at a numerical level this type of problem is often measured by *mean length of utterance* (MLU), the number of morphological units in a given utterance. For example, *he* *is* *eat-ing* *dinner* would be made up of five morphological units. At another level it is the type of utterance that he or she uses which characterises the output of the language-delayed child.

In the third year of life the child's ability to understand language out of context becomes of central importance to the differential diagnosis and treatment process. Although context-dependent comprehension remains central to the child's experience, a new type of comprehension emerges which allows the child to make deductions about the world from the language he or she hears around him or her. Inevitably this is based on the development of a receptive vocabulary or input vocabulary which the child is able to map on to the world of words with which he or she is surrounded. This, in turn, is based on a capacity to listen and decode language, skills which go back to the first year of life. Some children do not pick up these skills and this makes entry into the language extremely difficult. In some cases this may be due to specific conditions, such as language impairment associated with temporal lobe epilepsy (*see* Chapter 20), and clearly hearing loss and learning difficulties (Chapters 17 and 19) are likely to impact upon the development of comprehension.

However, some children are not very proficient in this area for what appear to be environmental reasons. Although some might say that it is all a matter of our fast-moving, 'sound bite' culture, it seems more likely that these children have difficulty focusing their attention anyway. In such cases parents need to play an active part in encouraging them to focus on what is important in what they hear around them. Those responsible for providing community health services have an active role to play in identifying such children and providing their parents with the necessary support. It is rarely a case of either a purely expressive or receptive language impairment. Many children with expressive delays also have delayed comprehension, albeit at a less severe level. Similarly it is comparatively rare for children to have isolated receptive impairments. It is, of course, possible for children to use language that they do not really understand. One example would be a small group of high-level autistic children who are able to repeat syntactic constructions well in advance of what would be expected for their receptive language age.

By three years or so it is also apparent that some children have reasonably intact syntactic skills but are experiencing specific difficulty with aspects of their speech or their fluency. Isolated phonological delays may be relatively benign in the young child. The differential diagnosis relative to other language domains must be made prior to this decision being reached. In particular the condition may depend on the level of anxiety associated with the lack of clarity on the one hand, and the severity and level of motor involvement on the other. Children who present with particularly severe or inconsistent patterns of speech difficulty, particularly in the context of feeding problems, drooling and poor control of the oral apparatus, may be dyspraxic and as such may be particularly vulnerable to persistent speech problems.

The level of intelligibility may also be affected by the degree of fluency in the child's speech. The reluctant, hesitant child or the child who exhibits effortful behaviour when trying to speak needs careful attention. It may be possible to reassure the parent that 'non-fluency' is comparatively normal in the young child. But for many the problems associated with dysfluency, *stammering* (UK) or *stuttering* (USA), are ones which need to be carefully monitored. Most of these children exhibit problems between two and three years of age, although for some there is a later onset. The course of the stammer may vary, with children experiencing alternating periods of fluency and dysfluency. Dysfluency is often, incorrrectly, considered to be a discrete problem, separate from other language impairments. On assessment dysfluent children may present with mild language difficulties which are likely to contribute to the child's hesitation as they struggle to process a request or formulate a new sentence. This is not always the case and dysfluency may also affect precocious speakers. In either case stammering can be very distressing and should be taken seriously.

The consolidation of language

One of the most alarming phenomena when considering the longitudinal development of children with language difficulties is the extent to which they can come to diverge in their skills relative to their non-affected peers. This divergence is accentuated as the skills of the latter develop apace alongside parental and societal expectations. By four years or so children without communication difficulties are able to use their language and cognitive skills to structure and retell a story accurately. With some exceptions, for example in morphology and verb usage, their attempts may approximate the adult model. Once children have acquired the basic language structures and find them functionally useful they go on to experiment with them, constantly refining their output and approximating closer and closer to the adult model. There may be a dissociation between the expectations of the family and the expectations of the social or preschool provision in which the child is placed. Initially children often imitate the style of speech of their elders and of other children around them. This may seem out of place in the very young child. But gradually these constructions become assimilated into the child's own system and they become a part of their linguistic culture. The same goes for speech, of course, and children become increasingly aware of how people speak rather than just what they say, for example noticing and imitating accents.

They also become increasingly aware of the social functions of communication. They need to learn to negotiate. To the two-year-old this may simply be a matter of pushing the other child out of the way and grabbing the toy. By the age of four years this process has usually become much more complex. The child has learned about the process of communication and how to manipulate it. For example, he or she can learn in groups of other children and can negotiate with others, using language to sort out problems and to build on prior learning. There are two interesting manifestations of this increased social use of language which coexist with the more obviously constructive aspects. We see an increase in the child's capacity to lie and to tell jokes. By three, many children know that it is possible to say something other than what happened but it is usually perfectly clear to the adult that the deception has taken place. By four, the deception can be concealed and the child has started to master the art of knowing how much to say and how much to conceal. We also see an increase in the child's capacity to joke, to use language to humorous effect. In many ways this reflects the other emerging linguistic abilities because it shows that the child has come to master the syntactic skills and is now putting them to use in a highly interactive way. The problem with jokes, as with lies, is that the intended recipient of the interaction may not perceive them in quite the same way as the one conveying the message.

It is important to recognise that language has both a public and a private function. We often pay more attention to the public aspect as we ask a child to carry out a particular task or to explain what he or she has done. But we must also see it from the child's point of view. Returning to the roots of the tree (*see* Box 1.1) with which we started this chapter, it is clear that motivation drives communication. It is not simply a matter of passively acquiring language or speech. The child must be engaged in the process. For most it is a delight but for some it is a very threatening experience, and as professionals we need to recognise this.

Difficulties arising in older children

It is apparent from discussion earlier in the chapter that by four or five years of age expressive and receptive language disorders have already manifested themselves. Indeed it seems relatively unlikely that a substantial number of new cases develop after this phase. However, the presenting symptoms do change with age. For example, it becomes more difficult to make a judgement about a child's vocabulary skills without formally assessing them as the child moves into school. Instead, the child's ability to retell a story, their narrative skills, becomes paramount. When asked to relate a story the child provides two or three key features of the event. For example, having just been to Disney World for a holiday a seven-year-old child with communication difficulties might say: *went for a ride ... Mickey Mouse and Goofy ... splash*. The child might be said to be experiencing expressive language delay but this label can obscure the presenting features of the difficulty. The older the child the more likely this is to be the case.

The older child might also be presenting with word-finding difficulties. These can only be readily identified once it is clear that the child has sufficient internal vocabulary from which to select the relevant word, a skill for which it may be necessary to formally probe using a standardised assessment of vocabulary. Thus the child, when asked to choose a picture of an umbrella from a set of pictures can do so accurately, but when trying to name the same object at a later date says: *raining ... put it up ... thing*. Where children do have difficulties of this nature it is especially important to observe the nature of the mistakes that they make because this can inform an understanding of the strategies that they are using. For example, some children, such as the one who produced the utterance above, are clearly using semantically relevant cues to help them access the word. Other children seem to approach the word using a phonological strategy. So for umbrella they might say 'under ... umba ... lella'.

For many older children one of the principal manifestations of early speech and language delays is not the speech or language, but the literacy skills. The majority of children who appear to have specific difficulties with reading or writing also had difficulties starting to speak. Given the close relationship between the spoken and the written word this is hardly surprising, but as Hoddell notes in Chapter 16 the relationship between early speech and language difficulties and literacy is often overlooked. Of course for some children the early speech difficulties are directly linked with persistent difficulties in this area. A small group of children – usually those with problems of a dyspraxic nature – continue to have considerable communication difficulties simply because they cannot make themselves understood.

Of particular importance in the older child is the capacity to interact effectively with peers. Many children with language impairments find this difficult. Their expressive difficulties create problems and they often do not have the strategies to disentangle themselves when the conversation breaks down and needs to be repaired. However, there is also a group of children for whom the primary difficulty is in the area of intervention. These children often have adequate expressive language in that they are able to formulate full sentences with relatively little difficulty. They appear to have adequate listening skills but the content of their expressive language is often bizarre and repetitive.

As already indicated, for part of the preschool period it is common for children to exhibit 'normal non-fluency'. For some of these children dysfluency continues and can make it very difficult for the child to integrate into the school environment. In some cases the child may be teased for his or her speech and may withdraw and avoid social interaction with peers. On the one hand there are the behaviours commonly associated with dysfluency, stammering or stuttering, notably sound and syllable repetitions, prolongations of syllables, pauses within words and, more worrying, the practice of 'blocking' on words and manifesting excessive tension leading to tics and distracting behaviours. On the other hand there is the individual child's response to these behaviours. These responses often exacerbate the initial difficulty.

There is also a group of children who present as silent in one situation but not in other contexts. Commonly the child does not speak in school but is reported to be fluent at home. This is a relatively common pattern when the child first goes into nursery but if it persists and it appears that the child is opting not to engage in the class it is possible that a diagnosis of *selective mutism* may be made (*see* Chapter 21). This condition is often construed as an emotional disorder but it is important to note that such children may present with co-occurring speech and language delays. However, it is the reluctance to engage in the process of the classroom which draws attention to them.

Individual differences in speech and language development

It is tempting to assume that because the majority of individuals learn to communicate with such consummate skill that everyone does this in the same way. However, while it is generally true that language has many more common properties than dissimilar properties across individuals, and indeed across languages themselves, there is an emerging body of evidence which suggests that in the very early years there are two or more styles which children adopt. Some select a highly imitative style which often appears to be following the intonation patterns of the more experienced speakers around them. These children are sometimes known as *expressive* language learners because they seem to emphasise the need to express themselves sometimes at the expense of content. By contrast there is a group of children who have come to be known as *referential* language learners who from a very early stage in their development seem to favour nouns and the process of labelling their world. In the early stages these children may appear less fluent because they speak less but they seem to emphasise the content of their utterance, perhaps at the expense of being less able as emerging conversationalists.

It remains something of a moot point as to whether these apparent differences in style persist through into school and beyond. It seems likely that for most children it is not a matter of one style or another. Rather the two styles are gradually combined so that the learning styles effectively converge on one another. Some authors have suggested that these styles are a function of the input the child receives from his or her linguistic environment. Others suggest that the children orientate themselves to information of one sort rather than another. Without splitting the population of language learners into two groups it is evident that all individuals have varying degrees of cognitive strengths and weaknesses which they bring to bear on the language learning process. Combined with the learning environments in which they develop both at home and in school, it is reasonable to assume that while children acquire the syntax of a language in a clearly defined and seemingly automatic fashion, there are many ways in which they come to use language to communicate. It is important that those charged with the task of identifying children with communication abilities keep this source of variability in mind.

The classification of language difficulties

Classification is important because it reflects current knowledge regarding disorder and because it allows clinicians and service providers to separate out groups that need different approaches to intervention. There have been a number of attempts to classify speech and language delays but to date no one system has received universal recognition. In part this is because of the wide range of disciplines involved in working with these children, orienting to them in different ways. For many the term speech and language impairment would be considered the overarching term and under it would be the distinction between speech and/or language delay and speech and/or language disorder. The distinction between delay and disorder can be somewhat confusing because the associated assumption is that delays are more benign than disorders, the former resolving spontaneously while the latter have more persistent and negative consequences for schooling, etc. In fact, while there is undoubtedly a group of children whose difficulties resolve spontaneously in the preschool years, there are many children who experience delays across a range of linguistic domains and continue to have difficulties well into the school years. Similarly children with disorders in specific linguistic domains – notably phonological disorders – may have a relatively good outcome. Nevertheless there are two groupings which are widely recognised, the distinction between primary and secondary language impairments and the broad brush classification system represented by the DSM-IV (*see* Box 1.4).[18]

Primary/secondary language impairment

Over recent years much has been made of the distinction between primary and secondary language impairment. The former refers to impairments or delays which are specific to speech or language development while the latter refers to speech or language delays which are clearly a product of other more pervasive developmental conditions, such as general learning disability, Down's syndrome, cerebral palsy, etc.

Box 1.4:   Differential diagnoses for speech and language disorders. From DSM-IV

Diagnostic criteria for Expressive Language Disorder

A The scores obtained from standardised individually administered measures of expressive language development are substantially below those obtained from standardised measures of both non-verbal intellectual capacity and receptive language development. This disturbance may be manifest clinically by symptoms that include having a markedly limited vocabulary, making errors in tense, or having difficulty recalling words or producing sentences with developmentally appropriate length or complexity.
B The difficulties with expressive language interfere with academic or occupational achievement or with social communication.
C Criteria are not met for Mixed Receptive–Expressive Language Disorder or a Pervasive Developmental Disorder.
D If mental retardation, a speech-motor or sensory deficit, or environmental deprivation is present, the language difficulties are in excess of those usually associated with these problems.

Diagnostic criteria for Mixed Receptive–Expressive Language Disorder

A The scores obtained from a battery of standardised individually administered measures of both receptive and expressive language development are substantially below those obtained from standardised measures of non-verbal intellectual capacity. Symptoms include those for Expressive Language Disorder as well as difficulty understanding words, sentences, or specific types of words, such as spatial terms.
B The difficulties with receptive and expressive language significantly interfere with academic or occupational achievement or with social communication.
C Criteria are not met for a Pervasive Developmental Disorder.
D If mental retardation, a speech-motor or sensory deficit, or environmental deprivation is present, the language difficulties are in excess of those usually associated with these problems.

Differential diagnosis

Expressive Language Disorder is distinguished from **Mixed Receptive–Expressive Language Disorder** by the presence in the latter of significant impairment in

Continued on next page

receptive language. Expressive Language Disorder is not diagnosed if the criteria are met for Autistic Disorder or another Pervasive Developmental Disorder. **Autistic Disorder** also involves expressive language impairment but may be distinguished from Expressive and Mixed Receptive-Expressive Language Disorders by the characteristics of the communication impairment (e.g. stereotyped use of language) and by the presence of a qualitative impairment in social interaction and restricted, repetitive and stereotyped patterns of behaviour. Expressive and receptive language development may be impaired due to **Mental Retardation**, a **hearing impairment** or **other sensory deficit**, a **speech-motor deficit** or **severe environmental deprivation**. The presence of these problems may be established by intelligence testing, audiometric testing, neurological testing and history. If the language difficulties are in excess of those usually associated with these problems, a concurrent diagnosis of Expressive Language or Mixed Receptive-Expressive Language Disorder may be made. Children with expressive language delays due to environmental deprivation may show rapid gains once the environmental problems are ameliorated. In **Disorder of Written Expression**, there is a disturbance in writing skills. If deficits in oral expression are also present, an additional diagnosis of Expressive Language Disorder may be appropriate. **Selective Mutism** involves limited expressive output that may mimic Expressive or Mixed Receptive-Expressive Language Disorder; careful history and observation are necessary to determine the presence of normal language in some settings. **Acquired phasia** associated with a general medical condition in childhood is often transient. A diagnosis of Expressive Language Disorder is appropriate only if the language disturbance persists beyond the acute recovery period for the etiological general medical condition (e.g. head trauma, viral infection).

Diagnostic criteria for Phonological Disorder

A Failure to use developmentally expected speech sounds that are appropriate for age and dialect (e.g. errors in sound production, use, representation or organisation such as, but not limited to, substitutions of one sound for another [use of /t/ for target /k/ sound] or omissions of sounds such as final consonants).
B The difficulties in speech sound production interfere with academic or occupational achievement or with social communication.
C If mental retardation, a speech-motor or sensory deficit, or environmental deprivation is present, the speech difficulties are in excess of those usually associated with these problems.

Differential diagnosis

Speech difficulties may be associated with **Mental Retardation**, a **hearing impairment** or **other sensory deficit**, a **speech-motor deficit** or **severe environmental**

deprivation. The presence of these problems may be established by intelligence testing, audiometric testing, neurological testing and history. If the speech difficulties are in excess of those usually associated with these problems, a concurrent diagnosis of Phonological Disorder may be made. Problems limited to **speech rhythm** or **voice** are not included as part of Phonological Disorder and instead are diagnosed as **Stuttering** or **Communication Disorder Not Otherwise Specified**. Children with speech difficulties due to environmental deprivation may show rapid gains once the environmental problems are ameliorated.

Diagnostic criteria for Stuttering

A Disturbance in the normal fluency and time patterning of speech (inappropriate for the individual's age), characterised by frequent occurrences of one or more of the following:
   1 sound and syllable repetitions
   2 sound prolongations
   3 interjections
   4 broken words (e.g. pauses within a word)
   5 audible or silent blocking (filled or unfilled pauses in speech)
   6 circumlocutions (word substitutions to avoid problematic words)
   7 words produced with an excess of physical tension
   8 monosyllabic whole-word repetitions (e.g. 'I-I-I-I see him')
B The disturbance in fluency interferes with academic or occupational achievement or with social communication.
C If a speech-motor or sensory deficit is present, the speech difficulties are in excess of those usually associated with these problems.

Differential diagnosis

Speech difficulties may be associated with a **hearing impairment** or **other sensory deficit** or a **speech-motor deficit**. In instances where the speech difficulties are in excess of those usually associated with these problems, a concurrent diagnosis of Stuttering may be made. Stuttering must be distinguished from **normal dysfluencies that occur frequently in young children**, which include whole-word or phrase repetitions (e.g. 'I want, I want ice cream'), incomplete phrases, interjections, unfilled pauses and parenthetical remarks.

While the distinction between primary and secondary makes sense from a clinical point of view there remains some discussion as to whether it is possible to define a category of primary or, as it is sometimes referred to, *specific speech or language impairment* (SLI). In the end the argument depends on the measures used. It seems fairly clear that it is possible to use the discrepancy between IQ and language quotient to determine a specific problem. However, when a group of children with SLI is examined across a range of measures, the distinction between language and other areas of development does not always seem so clear cut. For example, it has been shown that SLI children also experience difficulties in the development of symbolic play, in their hand/eye co-ordination and in their ability to carry out visual tasks. Indeed some have suggested that for many of these children there is an underlying neurodevelopmental lag.[2] It seems likely that Western societies are especially attuned to identifying these problems because of the value attributed to language development. Indeed it seems possible that many of these discrepancies may be a function of little more than normal variation or of the psychometric properties of the measures themselves.

Of course, the long-term impact of such difficulties also has implications for how we interpret the problem. The label SLI is useful if it helps us to identify a group of children who are at risk of resulting difficulties in school and beyond. If not, there is little need to identify them and label them in this way even if it is technically possible, by virtue of available psychometric measures, to pick them out. Indeed it is now clear that many of these children go on to experience marked literacy problems in school. The evidence seems to suggest that those with combined expressive/receptive language difficulties may be more vulnerable than those with speech difficulties.[19] Many of these children may also go on to present with challenging behaviours such that they interfere with their school performance. Some have suggested that these problems arise because the children are experiencing frustration in the classroom and indeed it is possible to demonstrate the positive effects of modifying the language level in the classroom. However, it is one thing to note the association but quite another to assume a causal relationship. It may be that the neurodevelopmental lag hypothesis would also explain both behavioural and literacy difficulties. For this reason it is imperative that the GP keeps a close eye on language development in young children, in part for what it tells us about the speech or language itself and in part for what it may signal in terms of other aspects of development.

DSM-IV classification

The DSM-IV captures the most commonly used terms and helps provide a common language with which to discuss these children. These are:

- expressive language disorder
- expressive/receptive language disorder

- phonological disorder
- stuttering.

See Box 1.4 for the differential diagnoses for these terms. This system provides a useful bottom line for classification but proves to be a relatively crude tool for the practitioner.

   Other classifications have been devised.[20] Speech and language therapists might also add a range of other diagnostic labels to subclassify these groups to help focus on the required therapeutic intervention. Many of these subclassifications arise out of the comprehensive and detailed assessment outlined at the beginning of this chapter and dealt with in greater detail in Chapter 5.

Summary

- All the different aspects of communication interact with one another. Any assessment must take this into consideration and ensure that the underlying skills are properly assessed before making assumptions about the more apparent aspects of communication, such as articulation or phonology.
- The development of communication starts from the moment the child is born. Initially the parent plays a central part as the interactive partner but the infant is soon actively involved. Other family members and peer groups play an increasing role in the process of the stimulation of speech and language development.
- At the end of the first year we see a shift to intentional symbolic communication on the part of the child. Language structures follow on from this. It is useful to see communicative intention driving the onset of language structure, pragmatics preceding syntax, rather than specific syntactic structures emerging out of the neurological blue.
- Vocabulary is often overemphasised as a measure of communicative skill. It is only one part of the overall picture and research shows considerable variation within the normal range. Nevertheless in the very young child it is bound to be one of the first indicators of delay and the clinician would be wrong to think that all children with slow vocabulary development at, say, two years, necessarily catch up.
- The shift to syntax, and in particular the development of verbs, is probably one of the best indicators of developmental progress. As language develops it may be that the child's capacity to use what he or she has is more important than the acquisition of specific syntactic forms.
- Speech and language difficulties may create anxiety in parents and distress in young children and may go on to influence the child's performance in school, both in terms of educational attainment and socialisation. For this reason all concerns should be taken seriously.

References

1   Bishop DVM (1997) *Uncommon Understanding*. Lawrence Erlbaum, Chichester.

2   Bishop D and Edmundson A (1987) Language impaired 4 year olds: distinguishing transient from persistent impairments. *Journal of Speech and Hearing Disorders* **52**: 156–73.

3   Naremore RC and Hopper R (1997) *Children Learning Language: a practical introduction to communication development*. Singular Press, London.

4   Trevarthen C and Marwick H (1986) Signs of motivation for speech in infants, and the nature of a mother's support for the development of language. In: P Lindblom and R Zetterstrom (eds) *Precursors of Early Speech*. Macmillan, Basingstoke, Hants.

5   Fenson L, Dale P, Reznick S, Thal D, Bates E, Hartung J, Pethick S and Reilly J (1993) *MacArthur Communicative Development Inventories*. Singular Publishing, London.

6   Bruner J (1981) Intention in the structure of action and interaction. In: L Lipsitt (ed) *Advances in Infancy Research*, vol. 1. Ablex Publishing Corp., Norwood NJ.

7   Rice M, Buhr J and Nemeth M (1990) Fast mapping word learning abilities of language delayed preschoolers. *Journal of Speech and Hearing Disorders* **55**: 33–42.

8   Dale P (1976) *Language Development: structure and function*. Holt Rhinehart and Winston, New York.

9   Locke J (1993) *The Child's Path to Spoken Language*. Harvard University Press, London.

10 Pine J (1994) The language of primary caregivers. In: C Gallaway and BJ Richards (eds) *Input and Interaction in Language Acquisition*. Cambridge University Press, Cambridge.

11 Snow C, Perlman R and Nathan D (1987) Why routines are different: towards a multiple factors model of the relation between input and language acquisition. In: K Nelson and A Van Kleeck (eds) *Children's Language*, vol. 6. Lawrence Erlbaum, Hillsdale, NJ.

12 Pinker S (1994) *The Language Instinct*. Penguin Press, London.

13 Dale P, Simonoff E, Bishop D, Eley T, Oliver B, Price T, Purcell S, Stevenson J and Plomin R (1998) Genetic influences on language delay in two-year-old children. *Nature Neuroscience* **1**(4): 324–8.

14 Crago M and Gopick M (1994) From families to phenotypes: theoretical and clinical implications of research into the genetic basis of specific language impairment. In: RV Watkins and ML Rice (eds) *Specific Language Impairments in Children*. Paul Brookes, Baltimore.

15 Rice M (1997) Specific language impairment: in search of diagnostic markers and genetic contribution. *Mental Retardation and Developmental Disabilities Research Reviews* **3**: 350–7.

16   Glascoe F (1991) Can clinical judgement detect children with speech-language problems? *Pediatrics* **87**: 317–22.

17   Baron-Cohen S, Allen J and Gillberg C (1992) Can autism be detected at 18 months? The needle, the haystack and the CHAT. *British Journal of Psychiatry* **161**: 839–43.

18   American Psychological Association (1994) *Diagnostic and Statistical Manual of Mental Disorders*. 4th edn. APA, Washington, DC.

19   Bishop D and Adams C (1990) A prospective study of the relationship between SLI phonology and reading retardation. *Journal of Child Psychology and Psychiatry* **31**: 1027–50.

20   Bishop D and Rosenbloom L (1987) Classification of childhood language disorders. In: W Yule and M. Rutter (eds) *Language Development and Disorders*. MacKeith Press, Oxford.

CHAPTER 2

The size of the problem

James Law and Rashmin Tamhne

Clinicians and health planners need to be able to identify vulnerable groups within their populations and determine which require intervention. As part of this process they need to know who is likely to present with communication difficulties and about the extent and severity of those difficulties and for how long they are likely to persist.

How common are communication difficulties?

Prevalence refers to the number of cases in a defined population at the given time point or across a given time period. It is useful as a means of giving some indication of the level of need in a given population. By contrast, *incidence* provides a measure of the number of new cases in a population and can be taken to have aetiological implications. A good knowledge of the experiences of the individuals prior to their becoming cases, their *exposure* in epidemiological terms, may help us understand the process by which they come to acquire the condition in question. Inevitably prevalence is a function of incidence and a consistent incidence in the absence of spontaneous recovery or death would result in ever-increasing prevalence. In the case of communication difficulties in childhood, the latter is only very rarely at issue but the former may be relatively common, at least in the early years. The impact of intervention is, as yet, uncertain but, given the results reported in Chapter 6, the possibility that prevalence may decline as a function of intervention is one which needs to be taken seriously.

The general consensus is that the percentage of children reaching school age with significant speech and language difficulties is around 5%, with the number of cases of very severe problems confined to speech and/or language being of the order of 1/500[1,2] or between 20 and 500 in 10 000. To put these figures in perspective it is worth considering the figures for one of the most pervasive communication disorders, autism. The figures for autism fall between 4.5 and 6.0 in 10 000 for the most serious forms of the disorder[2] to 26 in 10 000 for what are known as autistic spectrum manifestations of the disorder.[3]

Something of the detail is revealed in a recent systematic review of the literature.[4] Using a wide range of data sources these authors calculated median prevalence figures and reached a composite figure for speech and/or language difficulties of 5.95%. This is strikingly similar to the figure to which reference is commonly made. This makes communication difficulties the most common neurodevelopmental condition in early childhood and consequently of considerable public health interest.[5] Taking an average family practitioner list as 17 000, of which 15% fall below 16 years of age, this would lead to approximately 150 cases of pronounced primary speech and/or language delay. It has been suggested that as many as 250 000 school-aged children in Britain have some degree of speech and language impairment or disorder.[6]

The majority of studies meeting the criteria for Law *et al.*'s review[4] addressed the issue of prevalence rather than incidence and the figures quoted range relatively widely (*see* Table 2.1 taken from ref. 4). This range can largely be explained by differences in:

- the age that the population is sampled
- the type of problem within the overall category of communication difficulties which is identified
- the level of the problem identified.

Table 2.1   Prevalence estimates by type of speech and language delay by age

Age	% Speech/language delay Median of estimates [range]	% Language delay only Median of estimates [range]	% Speech delay only Median of estimates [range]
2;0 years	5.00[7]	16.0 [8.00–19.0][11]	–
3;0 years	6.90 [5.6–8][7–9]	2.63 [2.27–7.60][12–14]	–
4;6 years	5.00 [–][7]	–	–
5;0 years	11.78 [4.56–19.00][10]	6.80 [2.14–10.40][10,12,15–17]	7.8 [6.40–24.60][10,16,17]
6;0 years	–	5.50 [–][17]	14.55 [12.60–16.50][16,17]
7;0 years	–	3.1 [2.02–8.40][12,17]	2.300[17]

Superscript numbers refer to references.

Although there is considerable variation in these figures it is evident that all the studies suggest that the number of children with speech and or language delay is high. How is it possible to explain these differences? In some cases it is simply a matter of the level of difficulty counted as a 'problem'. If a relatively liberal cut off is adopted the prevalence figure rises. For example Beitchman and colleagues[10] targeted all children falling below what is conventionally determined as psychometric normality, i.e. one standard deviation or more below the mean on standardised speech and language measures and reached the figure of 19% in the Ottawa Carleton region in Canada. This is much higher than the figures quoted elsewhere, which have tended to adopt more conservative levels of case definition.

The type of communication measured is also an issue. The figures fluctuate according to whether difficulties are confined to speech or language separately or whether they are based on a composite of the two. The figure which is of most interest to the planner of services is this composite figure, including children who have speech and/or language difficulties. Over the age span considered there appears to be some degree of consistency and with the exception of the Beitchman *et al.* figure to which reference has already been made,[10] the message seems to be that the prevalence for this group remains relatively static.

By contrast, the isolated language delays and the speech delays pose problems of interpretation. Rescorla *et al.*[11] examined the prevalence of delay in acquiring vocabulary at two years and found a level of prevalence far in excess of most other researchers. Are these results simply discordant or is there an obvious explanation for the apparent imbalance? The explanation may be that they were basing their cut-off point on a single measure of parent-recorded vocabulary at a time when vocabulary is an extremely noisy developmental phenomenon. That is, it is difficult to distinguish normal variability from pathology on the basis of vocabulary alone. Whether a delay in vocabulary development alone really has clinical significance at this stage in a child's development remains uncertain. Those who have looked at expressive language delay after the age of two have tended to note less discrepancy, probably because they used more sophisticated measures of language, for example measures of the child's grammatical output.

The data show that estimates of speech delay on its own have not been considered a very useful concept before the age of five. This is almost certainly because there is a recognition that it is a very difficult matter to determine case status of speech difficulties in the preschool years. Children commonly make mistakes relative to the adult model in their pronunciation but these are not necessarily problems, and trying to differentiate problems from those that are simply normal immaturities can be very difficult at an epidemiological level. This problem is not fully resolved after the preschool period and the figures continue to vary considerably. Again this may be because there is little consensus as to what is a problem. Some studies assume that children should be 'normal' speakers once they reach school and thus that continuing immaturities amount to clinical levels of difficulty. Others maintain that a child has to have a severe problem before he or she is picked up as having speech difficulties in need of intervention.

How is prevalence affected by environmental conditions? Hart and Risley[18] have demonstrated convincingly the different opportunities offered to children from different social backgrounds and this is mirrored in studies which have demonstrated differential rates of vocabulary delay in children from different socioeconomic backgrounds.[11,19] Does this necessarily translate into socioeconomic status-dependent differences in the later years? The evidence here is more equivocal. Conti-Ramsden *et al.*,[20] for example, found no corresponding differences in children attending specialised educational facilities for speech and language-impaired children in the primary years. Is there evidence that children may be disadvantaged by having less access to the language in which the prevalence study was carried out? Presumably because researchers are aware of this issue and sample accordingly, this does not readily emerge from the prevalence literature. Wong, for example, found comparable levels in a Cantonese speaking community in Hong Kong,[14] as Stevenson and colleagues had done in urban London.[21] Similarly concern has been expressed that children from different ethnic or linguistic backgrounds are not over-identified. Although some authors have suggested that African-Americans may be over-represented, the data from other studies suggest otherwise.[15,22]

Are communication difficulties a real problem?

Whether the primary healthcare practitioner should be worried about communication difficulties depends on both the immediate impact of the problems experienced by the child and the family, and the long-term consequences of the condition in question. It is sometimes assumed that such difficulties resolve spontaneously to such an extent that they do not merit further attention. Clearly there is a grain of truth in this. Not all children who seem to be slower than others at two years of age go on to have problems.

There is some suggestion that early expressive language delays on their own will not necessarily lead to a poor outcome.[23] By contrast, children with expressive language difficulties in conjunction with delays in comprehension have a far worse prognosis. Some indication of the level of prediction for different subgroups of the communication delayed population is given in Tables 2.2 and 2.3. It should be noted that these studies refer only to speech and language outcomes and include only those studies where it was reported that no intervention took place. The studies below include both large-scale cohort studies and the follow-up of selected populations. It is not possible from this data to compare directly the level of difficulty experienced by the children within each group.

But it is possible that the children whose difficulties resolve were less severely affected in the first instance. One study in inner city London demonstrated a differential rate for serious and milder forms of speech and language delay.[7] The authors

Table 2.2 Persistence for individual studies: speech only, language only and speech and language

	Cases/ sample size	Persistence %	Age range (years;months)
Speech only			
Bralley and Stoudt[25]*	60/60	21.6	6;6–11;6
Felsenfeld et al.[26]	24/52	50	4;10–33;0
Renfrew and Geary[27]	150/150	54	5;0–5;6
Median		50	
Language only (expressive and receptive)			
Hall et al.[28]	5/9	100	4;7–7;0
Rescorla and Schwartz[29]	25/25	54	2;2–3;0
Richman et al.[21]	22/705	65	2;0–3;0
Scarborough and Dobrich[30]	4/16	0	2;6–5;6
Silva et al.[12]	23/1027	78.2	3;0–7;0
Thal and Tobias[31]	10/30	40	1;10–3;0
Ward[32]	119/321	82	1;0–2;0
Ward[32]	61/321	73	0;10–1;10
Ward[32]	23/321	50	0;10–1;10
Median		66	
Speech and language			
Fiedler et al.[33]*	46/138	38	3;0–7;0
Median		38	

*Persistence for the longest of three periods within the same study.
Superscript numbers refer to reference numbers.

found a relatively constant rate for severe cases between 2, 3 and 4;6 years [3–5–3%], but that the rate for less severe cases during the same period declined convincingly from 17 to 12 to 7%. Studies that have relied on standardised measures have often painted a rather different picture with the same proportion presenting across childhood.[24] What is not clear at this stage is which children in the earlier age groups are the ones who need to be identified because they are at greatest risk of ongoing problems. No attempt has been made to follow a population through to ascertain which children are failing at five or seven and then looking back to the earliest years to identify those most in need of intervention. One of the obstacles to such an approach is that, as we shall see below, relatively few of these communication difficulties truly exist in isolation and that given the nature of services to children in Europe or the USA, for example, it is unlikely that it is really possible to conceive of natural history in the sense that a patient is given a drug or is not. In fact many children will be in nursery and all will be in school at some point. In such circumstances children are identified as being in need of support services and, even if they

Table 2.3 Persistence for individual studies: receptive language only, expressive language only and expressive/receptive language

	Cases/ sample size	Persistence %	Age range (years;months)
Receptive language			
Silva et al.[12]*	23/1027	8.7	3;0–7;0
Expressive language			
Rescorla and Schwartz (1990)[29]§	25/25	54	2;2–3;0
Thal and Tobias[31]	10/30	40	1;10–3;0
Scarborough and Dobrich[30]	4/16	0	2;6–5;6
Silva et al.[12]	21/1027	28.6	3;0–7;0
Ward[32]	23/321	50	0;10–1;10
Median		40	
Receptive/expressive language			
Richman et al.[21]	22/705	65	2;0–3;0
Ward[32]	119/321	82	1;0–2;0
Ward[32]	61/321	73	0;10–1;10
Hall et al.[28]	5/9	100	4;7–7;0
Klee et al.[34]	6/36	67	2;0–3;0
Silva et al.[12]*	23/1027	78.2	3;0–7;0
Median		75.6	

*Persistence for the longest of three periods within the same study.
§Median between two expressive scales reported.
Superscript numbers refer to references.

do not receive those services, often elicit the additional attentions of their teacher. Their communication difficulties thus influence their environment such that those within it (parents, teachers, etc.) adapt to meet the needs of the child.

If this is the case then the concept of natural history is likely to become difficult to pin down with any certainty. It may be as useful to examine natural history irrespective of the intervention received. In order to account for the variability in the potential intervention, such a study would need to have a large population of children identified with the difficulty. One such study has reported the outcome for 71 children identified as being clinical cases in the preschool period and followed up first to 5;6, when they were classified as having resolved, as having persistent specific speech and language difficulties or as having general learning difficulties, and then followed up to 15 years.[35] The data indicate that 90% of children with confirmed difficulties at 5;6 still have marked problems at 15 years, 20% having general developmental delay. By contrast, some 34% of the children whose difficulties appeared to have resolved by 5;6 were found to have either specific speech and language delays

Table 2.4   Follow-up of children with primary speech and language delay at age 15 years[35]

		Satisfactory speech and language	Impaired speech and language	General delay	Totals
	Resolved	17	8	1	26
	SLI [%]	[65.4]	[30.7]	[3.8]	
Aged 5;6	Persistent	3	21	6	30
	SLI [%]	[10]	[70]	[20]	
	General	3	5	7	15
	delay [%]	[20]	[33.3]	[46.7]	
	Totals	23	34	14	71

or general delays at 15 years (Table 2.4), effectively demonstrating that speech and language difficulties picked up at the start of schooling are likely to still be affecting them when they leave. It is important to note that, in the first instance, this group was identified as having difficulties specific to speech and language. Children with other handicapping conditions of which speech and language impairments are a part had already been excluded from this sample. If they had been included it is highly likely that the persistence would have been higher.

The evidence suggests that the outcomes for many of these children can be poor. We do not yet have a clear picture of how these young people fare in adulthood. Felsenfield et al.[26] demonstrated that 50% of children who presented with speech falling below −1.5 standard deviations on a standardised test of articulation at preschool were still failing speech assessment when they were 33 years of age. Haynes and Naidoo[36] showed that the majority of children who had attended a residential school for children with severe speech and language difficulties found it difficult to get employment and when they did they tended to work in jobs that made few demands on their communication skills. The long-term outcomes from this study are discussed in greater detail in Chapter 8.

What are the determinants of outcome for communication difficulties?

In any epidemiological model it is necessary to establish the exposure and response variable. When discussing communication difficulties there are two types of outcome which need to be considered. In the first instance the outcome is the speech and language. What is it that predicts speech and language status at five or at ten years? In such cases speech and language status is the response variable and hearing difficulties, adverse birth history or social stress are the exposures of interest. Alternatively the outcome of interest may be the impact the communication difficulty may have on the child's well being. For example, behaviour difficulties are often strongly associated with speech and language difficulties. Reducing the frustration due to speech and language delay may well have an impact on the child's behaviour, their response to schooling or the nature of interaction in the family. Similarly it has been shown that there is a relationship between early speech and language difficulties and subsequent literacy skills. Increasing a child's language-processing skills in the preschool period is likely to influence the development of reading and writing skills and thus general school performance.

Tomblin and his colleagues, in a retrospective study,[37] calculated the odds ratios (OR) associated with case status of specific language impairment at five years and found that paternal rather than maternal history of speech and language difficulties was significantly associated with the occurrence of specific language impairment (OR = 2.1; CI 1.3–3.1). Maternal history of speech and language difficulties and paternal, rather than maternal, smoking during fetal development were particularly associated with specific language difficulties, once parental education had been controlled for (OR = 1.5; CI 1.0–2.1). Conversely breast-feeding (OR = 0.5; CI 0.4–0.7) and length of breast-feeding functioned as a protective factor, effectively reducing the risk of specific language impairment.

Another study to use this method examined the prediction of language and other outcomes at seven to eight years from population screening at five age points below the age of three years in two different designs – a case-controlled study and a selected prospective study.[38] Their findings turned up a number of interesting methodological issues not least of which was the difference between the strengths of association in the two designs adopted. The case-controlled design showed consistently higher levels of association than the prospective study. Expressive language problems in school were predicted from 15 months by an adaptive scale (OR = 1.51; CI 1.00–2.26), from two years by a screening measure of adaptive skills (OR = 1.54; CI 1.06–2.23), language skills (OR = 1.86; CI 1.2–2.89) and behaviour (OR = 1.50; CI 1.0–2.25). By three years the prediction had improved so that all aspects of the developmental screening predicted subsequent expressive language difficulties (motor skills OR = 1.64, CI 1.11–2.43; adaptive skills OR = 1.80, CI 1.24–2.62; language OR = 1.63, CI 1.14–2.34; behaviour OR = 1.60, CI 1.12–2.27; and neurological development OR = 2.44, CI 1.50–3.97).

There has been extensive discussion of factors associated with communication difficulties but relatively little attention has been paid to the extent to which these phenomena actually predict subsequent outcomes. Expressive language appears to exhibit a much weaker association with subsequent school performance than adaptive, motor or neurological screening.[38] Indeed the only area of difficulty that language screening predicted with any success was expressive language difficulties and reading problems (OR = 1.59, CI 1.08–2.34 at 2 years and OR 1.65, CI 1.17–2.34 at 3 years). It is likely that this relationship would become stronger still if language comprehension is introduced into the equation. It is important to recognise that these odds ratios are all adjusted for parental education level.

What are the implications of communication difficulties at a health services level?

The impact of communication difficulties is much less easy to quantify than it is for fatal and more clearly defined medical conditions. As a consequence it is difficult to make clear judgements about the implications for the providers of health services. There is no equivalent of the Quality Adjusted Life Year and no assessment of parental willingness to pay for the type of service that would support these children, both measures which are used in other areas of health service provision to denote level of concern. Nevertheless it is clear from the preceding discussion that communication difficulties represent a high-prevalence condition which puts children at risk of subsequent difficulties. Not all children go on to have difficulties but, as we shall see in Chapter 7, evidence is beginning to emerge of the positive impact of intervention. What we need to know is which children stand to benefit most from intervention such that the risk of subsequent difficulties can be minimised, and which will need ongoing support.

In terms of health priorities it would be most useful to move away from the concept of a specific prevalence figure upon which all services are based. Instead it would be appropriate to look at the potential for distinguishing risk groups. So rather than saying that services are planned around a prevalence estimate of 6% of the population at five years of age, the nature of the population in question is examined in relation to the relative risk of future difficulties. Thus it might be possible to establish risk groups – those with multiple difficulties, those from lower income families, those with pronounced medical histories, most notably birth histories or otitis media, and those who have experienced abuse or neglect, and to target those groups.

The issue is clouded from the point of view of the health services provider by the fact that communication difficulties are not the sole preserve of health services. Indeed the very essence of communication is its social and its educational role in the life of the child. Not surprisingly then, the question has been raised about where the responsibility for difficulties in this area lies. If the difficulties experienced are educational, should not educational services address them? This division between health and educational services is an operational matter which should not be allowed to get in the way of appropriate provision. The more important issue is what is the nature of such provision?

Finally, the way in which services respond to communication difficulties in childhood is a matter of concern to all those involved with identifying need in young children. In particular it is important to ascertain whether it is feasible to screen the whole population to identify cases or whether it is more appropriate to use other methods, such as opportunistic detection, response to parental concern or confirmatory screening only after concern has been expressed by a parent or public health practitioner. These issues will be discussed further in Chapter 3.

Conclusions

- The number of potential cases of children with communication difficulties is high. The more conservative estimates suggest 1–2%, but well-designed studies suggest that as many as 7% of children may have difficulties which warrant attention.
- Children with confirmed case status at school entry are clearly at risk of subsequent educational difficulties although the position is much less clear for younger children. Natural history is of central concern given the relatively high rate of spontaneous remission in the population.
- Early speech and language delays should be considered a risk factor both for subsequent speech and language difficulties and for other schooling and social problems, a risk which needs to be taken seriously.
- The epidemiological framework provides a useful starting point in establishing the most relevant data. As yet there remain a number of gaps in the literature which makes reliance on this methodology difficult for making judgements regarding the implementation of mass screening for communication difficulties.

References

1   AFASIC/ICAN (1995) *Principles for Educational Provision*. AFASIC 347, Central Markets, Smithfield, London EC1A 9NH.

2   American Psychological Association (1994) *Diagnostic and Statistical Manual of Mental Disorders*. 4th edn. APA, Washington, DC.

3   Gillberg IC and Gillberg C (1989) Asperger syndrome – some epidemiological considerations: a research note. *Journal of Child Psychology and Psychiatry* **30**: 631–8.

4   Law J, Boyle J, Harris F, Harkness A and Nye C (1998) Screening for Speech and Language Delay: a systematic review of the literature. *Health Technology Assessment* **2**(9).

5   Drillien CM and Drummond MB (1983) *Developmental Screening and the Child with Special Needs*. William Heineman, London.

6   Enderby P and Phillip R (1986) Speech and language handicap: towards knowing the size of the problem. *British Journal of Disorders of Communication* **21**: 151–65.

7   Bax M, Hart H and Jenkins S (1983) The behaviour, development and health of the young child: implications for care. *BMJ* **286**: 1793–6.

8   Burden V, Stott CM, Forge J and Goodyer I (1996) The Cambridge Language and Speech Project (CLASP). 1. Detection of language difficulties at 36–39 months. *Developmental Medicine and Child Neurology* **38**(7): 613–31.

9   Randall D, Reynell J and Curwen M (1974) A study of language development in a sample of 3 year old children. *British Journal of Disorders of Communication* **9**(1): 3–16.

10   Beitchman JH, Nair R, Clegg M, Patel PG, Ferguson B, Pressman E *et al.* (1986) Prevalence of speech and language disorders in 5-year-old kindergarten children in the Ottawa-Carleton region. *Journal of Speech and Hearing Disorders* **51**(2): 98–110.

11   Rescorla L, Hadicke-Wiley M and Escarce E (1993) Epidemiological investigation of expressive language delay at age two. Special Issue: Language development in special populations. *First Language* **13**(37, Pt 1): 5–22.

12   Silva PA, McGee R and Williams SM (1983) Developmental language delay from three to seven years and its significance for low intelligence and reading difficulties at age seven. *Developmental Medicine and Child Neurology* **25**: 783–93.

13   Stevenson J and Richman N (1976) The prevalence of language delay in a population of three-year-old children and its association with general retardation. *Developmental Medicine and Child Neurology* **18**(4): 431–41.

14   Wong V, Lee PWH, Mak-Lieh F, Yeung CY, Leung PWL, Luk SL *et al.* (1992) Language screening in pre-school Chinese children. *European Journal of Disorders of Communication* **27**(3): 247–64.

15   Tomblin JB, Records N, Buckwalter P, Zhang X, Smith E and O'Brien M (1997) Prevalence of specific language impairment in kindergarten children. *Journal of Speech, Language and Hearing Research* **40**(6): 1245.

16   Tuomi S and Ivanoff P (1977) Incidence of speech and hearing disorders among kindergarten and grade 1 children. *Special Education in Canada* **51**(4): 5–8.

17   Dudley JG and Delage J (1980) Incidence des troubles de la parole et du langage chez les enfants franco-quebecois. *Communication Humaine* **5**: 131–42.

18   Hart B and Risley TR (1995) *Meaningful Differences in Everyday Experiences of Young American Children*. Paul Brookes, Baltimore.

19   Arriaga RI, Fenson L, Cronan T and Pethick SJ (1998) Scores from the MacArthur Communicative Development Inventory of children from low and middle income families. *Applied Psycholinguistics* **19**(2): 209–23.

20   Conti-Ramsden G, Crutchley A and Botting N (1997) *Educational Transitions of Children with Specific Language Impairments Attending Language Units: findings from Nuffield Foundation/University of Manchester research project*. Available from Centre for Educational Needs, University of Manchester.

21   Richman N, Stevenson J and Graham PJ (1982) *Preschool to School: a behavioural study*. Academic Press, London.

22   Stewart JM, Hester EJ and Taylor DL (1986) Prevalence of language, speech and hearing disorders in an urban preschool black population. *Journal of Childhood Communication Disorders* **9**(2): 107–23.

23   Whitehurst GJ and Fischel J (1994) Practitioner review: early developmental language delay: what, if anything, should the clinician do about it? *Journal of Child Psychology and Psychiatry* **35**: 613–48.

24   Silva PA, Williams SM and McGee R (1987) A longitudinal study of children with developmental language delay at age three: later intelligence, reading and behaviour problems. *Developmental Medicine and Child Neurology* **29**: 630–40.

25   Bralley RC and Stoudt RJ (1977) A five year longitudinal study of development of articulation. *Language, Speech and Hearing Services in Schools* **8**(3): 176–80.

26   Felsenfield S, Broen PA and McGue M (1992) A 28-year follow-up of adults with a history of moderate phonological disorder: linguistic and personality results. *Journal of Speech and Hearing Research* **35**: 1114–25.

27   Renfrew CE and Geary L (1973) Prediction of persisting speech deficit. *British Journal of Disorders of Communication* **8**(1): 37–41.

28   Hall NE, Yamashita TS and Aram DM (1993) Relationship between language and fluency in children with developmental language disorders. *Journal of Speech and Hearing Research* **36**: 568–79.

29   Rescorla L and Schwartz E (1990) Outcome of toddlers with specific expressive language delay. *Applied Psycholinguistics* **11**(4): 393–407.

30   Scarborough HS and Dobrich W (1990) Development of children with early language delay. *Journal of Speech and Hearing Research* **33**(1): 70–83.

31   Thal DJ and Tobias S (1992) Communicative gestures in children with delayed onset of oral expressive vocabulary. *Journal of Speech and Hearing Research* **35**: 1281–9.

32   Ward S (1992) The predictive validity and accuracy of a screening test for language delay and auditory perceptual disorder. *British Journal of Disorders of Communication* **27**: 55–72.

33   Fiedler MF, Lenneberg EH, Rolfe UT and Drorbaugh JE (1971) A speech screening procedure with three-year-old children. *Pediatrics* **48**(2): 268–76.

34   Klee T, Carson DK, Gavin WJ, Hall L, Kent A and Reece S (1997) Concurrent and predictive validity of an early language screening program. (Unpublished.)

35   Stothard SE, Snowling MJ, Bishop DVM, Chipchase BB and Kaplan CA (1999) Language impaired pre-schoolers: a follow-up into adolescence. *Journal of Speech, Language and Hearing Disorders* **41**: 407–18.

36   Haynes C and Naidoo S (1991) *Children with Specific Speech and Language Impairment*. Blackwell Scientific, Oxford.

37   Tomblin JB, Smith E and Zhang X (1997) Epidemiology of specific language impairment: prenatal and perinatal risk factors. *Journal of Communication Disorders* **30**: 325–44.

38   Drillien CM, Pickering RM and Drummond MB (1988) Predictive value of screening for different areas of development. *Developmental Medicine and Child Neurology* **30**: 284–305.

CHAPTER 3

Surveillance and screening

Frances Page Glascoe and Ray Sturner

Untreated speech and language problems are one of the most common reasons for school failure. If language problems are not only treated but treated early, children have a much greater chance of school success. Well-delivered, early intervention, of which the facilitation of language skills is a major component, has been shown to have long-term effects for socially disadvantaged groups in that it reduces drop-out, teenage pregnancy rates, increases the likelihood of employment and decreases criminal behaviour in the long term. Similarly, early intervention has been shown to have positive effects for children with both general developmental delays[1] and more specific speech and language difficulties.[2] It has been demonstrated that such interventions can demonstrate marked economic benefits.[3] Yet early intervention and its numerous benefits can only be offered when children with problems are detected early. Early detection is usually dependent on doctors and health visitors – the only professionals with knowledge of development who are in routine contact with families of young children. The focus of this chapter is on approaches to early detection in healthcare settings. It begins with an outline of 'trigger questions' appropriate for the use in opportunistic screening[4] to ascertain the level of the child's current performance and goes on to look at validated methods for identifying early communication difficulties. The latter includes questions addressed to parents to elicit the level of concern and screening tests designed to access the current level of child's speech and language functioning.

Developmental surveillance

Developmental surveillance is a process by which child health professionals carefully note, during the course of well-child visits, the developmental progress of each patient. One approach to surveillance is to ask parents developmentally appropriate trigger questions. These can be supplemented by 'opportunistic observations' throughout the visit and during the physical examination. Specific trigger questions and the range of clinically problematic or optimal responses are described below.

Surveillance of hearing and underpinning skills: the first few months

As can be seen in Box 3.1, developmental surveillance during the first few months of life should focus mainly on the detection of hearing impairment via a combination of eliciting parents' perceptions and observation of infant behaviour during the physical examination. It must be stressed that risk factors for hearing impairment (*see* Chapter 4) are evident in only half of all children with significant congenital hearing loss and that screening only in the presence of risk factors will underdetect by 50%. Indeed, in some countries, formal hearing screening is available and recommended for all neonates prior to hospital discharge (via otoacoustic emissions and/or automated brainstem response).

It should also be noted that observation during a visit is an unreliable way to detect hearing problems (e.g. the baby may be momentarily unresponsive because of sleep or hunger states, or may appear alert but be relying heavily on visual cues). Parents, in contrast, have many occasions to observe their infants' response to environmental

---

Box 3.1:   Hearing and underpinning abilities in the first few weeks of life

First week
- Responds to sound by blinking, crying, quieting, changing respiration or showing a startle response (observation)
- Responds to parents' voice (observation)
- '*How is feeding going?*' (elicit parents' perceptions)

At one-month
- When crying, can be consoled most of the time by being spoken to (or held) (observation)

At two-months
- Coos and vocalises reciprocally (observation)
- Is attentive to voices (observation)
- Smiles responsively (observation)
- '*Do you think your child hears all right?*' (elicit parents' perceptions)

---

noises. Parental uncertainty about their infant's hearing should be promptly met with follow-up hearing testing.

In some cases, infants will pass hearing screening despite parental concerns. This should not be dismissed as simply a 'false positive'. Such parents may not be engaged enough with their baby to notice responses to sound or acute anxiety may cause parents to distrust their own observations. A third explanation is that these infants have challenging temperaments and are thus under- or over-responsive to sound. In all such cases, parents need assistance. A referral to a child development team or to local child psychological or speech and language therapy services may be appropriate. Alternatively a health visitor may be helpful in showing parents how to respond to their baby's cues and preferences (e.g. for tactile stimulation).

Early feeding difficulties are a 'red flag' for possible communication disorders. Most severe oral-motor problems that cause subsequent difficulties with expressive language and articulation skills first present as feeding difficulties. Some speech and language therapists (usually those associated with a rehabilitation service) have expertise that may help with evaluation and treatment of oral-motor and swallowing difficulties as well as the speech difficulties which are apparent later.

Early observations of expressive language include the small throaty sounds heard at one month. These evolve into 'cooing' by two months of age – two distinct vowel sounds (e.g. ah, eh, or uh) – but the full range of vowel sounds doesn't usually appear until five months.[5] Cooing develps into prolonged vocal-social exchanges around three and four months. Thus, the ideal two-month-old 'snapshot' is mutual parent/infant interest and joy (between colic episodes of course!).

Expressive language: four months to four years

Ideally infants will demonstrate a range of affect. Early signs of this may be seen by two months, such as when a baby begins to take pleasure in social interactions or when observing an object such as your stethoscope. You may also see displeasure (not crying) or sadness when the baby's head is restrained as for an ear exam. By four months, pleasure is usually expressed by a real belly laugh and excitement, accompanied by heavy breathing (e.g. when interested in an object). Although smiling is expected around two months, by four to five months, joyful squealing or high-pitched sounds generally appear. Acute displeasure is more typical of six-month-olds (e.g. when an object is removed from the baby's hand).

Box 3.2 lists vocalising as a four-month level skill. This can be a bit confusing since infants by two months of age generally begin to vocalise when you smile or speak.[6] It is necessary to know that 'babbling' refers to syllables with consonants and that this typically emerges at six months.[7] Repetitive incantations of 'dada' and 'baba' are not generally expected until eight months. Cooing refers to a strictly vowel sound utterance first seen at two to three months.[7] Pointing is expected by ten months of age but 'no', accompanied by a shaking of the head may not appear before 12 months.

Box 3.2:   **Expressive language skills: routine trigger questions, content and sequence of parental responses**

'How does your child communicate what he wants?'

Demonstrates range of AFFECT	2–6 months
VOCALISES (babbles, 'dada', 'baba')	4–6 months
GESTURES (points, shakes head)	10–14 months
SPEAKS WORDS specific 'mama', 'dada' and 1–3 other words	12 months
3–6 words	15 months
2–3 word phrases	18 months
rapidly expanding vocabulary	15–24 months
sentences of 3–4 words	3 years
4–5 word sentences and can describe recent experiences; can sing a song; gives first and last names	4 years
Speaks INTELLIGIBLY to:	
family	18–24 months
strangers (25%)	2 years
strangers (75%)	3 years
almost completely intelligible but may show some dysfluency	4 years
Uses GRAMMATICAL forms:	
plurals, pronouns	3 years
past tense	4 years

Nodding of the head to indicate 'yes' is more typical of 14-month-olds. However, a few gestures are expected by eight months, including 'extending arms upward to signal a wish to be picked up' and 'smacking lips to indicate something tastes good'.[8] Parent reports of gestures or your observations of these are an excellent clinical marker deserving of careful attention.

As we have seen in Chapter 1 the second year sees an explosion in the child's communication skills. Initially the child points, then points and names, and then names the objects around him or her without pointing. Clearly the more attentive the parent is to this type of activity the more rewarding it will be and the more likely the infant will want to carry on doing it. There is no set pattern for the emergence of words and parents often report the use of quite sophisticated first words which are commonly used within the family context. However, in general, the child refers to common objects in the immediate environment or that have recently moved out of it. Verbs emerge more slowly. Some parents express concern about speech in the second year of life and this usually suggests that they are making comparisons with adult norms rather than the great range of intelligibility commonly found in such young children. In general, speech (as opposed to language or other communication) difficulties in this early period are only clinically significant if there is accompanying oro-motor, cranio-facial or feeding difficulties.

By the beginning of the third year the clinician should note use of 'a few grammatical forms'. There is a steady increase in the use of suffixes to designate plurals and other grammatical meanings (e.g. possessive (-s), progressive (-ing) and past tense (-ed)) between 16 months and 30 months. At 16 months few children are reported to use these forms but by 30 months most children are using all four of them.[8] Use of pronouns follows a similar pattern. Commonly used pronouns such as 'I', 'me' and 'you' are expected by 24 months, although the child may not refer to himself as 'I' or 'me' for another six months.[8]

Receptive language: four months to four years

Receptive language is often more difficult to ascertain from trigger questions (*see* Box 3.3). Parents develop many different ways of communicating with their child and may find it difficult to distinguish a response which results from the child's familiarity with the context from the child's interpretation of what is expected from the impact of the utterance that he or she has heard. However, at the four-month visit infants should demonstrate a recognition of their mother's voice. This can be tricky because babies visually recognise their mothers at two months and it is not clear whether parents can discriminate the infants' visual from auditory response. The kind of robust excitement upon hearing the mother's voice versus that of a stranger's is not expected until eight months.[6] The clinical indicator one is looking for at the four-month visit is subtler, a change of expression or slight turning of the head with the mother's voice that does not occur with anybody's voice and is first seen at two months. At six months of age, if at eye level and to the side of the baby, he or she will turn to your voice. If standing above the baby, such a response is not expected until nine months of age. By eight months, most children respond to simple phrases such as 'no-no' and 'bye-bye' and by 12 months they also respond to 'peek-a-boo' and 'all gone'.[8]

At one year of age, children understand simple requests if accompanied by a gesture (e.g. ask the child for the toy or tongue depressor he is holding and prompt him by holding out your hand or accept a parent report of a similar response). By 15 months, some children respond to such requests without gestures and by 18 months about 50% can respond to 'put it on the table'. It is important to note that the level of the request depends on the number of information-carrying words in that utterance. So 'put it on the table' may only require the child to understand one word (table) if the object (it) and the action (put) are explicit from the gesture. By 24 months, all children should be able to respond to some instruction without help from the context, although this depends on a high degree of interest and attention to what is being requested – an inconsistent phenomena in two-year-olds! However, not until four years of age can children follow two- to three-step instructions. This may be an

---

Box 3.3: Receptive language skills: routine trigger questions, content and sequence of parental responses

'What do you think your child understands?'

Recognises MOTHER'S VOICE	2 months
NAMES	
own; names of family members	8 months
most common objects	3 years
PHRASES simple ('no-no', 'bye-bye', 'peek-a-boo', 'no more')	8 months
COMMANDS	
simple requests ('give me the ball')	12 months
simple instructions without gestured cues ('sit down', 'got and get your shoes')	18–24 months
2-step instructions (*'go and get your coat and put it on*)	3 years
3-step instructions (*'find your crayons, put them away and go upstairs'*)	4 years
BODY PARTS	
points to when named	18 months
7 named parts	24 months
BASIC CONCEPTS	
understands two prepositions ('in', 'on', 'under')	3 years
points to boys versus girls	3 years
points to same versus different	4 years

---

important point for anticipatory guidance since parents may have inappropriately high or low expectations of the language development of young children. Likewise they may attribute inconsistent compliance to stubbornness.

By 15 months of age almost all children can point to body parts, especially those of the face. Absence of this skill at 18 months clearly constitutes a developmental lag. By 24 months, children should be able to point to between seven and 14 body parts.[8]

Play: nine months to four years

Much communication takes place within the context of play. Accordingly it is very important that the health professional examining the child's speech and language has a clear picture of the child's play skills. As with speech and language it is often difficult to elicit these skills within the context of a busy clinic and this means that the clinician is heavily dependent on the report of the parent. The important feature to look out for is the child's interest in play materials in the first instance and subse-

---

Box 3.4:   Play: occasional trigger questions and responses

'*Tell me about your child's typical play*'
    IMITATES a cough or razzing noises; imitates vocalisation   9 months
        makes these sounds spontaneously at earlier ages
        engages in simple REPRESENTATIONAL PLAY
            with doll (e.g. pretends to feed)   18 months
        participates in social play   18 months
    LISTENS TO STORIES
        looking at pictures and naming objects   18 months
        engages in simple FANTASY PLAY   2 years
        elaborate play (with people); takes a chosen role   3 years
        elaborate fantasy play   4 years
    INTERACTIVE GAMES with peers (takes turns)   3 years

---

quently whether the child is moving on to using materials symbolically – using a common object such as a comb as if it is something else. It is also important to ask about the child's ability to play with others (*see* Box 3.4). Obviously children are very egocentric in their early attempts at play, but just as they need to understand the social nature of communication so they need to learn to co-operate with other children in their games. Clearly it would be unrealistic to expect children to co-operate at the age of two or even three years but by the age of four this should be becoming an element of their games. There are many reasons why it might not be the case and the report of concern in this area should lead the clinician to further investigations. It is important to note that children play with whatever materials they are familiar with and may find it difficult to respond to unfamiliar objects in the clinic.

Advantages and disadvantages of developmental surveillance

Surveillance should actively engage parents in discussions about their child's development. Such dialogue provides the opportunity and context for discussions that promote normal development. For example, with parents who seem reserved and disinclined to talk to their babies, clinicians might take the time to model the joy of talking and smiling to infants. Such modelling has a known, positive impact on parent–child interaction compared to routine visits without such demonstrations.[9] For other parents, the trigger question regarding what the child seems to understand, may naturally lead to the comment that toddlers can only be expected to comprehend a one-step command (even if parents have caught their attention) and that toddlers should not be punished for failing to comply with complex requests. As an aside, behavioural concerns are the most common of all psychosocial complaints and are raised by almost 60% of parents. However, behavioural and developmental problems have an almost 50% overlap with one another. By addressing developmental problems first, health professionals may identify the source of the frustrations which lead to behavioural problems. If they only respond to the parents' concern about behaviour they may find that they have missed possible causal factors, such as untreated speech-language or other developmental problems (e.g. ref 10). Developmental surveillance also benefits child health clinicians by sharpening their clinical skills. When clinicians begin to systematically observe normal communicative functioning and the range of related parent perceptions, deviant functioning becomes more evident – just as looking at normal ear drums makes ear pathology stand out. The trigger questions and related observations then become the clinical instrument or 'otoscope' for routine checks of the speech-language system.

However, relying on informal developmental surveillance methods can be problematic. For example, it depends entirely on the skills and judgement of physicians who must decide when to screen or refer. The challenges of this approach are many and are highlighted in studies of the inaccuracy of physicians' clinical judgement which suggest that there may be high levels of underdetection of children with disabilities. Recent research from the UK revealed that only 45 to 55% of children with developmental problems are detected prior to school entrance.[11,12] Such appalling findings illustrate that informal methods routinely err in the direction of 'let's wait and see' rather than 'this could be serious and let's explore it carefully'. While underdetection is understandable because developmental problems in childhood are subtle, i.e. most children with language impairments do talk, they just do not talk well, the consequences are very troubling, given what we know about the effectiveness of early intervention and the adverse outcomes experienced by children who do not receive treatment. It is thus reasonable to ask why we treat detection of language and other development difficulties in a manner differently than blood lead levels, anaemia, hypercholesterolaemia and so forth. We would never simply eyeball such potential problems and deem our observations sufficient. Testing with high-quality tools that have proven levels of accuracy is demanded and routinely used by healthcare professionals. Should we not maintain such high standards of professionalism when it comes to detecting developmental problems?

This question leads us to wonder why physicians don't use developmental screening tests with much frequency. In one survey, physicians noted that many screening tools are too long for routine use and that there is little time to administer them. Another deterrent is the challenge of trying to manage children's behaviour during testing (e.g. children may be fearful, sick, asleep or, in many cases, not available for well-child visits). Finally, physicians also question the accuracy of popular measures such as the Denver-II and its predecessor, the Denver Developmental Screening Test.[13]

Recently, however, several measures have been published that consider the exigencies of primary care. The most applicable of these rely on information from parents. The advantages of using information from parents are many. They have prolonged opportunities to observe their children and are known to be highly accurate in describing what their children can and cannot do (although professionals must tolerate some incongruity between their own observations and those of parents, because parents often describe skills that are emerging and not yet fully mastered – meaning that children demonstrate them only in familiar environments). Further, parents' information can be gathered over the telephone, in waiting rooms or by mail. This offers a substantial time-saving for clinicians and much flexibility in how and when surveillance is conducted.

Validated approaches to surveillance: PEDS

One of the most promising new measures is a validated and standardised approach to developmental surveillance, called Parents' Evaluations of Developmental Status (PEDS).[14] PEDS operates not by asking parents about what the child is able to do at that point in time but by specifically eliciting the parents' level of concern about a range of specific categories of behaviour, such as development, socialisation, and speech and language. Unlike screening tests that usually offer only a binary answer, i.e. refer/don't refer, PEDS assists with a range of decisions, including when to monitor children more vigilantly, when to counsel parents on child-rearing or developmental promotion, and when to refer for mental health services versus speech-language or intellectual/educational assessment. Its accuracy in detecting developmental problems ranges from 74 to 80% (depending on the age of the child) and identifies children as normal with 70 to 80% accuracy. Over-referrals tend to be of children who perform well below average (at or below the 16th percentile on measures of language, intelligence or academic skills) but who are not so low as to be considered a clinical case. Such over-referred children may also benefit from assessment because, although their difficulties may not warrant the drawing up of statements of special educational needs, other forms of provision can be made for them. For example, additional testing can define difficulties, pinpoint goals and techniques, and lead to other kinds of helpful services such as early stimulation or preschool programmes. The concept of screening as it is discussed here reflects a predominantly medical 'case-based' approach. In practice in the UK the emphasis is for developmental needs to be identified in a less formal fashion through all forms of childcare in the early years.

PEDS simulates the kinds of questions routinely asked during well visits. Figure 3.1 shows a sample protocol from PEDS. The questions are written at the reading level of the average 10-year-old so that 90% of parents can complete the questionnaire independently while waiting for their appointment. This leaves the clinician to score and interpret the results which takes about two minutes. Although the questions appear simple, appearances (like development) are deceptive! Alternative wordings

PEDS: Parents' Evaluations of Developmental Status

Child's name _____ *Billy Morris* _____ Parents' name _____ *Linda Morris* _____

Child's birthday _____ *4/7/95* _____ Child's age _____ *3 yrs* _____ Today's date _____ *4/12/98* _____

1. Please list any concerns about your child's learning, development and behaviour.

I don't think he talks as well as he should for his age. Otherwise, he's a great little boy, very loving, watches everything carefully. Figures things out fast. Very bright!!!

2. Do you have any concerns about how your child talks and makes speech sounds?

Circle one: No   Yes   (A little)   COMMENTS
Doesn't talk much.

3. Do you have any concerns about how your child understands what you say?

Circle one: (No)   Yes   A little   COMMENTS
He understands everything.

4. Do you have any concerns about how your child uses his or her hands and fingers to do things?

Circle one: (No)   Yes   A little   COMMENTS

5. Do you have any concerns about how your child uses his or her arms and legs?

Circle one: (No)   Yes   A little   COMMENTS
He's very co-ordinated.

6. Do you have any concerns about how your child behaves?

Circle one: (No)   Yes   A little   COMMENTS
Very helpful and co-operative.

7. Do you have any concerns about how your child gets along with others?

Circle one: (No)   Yes   A little   COMMENTS
Plays well, just too quietly.

8. Do you have any concerns about how your child is learning to do things for himself/herself?

Circle one: (No)   Yes   A little   COMMENTS

9. Do you have any concerns about how your child is learning pre-school or school skills?

Circle one: (No)   Yes   A little   COMMENTS

10. Please list any other concerns:

None.

Figure 3.1   PEDS: Parents' Evaluation of Developmental Status.

attempted in pilot studies showed that only 50% of parents understand the meaning of the word 'development' so it must be paired with more common synonyms. Similarly, parents do not respond well or often to questions such as 'do you have any worries about your child?' or 'do you think your child has any problems?'. These are too ominous and negative whereas the word 'concerns' is interpreted more innocuously. Parents also need prompting to think through the range of developmental domains. For example, the parent who complains that his or her child does not behave well, is encouraged through the PEDS protocol to consider whether his or her child hears, has the language skills to understand commands, the motor or cognitive skills to execute them, etc.

How is it that parents, with little training in child development and often little experience, can raise concerns that are accurate indicators of developmental and behavioural status? Research shows that parents tend to compare their children to others. They use contact with other parents and children (e.g. at the supermarket, in physicians' offices, play groups or church) to observe what other children can do and to judge their own child accordingly. The intellectual skills required to make comparisons are not great (e.g. most people with severe learning disabilities can tell when two things are or are not alike). This phenomenon seems to explain why parents regardless of their level of education are equally accurate in appraising their child's development.[15–17]

Nevertheless, professional skill is required not only to elicit but also interpret parents' concerns. For example, parents' concerns in a particular area do not necessarily mean that children have problems in that area (e.g. a concern about speech-language development may reflect global developmental delays and not just a speech-language deficit). Further, only some concerns are predictive of problems. Finally, the predictive value of concerns changes with children's ages. Figures 3.2 and 3.3 illustrate the application of the PEDS. Figure 3.2 shows the PEDS longitudinal score form. The shaded boxes show concerns that are predictive of developmental problems at the various age ranges.

Figure 3.3 shows the PEDS interpretation form for the same child. This leads clinicians to one of five paths depending on the type and frequency of concerns raised:

1 Multiple predictive concerns (typically raised by about 10% of parents seeking paediatric care) are especially strong indicators of problems. Indeed when parents have two or more such concerns their children have a 70% chance of disabilities or substantial delays. This suggests the need for further testing. Specific types of concerns predict the need for speech-language versus intellectual/educational testing with a high degree of accuracy, enabling clinicians to make focused referrals.
2 A single predictive concern (typically raised by 20% of all parents and mostly concerning speech-language) produces a 30% chance of disabilities and should be responded to with additional screening to determine whether referrals are needed or whether children should be watched vigilantly and their parents' advised about how to stimulate their development.

PEDS SCORE FORM

Child's name _____*Billy Morris*_____   Parents' name _____*Linda Morris*_____

Child's birthday _____*4/7/95*_____   Child's age _____*3 yrs*_____   Today's date _____*4/12/98*_____

Directions: Find appropriate column for the patient's age. Place a check mark in the appropriate box to show each concern mentioned on the PEDS Response Form.

Age of patient	0–1½	1½–3	3–4½	4½–7
1. Global/cognitive	☐	☐	☐	☐
2. Expressive language/ articulation	☐	☐	✓	☐
3. Receptive language	☐	☐	☐	☐
4. Fine motor	☐	☐	☐	☐
5. Gross motor	☐	☐	☐	☐
6. Behaviour	☐	☐	☐	☐
7. Social/emotional	☐	☐	☐	☐
8. Self-help	☐	☐	☐	☐
9. School	☐	☐	☐	☐
10. Other	☐	☐	☐	☐

Directions: Total the number of marked shaded boxes and place this figure in the large shaded box below. If any non-shaded boxes are marked, place a check in the large non-shaded box below.

Number of significant concerns   ⟶   ☐   ☐   *1*   ☐

If two or more significant concerns, follow Path A on PEDS Interpretation Form. If one significant concern, follow Path B.

Non-significant concerns   ⟶   ☐   ☐   ☐   ☐

If any non-significant concerns (and no significant concerns), follow Path C. If no concerns (either significant or non-significant), consider Path D if relevant. Otherwise, follow Path E.

Figure 3.2 PEDS score form.

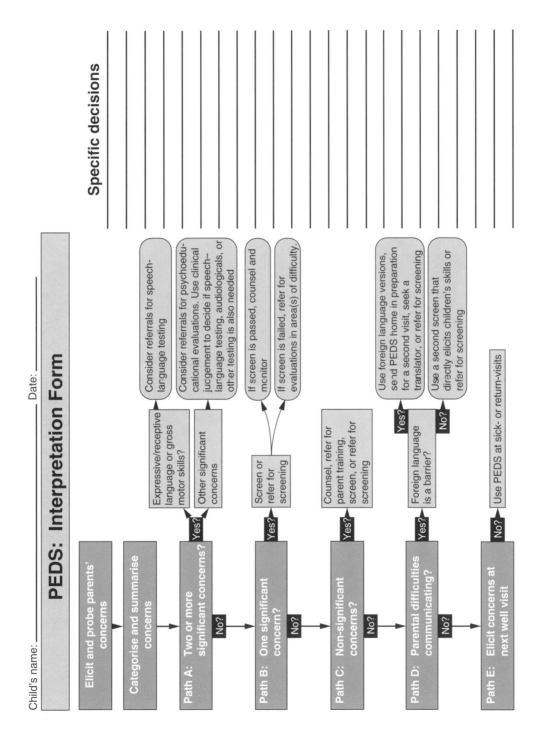

PEDS: Interpretation Form

Child's name: _____ Date: _____

Specific decisions

Elicit and probe parents' concerns	
Categorise and summarise concerns	

Path A: Two or more significant concerns? — Yes?
- Expressive/receptive language or gross motor skills? → Consider referrals for speech-language testing
- Other significant concerns → Consider referrals for psychoeducational evaluations. Use clinical judgement to decide if speech-language testing, audiologicals, or other testing is also needed

No? ↓

Path B: One significant concern? — Yes?
- Screen or refer for screening → If screen is passed, counsel and monitor / If screen is failed, refer for evaluations in area(s) of difficulty.

No? ↓

Path C: Non-significant concerns? — Yes?
- Counsel, refer for parent training, screen, or refer for screening

No? ↓

Path D: Parental difficulties communicating? — Yes?
- Foreign language is a barrier?
  - Yes? → Use foreign language versions, send PEDS home in preparation for a second visit, seek a translator, or refer for screening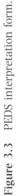
  - No? → Use a second screen that directly elicits children's skills or refer for screening

No? ↓

Path E: Elicit concerns at next well visit — No?
- Use PEDS at sick- or return-visits

Figure 3.3 PEDS interpretation form.

3 Non-predictive concerns (unshaded boxes) are almost always about behaviour and are raised by about 20% of parents. These children have a very limited likelihood of developmental disabilities. Their parents need advice about child-rearing and follow-up to assess the effectiveness of this advice. When results are poor, behavioural/emotional screening is recommended with referrals to mental health services or parenting classes as indicated.

4 A small group of parents (about 3%) fail to raise concerns even though their children have a moderate likelihood of disabilities. Often these were parents who could not communicate in English either by interview or in writing. Other communication barriers include parents who are not the primary caretakers (e.g. a teen mother whose own mother provides most of the child's care, or parents with serious mental health problems of their own). Referrals for screening are warranted for the children of such parents.[16]

5 Fortunately more than 40% of parents have no concerns and their children have little chance of disabilities. Routine monitoring and reassurance are sufficient.

Thus, PEDS, in only a few minutes, enables clinicians to make a wide range of evidenced-based decisions about psychosocial issues. It also builds a collaborative relationship with parents and offers encouragement to those who are reluctant to raise their concerns. Indeed, failure to clearly and carefully elicit parents' concerns means that about 40% of parents whose children have disabilities fail to mention their legitimate worries.[17] Although some parents remain reluctant to discuss their concerns, it is likely that by repeatedly asking them at each well-visit they will come to understand that their perspective is important and worthy of the doctor's attention.

Standardised screening tests

Screening is a brief method for sorting those who probably have problems from those who probably do not. Those with apparent problems should be referred for diagnostic evaluations and, if diagnosed, referred for treatment. Due to its brevity, screening cannot be error-free but should be as accurate as possible in order to reduce over-referrals, with their concomittant expense and anxiety for parents, or under-referrals, with their loss of critical learning opportunities for children and expense to society. A screening test's accuracy is defined by its sensitivity, specificity and positive predictive value (Box 3.5). For a test to be valid, sensitive and specific, it has to be standardised. This means that measures must include a sufficiently clear set of directions that they can be administered in exactly the same way by different examiners working in different settings. Only then can a child's score be interpreted confidently – compared to the test's norms (the performance of the large group of children administered the test under similar conditions, prior to publication). Another question that must be answered prior to confident score interpretation is, how like the normative sample was the child you plan to test? If the child is from an impoverished background, is it

Box 3.5:   Critical standards for screening tests

Sensitivity indicates the proportion of children with true problems correctly identified by a screening test (e.g. by failing, abnormal or positive results). Ideally, at least 70 to 80% of those with difficulties should be identified.

Specificity is defined as the percentage of children without true difficulties correctly identified by passing, normal or negative findings on screening. Because there are many more children developing normally than not, specificity should fall in the 70 to 80% range but preferably towards the higher end so as to minimise over-referrals.

Positive predictive value. When a child fails a screening test, he or she *probably* has a problem. Still there is always a chance that the screening test is in error. Positive predictive value is the percentage of children with failing scores on screening tests who have a true problem.

For both specificity and positive predictive value, it is important to know something about the children who are over-referred. Thus, screening tests should assess this group to determine if they are indeed truly normal or instead fall into the 'grey zone' between normal and disabled. The latter are children who need careful attention from their healthcare provider and will benefit from referrals to stimulation programmes, tutoring or other kinds of assistance.

Other characteristics of accurate screening tests

Validity. Accurate tests contain proof of various types of validity. *Content validity* refers to how well a test samples aspects of development. Items should cover a range of realistic behaviours that clearly reflect the domains measured and which are drawn from a wealth of research on developmental sequences. For example, a screening test that measures language should have items measuring both receptive and expressive language skills (and preferably articulation as well). Screening tests should provide evidence of *concurrent validity* and show a high degree of correlation (0.60 or greater) between the screen and diagnostic measures. Although screening tests need not provide evidence of *predictive* or *criterion-related validity*, it is extremely helpful for measures to sample heavily tasks which are most predictive of school success (i.e. language and pre-academic skills such as letter recognition in 4–5-year-olds).[18]

Reliability. Screening tests should produce the same score administered by different examiners, or when the same child is tested at different times. Reliability is usually expressed as a percentage of agreement (ideally 80% or greater) or as correlations (ideally 0.90 or higher). There is, even with the best tests, some variability across domains (motor skills are more inconsistently expressed and hence less reliable than language, academic or cognitive skills).

Box 3.6:   Features of good screening tests

- Materials should be interesting to children but sufficiently minimal in number that examiner's can find them easily in the test kit
- Directions for item administration should be bold-faced or printed in colour so they are easy to locate during testing
- Scoring procedures should be clear and simple so that computational errors are minimised
- The amount of training required and training exercises should be included in the manual
- Directions for interpreting test results to families should be included (e.g. examiners should be advised to avoid diagnostic labels, offer ongoing support, telephone numbers, additional opportunities to discuss the results, etc.) and guidance should be given for the kinds of referrals that may be needed based on various profiles (e.g. falling scores on language domains but average performance in other areas should dictate a referral for speech-language evaluations, while deficits in motor development areas only should suggest referrals to a neurologist or physical therapist)
- It is helpful to have a prescreening subtest built into the test so as to facilitate applicability in medical settings
- Alternative methods for administering items are desirable (e.g. via parental report, observation and/or direct elicitation) so that examiners can circumvent child recalcitrance, limited English on the part of parents or children, or parents with minimal knowledge of their child's development, such as when a parent is not the primary care-taker

---

reasonable to compare his or her performance to a sample that included only children from wealthy, educated families? Ideally, tests should be standardised on a large group of children, stratified geographically and on the basis of ethnicity and socioeconomic status. The absence of appropriate stratification does not mean a test should not be used, provided there is subsequent validation work by the author or by other researchers that supports the application of the measure with different populations.

There are many screening tests on the market. None meets all the recommendations in Box 3.5 but some approach the standards. Below is a critical discussion of several tests. A list of such screening tests is provided in Appendix 1. Box 3.6 shows the features of the best screening procedures. Several existing screens are devoted only to measuring language skills, although these should be approached with particular caution for the following reasons: (a) of the more than 50 speech and language screening tests on the market, only one approaches the standards for screening tests and this one has only been validated on a relatively small sample of kindergarten students.[19] All others either failed to provide evidence of accuracy (e.g. Bankson

Table 3.1 High quality broad-band developmental screening tools

Measure	Age range	Description	Scoring	Accuracy	Time frame
Child Development Inventories (formerly Minnesota Child Development Inventories) (1992) Behavior Science Systems, Box 580274, Minneapolis. MN 55458 (612-929-6220)	3–72 months	Three separate instruments each with 60 yes–no descriptions. Can be mailed to families, completed in waiting rooms, administered by interview or by direct elicitation. A 300-item assessment level version may be useful in follow-up studies or subspeciality clinics and produces age equivalent and cutoff scores in each domain.	A single cutoff tied to 1.5 standard deviations below the mean.	Sensitivity in detecting children with difficulties is excellent (greater than 75% across studies) and specificity in correctly detecting normally developing children is good (70% across studies).	About 10 minutes.
Parents' Evaluations of Developmental Status (PEDS) (1997) Ellsworth & Vandermeer Press Ltd. 4405 Scenic Drive, Nashville. Tennessee (615-386-0061; fax: 615-386-0346) http://edge.net/~evpress	Ages birth to 8 years	Both a screen and a surveillance system, PEDS has 10 questions eliciting parents' concerns. Waiting room, interview and Spanish versions. Written at the 5th grade level. Determines when to refer, provide a second screen, counsel, or monitor development, behaviour, and academic progress.	Identifies levels of risk for various kinds of disabilities and delays.	Sensitivity ranging from 74% to 79% and specificity ranging from 70% to 80% across age levels.	About 2 minutes.
Ages and Stages Questionnaire (formerly Infant Monitoring System) (1994) Paul H Brookes Publishers, PO Box 10624, Baltimore. Maryland 21285 (1-800-638-3775)	0 to 60 months	Clear drawings and simple directions help parents indicate children's skills. Separate copyable forms of 30–35 items for each age range (tied to well-child visit schedule). Can be used in mass mail-outs for child-find programs.	Single pass/fail score.	Sensitivity ranged 70% to 90% at all ages except the 4-month level. Specificity ranged from 76% to 91%.	About 5 minutes.

Table 3.1: Continued

Measure	Age range	Description	Scoring	Accuracy	Time frame
Brigance Screens (1985) Curriculum Associates Inc., 5 Esquire Road, N Billenca, MA. 01862 (1-800-225-0248)	21–90 months	Seven separate forms, one for each 12-month age range. Taps speech-language, motor, readiness and general knowledge at younger ages and also reading and maths at older ages. Uses direct elicitation and observation.	Cutoff and age equivalent scores in three domains.	Sensitivity and specificity to giftedness and to developmental and academic problems are 70% to 82% across ages.	About 10 minutes.
Battelle Developmental Inventory Screening Test (BDIST) (1984) Riverside Publishing Company, 8420 Bryn Mawr Avenue, Chicago, Illinois 60631 (1-800-767-8378)	12–96 months	Items use a combination of direct assessment, observation, and parental interview. The receptive language subtest may serve as a brief prescreen. Difficult to administer and takes 15 minutes for younger children and 35 for older ones. Well standardised and validated.	Age equivalents (somewhat deflated), cutoffs at 1.0, 1.5, and 2.0 standard deviations below the mean.	Sensitivity and specificity are 70% to 80% across ages.	25–35 minutes.
Bayley Infant Neurodevelopmental Screen (BINS) (1995) The Psychological Corporation, 555 Academic Court, San Antonio, TX 78204 (1-800-228-0752)	3–24 months	Uses 10–13 directly elicited items per 3–6-month age range, assess neurological processes (reflexes and tone), neurodevelopmental skills (movement and symmetry) and developmental accomplishments (object permanence, imitation and language).	Categorises performance into low, moderate or high risk via cutoff scores. Provides subtest cutoff scores for each domain assessed in order to focus referrals.	Specificity and sensitivity are 75% to 86% across ages.	10–15 minutes.

Language Screening Test, Stephenson Oral Language Screening Test) or had sensitivity and specificity that was unacceptably low (e.g. Fluharty Preschool Speech and Language Screening Test; and The Speech and Language Screening Questionnaire); (b) children who present with language delays or whose parents are concerned about language are often children with global developmental difficulties; and (c) children who present with behavioural or psychiatric problems (for whom it might seem logical to measure behavioural status or to refer for counselling or parent training) are often those with unidentified language or global delays. Consequently, it is most advisable in medical settings to administer broad-band measures – those that tap multiple developmental domains. A list of the more accurate broad-band tools is provided in Table 3.1.

A second word of caution has to do with the fact that children manifest language and behaviour that can be highly context-dependent and this may be particularly relevant in more formal, unfamiliar situations such as those in which a child is being tested. In medical settings, they are often too fearful or ill to demonstrate skills willingly. This phenomenon sometimes leads medical professionals to discount parental descriptions and concerns when in fact, it is the professionals' observations that are misleading or simply incorrect.[20] At no time is this potential conflict greater than when parents complain about children's behaviour and emotional status. Children may be extremely co-operative or well-behaved in the medical offices and quite the opposite at home. Children with communication and other developmental problems arc often aware of their difficulties. Since they are often given tasks which are too difficult for their level of skill development, they may be inherently frustrated, anxious about the effectiveness of their communication attempts or excessively dependent on those who understand them best, i.e. their primary carer. Although children with language difficulties are likely to be quiet and extremely co-operative during the medical encounter, their parents may offer descriptions of troubling behaviour at home. These children should receive careful scrutiny for the possibility of developmental as well as behavioural impairments.

Summary

- Surveillance is an important issue for everyone who works closely with young children, especially those with a responsibility for overseeing the needs of the whole population.
- There are good reasons for identifying young children with communication difficulties. As a group, they are at risk for a number of educational, behavioural and social difficulties which are amenable to early intervention. Speech and language difficulties may also be markers of other conditions.
- However, the process of identification is not one which can be treated casually. It is possible to generate a number of questions for parents and carers pertaining to a range of both the skills underlying speech and language development and to the

skills themselves. While they are evidently highly relevant it is difficult to establish how accurate they are because the clinician has to interpret the responses to them.

- An alternative is a more formalised, yet easy-to-administer, questionnaire system such as the PEDs. Although language-only developmental screens have not proven generally effective, there is a range of broad-band tools that have high levels of accuracy.

- The key to effective surveillance is good observational skills, a sound knowledge of developmental expectations, the use of effective trigger questions to tap the observational skills of parents and preferably the use of an accurate, validated broad-band screening test.

References

1   Farran DC (1990) Effects of intervention with disadvantaged and disabled children: a decade review. In: SJ Meisels and JP Shonkoff (eds) *Handbook of Early Childhood Intervention*. Cambridge University Press, Cambridge.

2   Law J, Boyle J, Harris F, Harkness A and Nye C (1998) Screening for Speech and Language Delay: a systematic review of the literature. *Health Technology Assessment* **2**(9).

3   Barnett WS and Escobar CM (1990) Economic costs and benefits of early intervention. In: SJ Meisels and JP Shonkoff (eds) *Handbook of Early Childhood Intervention*. Cambridge University Press, Cambridge.

4   Green M (ed) (1994) *Bright Futures: guidelines for health supervision of infants, children, and adolescents*. National Center for Education in Maternal and Child Health, Arlington, VA.

5   Bayley N (1994) *The Bayley Sales of Infant Development II*. Psychological Corp., San Antonio, TX.

6   Gesell A and Armatruda C (1964) *Developmental Diagnosis*. Harper & Row Publishers, New York.

7   Capute AJ, Palmer FB, Shapiro BK, Wachtel RC, Schmidt S and Ross A (1986) Clinical linguistic and auditory milestone scale: prediction of cognition in infancy. *Developmental Medicine and Child Neurology* **28**(6): 762–71.

8   Fenson L, Dale PS, Reznick JS, Bates E, Thal DJ and Pethick SJ (1994) Variability in early communicative development. *Monographs of the Society for Research in Child Development* **59**, no. 5.

9   Casey P and Whitt J (1980) The effect of the pediatric clinician in child health supervision on the mother–infant relationship and infant cognitive development. *Pediatrics* **65**: 815.

10   Beitchman JH, Nair R, Clegg M, Patel PG, Ferguson B, Pressman E *et al.* (1986) Prevalence of speech and language disorders in 5-year-old kindergarten children in the Ottawa-Carleton region. *Journal of Speech and Hearing Disorders* **51**(2): 98–110.

11   Dearlove J and Kearney D (1990) How good is general practice developmental screening? *BMJ* **300**: 1177–80.

12   Bowie D and Parry JA (1984) Court come true – for better or for worse. *BMJ* **299**: 1322–4.

13   Frankenburg N, Dodds J and Archer P (1990) *Denver-II: technical manual.* Denver Developmental Materials, Denver.

14   Glascoe FP (1997) *Parents' Evaluations of Developmental Status (PEDS).* Radcliffe Medical Press, Oxford.

15   Glascoe FP, Maclean LE (1990) How parents appraise their child's development. *Family Relations* **39**: 280–3.

16   Glascoe FP (1997) Parents' concerns about children's development: prescreening technique or screening test? *Pediatrics* **99** 522–8.

17   Glascoe FP (1997) Do parents discuss concerns about children's development with health care providers? *Ambulatory Child Health* **2**: 349–56.

18   Simner ML (1983) The warning signs of school failure: an updated profile of the at-risk kindergarten child. *Topics in Early Childhood Education* **2**: 3–11.

19   Sturner RA, Layton TL, Evans AW, Heller JH, Funk SG and Machon MW (1994) Preschool speech and language screening: a review of currently available tests. *American Journal of Speech-Language Pathology* **3**: 25–36.

20   Bricker D, Squires J, Mounts L *et al.* (1999) *Ages & Stages Questionnaires (ASQ): a parent-completed, child-monitoring system.* Paul Brookes Publishing, Baltimore.

CHAPTER 4

The medical context

Rashmin Tamhne

The transformation of a newborn baby, whose only form of communication is probably crying, into a 4–5 year-old using sophisticated means of communication (verbal and non-verbal, including crying!) in negotiating his or her way, is a remarkable feat of human development.

Children acquire language for sharing what they have in their mind through expression and interpretation, and language development connects with all aspects of a child's physical, cognitive, perceptual-motor, emotional, social and cultural development. It influences all these aspects, acting as a driving force, and is in turn influenced by them. This model of 'intentionality and language development' proposed by Bloom integrates different perspectives and provides a holistic foundation for understanding not only normal language development, but also the reasons why it might not develop normally.[1]

That in the vast majority of children, language and communication develop in a manner that does not lead to concerns is partly a measure of 'evolutionary ingenuity', as expressed through their genes, as well as positive attributes in a child's physical and social environment. However, a significant number, anywhere up to 15%, of children do present with difficulties in communication development, as was discussed in Chapter 2. The medical context, at whatever level, provides an excellent opportunity for a holistic view of children's communication difficulties, through both the medical evaluation *per se* and as a result of the networking of medical practitioners with other childcare professionals. Such an approach, based on the biopsychosocial concept of health,[2] is essential in the light of Bloom's conceptual framework of language development, whether in promoting children's language development or helping those who encounter problems.

Case study 1

Darren's parents were quite pleased with his language development until he was about one year old, when he was alert, responsive and able to say three or four words with

---

Box 4.1:   Communication disorders in children: paediatric roles

1 Clinical – as diagnostician
2 For networking with:
   – other health professionals
   – the education department
   – social services, when appropriate
   – voluntary agencies
3 Ongoing healthcare of emerging problems
4 As the advocate for the child and family, e.g. in obtaining benefits
5 Ongoing support to the family
6 As co-ordinator of health service interventions

---

meaning. He then started going to the local day nursery and appeared not to be making any further progress, contrary to his parents' expectations. By the time he was 16 months of age, his parents were so concerned that they contacted the health visitor who shared their concern. Darren was saying virtually no clear words. In accordance with the practice guidelines, the health visitor arranged for Darren to see his GP who noted that Darren had been seen by him and his other partners at the surgery quite a few times for ear infections during the preceding months. On examination he was noted to have otitis media with effusion (glue ear). He was promptly referred for a hearing test that confirmed a hearing loss and a few weeks later the local ENT surgeon performed an operation for the insertion of grommets. His hearing improved, leading to a resolution of the communication problem.

Case study 2

Jenny's mother had been concerned about her daughter since she was a few weeks old. She was always in her own world and never responded to her mother's social overtures. Deep down, she was worried that Jenny had something quite drastically wrong with her. Now, at the age of 18 months, Jenny was hardly saying a word and she expressed no interest in communicating with others. At the 18-month check, the family health visitor was also very concerned about Jenny. The screening tool, the Checklist for Autism in Toddlers (CHAT), strengthened her suspicion that Jenny was likely to have an Autistic Spectrum Disorder. The health visitor discussed the matter with her GP who referred Jenny to the local paediatrician, while simultaneously making a referral to the speech and language therapist. The paediatrician took a detailed developmental history as well as examining Jenny physically for any neurological problems. Arrangements were made for Jenny to have investigations which led to a finding of Fragile X syndrome. The paediatrician's and speech and language therapist's assessments led to a diagnosis of Autistic Spectrum Disorder and formal notification was made to the local education department that Jenny was likely to go on to have special educational needs. She was placed at a local specialist pre-school nursery following further assessment from the educational psychologist. Jenny's parents needed considerable counselling and social support provided by social services, specialists and family health visitors. The local geneticist advised the parents about the risk of Autistic Spectrum Disorder and Fragile X syndrome in future pregnancies.

Case study 3

Nathan was a boisterous three and a half-year old boy who became well known for his aggressive manner, especially towards his siblings and peers at the nursery. He was quite a big boy with good motor development but his expressive language development was quite delayed, in that he was unable to say full sentences. There were no problems with his hearing and the paediatrician's assessment showed no evidence of neurological problems. The social circumstances were satisfactory and he received a fair deal of stimulation both at home and at the nursery. The speech and language therapist's assessment confirmed a diagnosis of specific language impairment, leading to referral by the paediatrician to the education department. Nathan was eventually statemented for special educational needs, with continuing paediatric monitoring and speech and language therapy until he started junior school.

Case study 4

Vijay, a five-year old boy, had moderate learning difficulties associated with delayed language development. His early development was uneventful and when, at the age of three, he was thought by his parents to have slow language development, it was believed that this was a result of his bilingual upbringing; Gujarati was spoken at home and English at the pre-school nursery. Vijay then developed epilepsy and his learning difficulties became more obvious. At the age of five he had a number of problems requiring co-ordinated management of educational professionals - psychologists and teachers - as well as the speech and language therapist and the neurologist. He was placed at a local assessment unit for further delineation of his communication problems and his need for augmentative forms of communication. His management necessitated regular contact between all the listed professionals and his parents.

These case studies, as well as describing medical involvement, illustrate the principle of partnership in the professional care of children with communication difficulties. Effective multi-disciplinary (within the health agency) and multi-agency working is at the heart of a care package for these children, and a mutual understanding of professional roles in this respect is essential.

Medical care: a service delivery framework

In the UK, a well-developed structure of primary care is intended to provide general medical care to *all* children. General practitioners, who may or may not have paediatric or developmental training, are joined in this task by health visitors, who do receive specific training in developmental issues. In the event of there being significant developmental concerns about a child, referral to secondary care professionals is

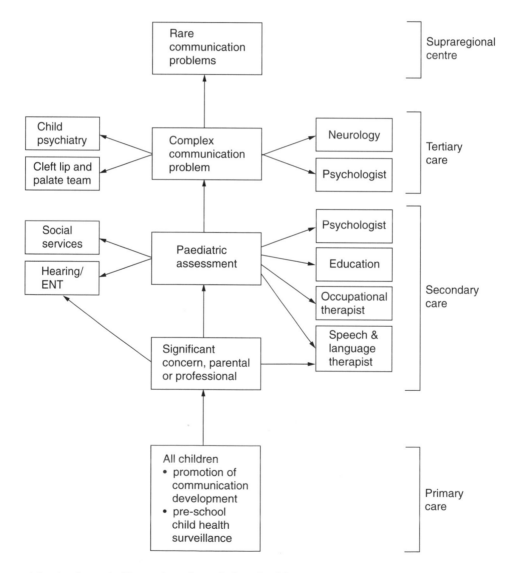

Figure 4.1 A schematic illustration of interlinking healthcare services at various levels for the identification of children with communication problems.

made, generally paediatricians and speech and language therapists or other professionals. Paediatricians who are developmentally trained, especially those practising in
the community, then help define a child's developmental problem and take the necessary actions to enable multi-disciplinary and inter-agency networking. Details of the
paediatric role are described later in this chapter. For complex cases, tertiary level
care involving the paediatric neurologist and child psychiatrist is needed. Such a
tiered approach is aimed at making the use of healthcare resources effective and cost
beneficial (*see* Figure 4.1).

However, in the USA and most of continental Europe, paediatricians with specialist
training in child development are primary care providers to *all* children (although this
pattern may be changing). The advantage of such a system is, of course, immediate
access to specialist level care for children with developmental problems at the primary
care level. In the UK, with the recent development of PCGs/Trusts, a tendency among
GPs to specialise in specific clinical areas such as paediatrics is likely to grow.

The primary healthcare context

By the nature of their generalist clinical role, GPs and health visitors are able to influence children's communication development. At this level two main components, in
addition to general medical care, are significant.

Promotion of communication development

Parents, especially with their first child, often seek advice from their GP or health
visitor on ways in which to promote their child's communication development. Box
4.2 summarises the principles involved in this aspect of health promotion.

Child health surveillance (CHS)

Health surveillance of pre-school children (*see* Chapter 3), part of the overall child
health promotion programme, is a key feature of child healthcare in every UK health
district. The content of the programme, based on the recommendations of a national,
multi-disciplinary working party on CHS,[6] is generally evidence based with an
emphasis on developmental surveillance using selected screening tests. GPs, who need
appropriate training to provide CHS, and health visitors together provide a focus on
children's development including communication.

In addition to the overview of CHS in Chapter 3, there are certain contemporary
issues in the UK affecting communication development surveillance that require
mention.

Box 4.2:   Promoting language development of young children

Practical advice for parents

Context
- At the developmental level of the child
  – avoid overwhelming
- Emotional engagement/attunement with child
- Setting aside separate time, e.g. for reading stories *or* making the most of everyday situations
- Making communication fun - for both the child and parent

Content
- Balance of being supportive (encouragement, patience, listening) and challenging (cognitively) (use of Vygotsky's principle of Zone of Proximal Development)[3]
- Motherese (child directed speech - Chapter 1)
- Recast (phrase the same meaning in a different way)[4]
- Echo (repeat what the child says, especially if incomplete)
- Expand (restate child's phrases in a linguistically more sophisticated and clear manner)
- Corrective feedback to the child
- Provide a model to the child, e.g. turn taking, listening

General
- Increase opportunities for peer interactions, e.g. playgroups
- Recognise potential impediments to language development, e.g. hearing loss

Specific programmes
- OWLing (Observe Wait Listen)
- Parenting skills training (if appropriate)
- Parent support through voluntary organisations, e.g. Home Start[5]

Hearing screening

The health visitor distraction test, carried out at 7–9 months, has been the mainstay of screening for sensori-neural hearing loss in the UK. While its sensitivity can approach 90% for hearing impairment of > 50db, it is possible for it to dip well below 50% if coverage and levels of professional expertise are not maintained.[7] A recent systematic review recommended universal adoption of electrophysiological techniques for neonatal hearing screening rather than the targeted screening of high-risk neonates (as currently practised in some centres).[8] This recommendation has considerable resource implications and its practical implementation awaits the outcome of further debate.

Screening for autism

Early diagnosis of autism (*see* Chapter 11) has many potential benefits and population screening tests are therefore being developed. Results of the evaluation of a recently developed screening test, Checklist for Autism in Toddlers (CHAT),[9] which is applied at 18 months are soon to be published. CHAT has the merit of bringing the issue of social communication in young children to the attention of health professionals and parents. Whether it is robust enough in its present form to be a screening test for universal application is not certain.

Immunisation

Immunisation, an important part of the child health promotion programme, produces a considerable, if indirect, impact on the occurrence of communication difficulties. Haemophilus b (Hib) vaccination, introduced in the UK in 1987, has led to a marked reduction in the incidence of *Haemophilus meningitis*, thereby reducing complications of hearing loss and developmental disability, each of which is associated with delays in communication development.

There has been recent controversy concerning the administration of measles, mumps, rubella (MMR) vaccination in children following a reported link between MMR (given as a triple vaccine) and autism and Crohn's disease. Subsequent reports have, however, failed to show any objective evidence for such an association. In a study by Taylor *et al.* (quoted by Bower[10]), 498 children with autism born since 1979 in the North Thames region were investigated, and no difference was found in the age of diagnosis, whether the children had received the MMR vaccine before or after 18 months of age, or had never been vaccinated. In the meantime, the uptake of MMR in England and Wales fell to 88% from the previous figure of 92%, and considerable efforts will be needed to restore parental confidence in this procedure.[11]

Personal child health records (PCHR)

Initiated in the early 1990s, a national version of the PCHR (*Red Book*) is given to parents soon after the birth of their children, and is now in use in most districts in the UK. It is a potentially effective tool for communication between parents and professionals, and a recent randomised controlled study aimed at examining the impact of 'add-on' sheets in PCHR for the care of children with special needs, has shown some evidence of their usefulness.[12]

Referral issues

An important issue in primary healthcare is whether to refer a child with concerns about communication development, to professionals in secondary care, be it a speech and language therapist, paediatrician or others. The wide range of normal communication development means that a potentially large number of children – possibly as many as 10–15 from a health visitor's typical caseload of 100 births per year – is likely to need to be considered for referral. The situation is complex. On the one hand, there are the socio-cultural perspectives of parents, their expectations for the communication development of their child and, at times, media-, especially Internet-, generated anxiety. On the other hand, a significant number of these children, particularly those with concerns about expressive language, show spontaneous improvement in communication development.[13] Significant problems such as Autistic Spectrum Disorder, while showing an apparent rise in prevalence, are still quite rare, as is specific language impairment.

On the whole there are no easy answers about who and when to refer but as Glascoe has shown, parental concern predicts significant problems more effectively than clinical judgement alone (and the PEDS is a practical tool for translating this into a clinical setting).[14] Parental concern regarding the emergence of social communication, particularly towards late infancy and throughout the second year, is quite significant and should always lead to a referral. Hall describes a useful approach to distinguish 'normal' shyness from more pervasive social communication problems, through the observation of social and emotional behaviours in children, and advises referral to a paediatrician or child psychiatrist on any suspicion of such problems.[15] Checking hearing and ears prior to the referral is important. Quite commonly, a normal HVDT at 7–9 months is taken as evidence of normal hearing thereafter but it is possible for conductive hearing loss to arise after 7–9 months and, hence, continuing surveillance for hearing loss is essential (*see also* Chapter 3).

The secondary healthcare context

Communication development is the result of diverse factors and as such the first evaluation at the secondary healthcare level of a child experiencing communication difficulties needs to be a broad one, but also one capable of generating a swift clinical and inter-agency response. Since the publication of the Court Report in 1976 on child health services, the UK has seen a gradual development of community-based consultant-led paediatric services that operate in conjunction with hospital-based clinical paediatric specialists, therapy and mental health professionals and education and social services.[16] In all except those cases of communication difficulty where assessment and intervention needs are met in the primary care setting, community-based paediatric services offer the required 'whole child' approach to assessment, combined with a developmental, preventative and evidence-based focus. From this initial assessment the need may arise for more detailed assessment involving a number of professionals depending on the child's difficulty (*see* Box 4.3).

Routes of referral

There are several routes leading to paediatric evaluation:

- referral from child health promotion programme, either from a set stage of developmental surveillance, usually at two years, or as a result of parental concern at any time (part of the broader concept of surveillance)
- as part of planned neuro-developmental follow-up programmes for high-risk neonates
- during the course of evaluation for adoption or fostering purposes
- following school-based concerns, especially with regard to reading, attention problems etc
- at any age following significant illness, e.g. meningitis, trauma etc
- during evaluation of a child for *any* problem.

Setting

This is most commonly an outpatient setting, hospital or community based, with an adequately sized room and toys for children to play with. A 30 to 45 minute appointment is usual, but flexibility is essential. A directory of Child Development Centres in the UK is available.[17]

A framework for the initial paediatric evaluation
(applicable for the evaluation of any developmental concerns)

This is essentially clinical, comprising:

- A history (from the parents/caregivers):
  - to explore concerns
  - to obtain information about the social, environmental and family context
  - to seek the chronology of the child's health-related milestones, and a description of relevant issues/problems.

Box 4.3:   Communication difficulties

Differential diagnosis
- Normal variation
- Social affective disorders
  - autistic disorder (*see* Chapter 11)
  - selective mutism (*see* Chapter 21)
- Cognitive developmental delay (pre-, peri- and post-natal causes)
  - learning disability (*see* Chapter 19)
  - auditory processing disorder
- Specific developmental problems
  - dyslexia
- Motor impairment
  - cerebral palsy (*see* Chapter 14)
  - spina bifida (*see* Chapter 18)
  - developmental co-ordination disorder
- Sensory impairment
  - hearing
       i congenital sensorineural
       ii acquired
  - vision
- Congenital malformation
  - cleft palate (*see* Chapter 15)
- Acquired brain damage
  - cerebrovascular accident
  - traumatic brain injury (*see* Chapter 23)
- Neurological
  - seizure disorder, e.g. Landau-Klefner syndrome (*see* Chapter 20)
- Environmental
  - maltreatment (*see* Chapter 9)
- Substance abuse
  - fetal alcohol
  - prenatal cocaine
  - glue-sniffing/drugs especially in adolescents
- Socioeconomic disadvantage
  - poverty (*see* Chapter 22)
  - cultural diversity (*see* Chapter 6)
- Specific language impairment

Comorbid conditions
- Psychiatric problems
  - ADHD (*see* Chapter 12)
  - childhood schizophrenia
- Disintegration of speech

Information from the history is useful in establishing the presence of any risk factors in communication development.

- Developmental review (*see* Box 4.4):
  - mainly from parental report
  - using developmental tests for rapid screening, e.g. draw-a-man test,[18] rather than detailed assessment.

Box 4.4:   Developmental overview during the initial paediatric evaluation

- Motor
  - gross motor
  - fine motor/adaptive
- Communication
  - verbal comprehension
  - expression
    - i language, e.g. vocabulary, grammar, pragmatics
    - ii speech
- Cognitive development
- Emotional development
- Social development
- Sensory
  - vision
  - hearing
- Control of body functions
  - continence of bowels and bladder

The aim of this review is to note if there is any developmental delay. If there is a delay:
  - is it global?
  - is there any dissociation:
    - i between different spheres of development?
    - ii within the communication sphere, e.g. expressive language and comprehension?

It is important to recognise that the initial paediatric evaluation is not intended to provide a detailed assessment of the child's development.

- Informal observations of the child and the parent–child interaction, including:
  - the social behaviour/emotional response of the child
  - spontaneous play
  - attention span and activity level
  - any abnormal behavioural pattern.

- A clinical examination:
  - general examination, looking for dysmorphism, growth problems etc
  - a neurological and neuro-developmental evaluation to assess the presence of any specific problems such as dyspraxia etc.

- A review of any other available information, including:
  - hearing test reports
  - nursery/school reports.

At the conclusion of the initial review, the presence of a significant communication problem is usually apparent and an indication of the need for further investigation and assessment is obtained.

Some important issues in the initial evaluation in relation to children's communication difficulties presenting as a primary concern are summarised below. (For more detailed paediatric and child psychiatric assessment, *see* Bax, Rutter, Rosenbloom and Newton and Wraith.[19–22])

Clinical evaluation and investigations

Exploring concerns

Time spent on a detailed exploration of concerns is well spent not only because it helps to set the scene and may offer aetiological clues, but also because concerns need to be addressed at the end of the evaluation. As described by Pinnock and Wolraich, an awareness of the link between poverty and developmental difficulties and the recognition of socio-economic disadvantage in the individual clinical situation, is an important first step (*see* Chapter 22). Waterstone has discussed identification and interventions in relation to child poverty in the UK and found that parental employment and housing are significant factors.[23]

Family context

The place of the child in the family, his or her relationship with parents/other adults and siblings, the 'linguistic environment' in the household and expectations of the child, are all important considerations. Myths are often built round the birth order of the child – there is no evidence to support these and the second child will not be put off talking because the first child does all the talking.

While single parenthood *per se* is not likely to be the cause of communication difficulties, it may exacerbate stress, and consequently affect parental coping ability. The availability of a social support network should be looked into.

Parental mental health is an important factor influencing the development of young children, particularly in the cognitive, emotional and social developmental spheres. Murray and Cooper, in a recent annotation on the subject, described two studies showing significant adverse effects on the developmental outcome early in the second year of exposure to maternal postnatal depression.[24] For a review of the long-term impact of parental strife *see* Wallerstein and Harthup.[25,26] The impact of maltreatment on communication development is discussed in Chapter 9.

Parenting problems with any combination of the above factors – or even without them – may deprive the child of 'good enough parenting' and jeopardise his or her development.

Gender

Boys are at higher risk of developing communication problems, and specific problems such as autism and ADHD are more common in boys. However, stereotypes such as 'emotional' female and 'tough' boy are no longer accepted as arising from purely biological factors. From an educational perspective, only in maths and visuo-spatial skills do boys narrowly outperform girls.[4]

Periconceptional and prenatal factors

The incidence of spina bifida has declined since the folic acid supplementation programme was initiated. The use of folic acid may be necessary in early pregnancy in mothers taking anticonvulsant valproate.

The impact of alcohol and other drugs, e.g. cocaine in the prenatal period is well recognised. Fetal Alcohol Syndrome, in addition to the dysmorphic features, is associated with reduced speech production skills and comprehension skills, the latter secondary to reduced working memory and various forms of hearing loss. Difficulty with pragmatic skills may persist into adulthood.[27] In cocaine exposure, the problem is biological and one of arousal and attention regulation, disrupting the communicative interactions of the child. This may, of course, be accompanied by social adversities.[27] Maternal smoking during pregnancy affects cognitive development, especially the concentration and attention span of children, in combination with the adverse social and environmental maternal circumstance that it usually signifies.[28]

Other teratogens such as infections (TORCHS) and irradiation have a significant impact on later development, especially if exposure occurs during the first 12 weeks of pregnancy.

Perinatal factors

Hagberg and Hagberg in their review of the origins of cerebral palsy clarify the aetiological factors and cerebral pathophysiology involved in different types of cerebral palsy, and particularly the differences between the term and pre-term babies.[29]

With the advent and wide availability of high-quality neonatal care over the last

20 years, there has been an increased survival rate of high-risk neonates. Limits of viability are gradually being pushed to earlier gestations. There is also increased awareness of the 'developmental cost' of survival, as shown in long-term outcome studies (mostly of neonatal survivors prior to the availability of surfactant therapy).

Wolke in a review of the literature on the long-term psychological outcomes of very low birth weight (VLBW) (< 1500 g) and extremely low birth weight (ELBW) (< 1000 g), found that 10–25% of VLBW children had severe cognitive impairment (IQ < 2SD), compared with an expected 2.3% in the normal population.[30] There was a negative correlation between the degree of fetal growth retardation and cognitive ability. Similar findings in VLBW children were reported from New Zealand.[31] Luoma et al. in a control-led study of speech and language comprehension and production at the age of five years in a cohort of children born at ⩽ 32 weeks gestational age, found a significantly lower performance in the entire pre-term group.[32] When children with major neurological disabilities were excluded from the pre-term group, statistically significant differences were found in four of the 12 speech and language measures, especially rapid word retrieval. Hutton et al. demonstrated a differential effect of pre-term birth and 'being small for gestational age' on cognitive and motor ability in their study of 8–9 year old children born at ⩽ 32 weeks.[33] Cognitive ability as measured by IQ and reading comprehension was negatively associated with the degree of fetal growth retardation, while motor ability was better with increasing gestational age, and negatively associated with the degree of fetal growth retardation. The developmental outcome at 12 years in 138 VLBW children was studied by Botting et al. who found lower IQ scores and poorer educational scores in VLBW children, in comparison to a control group.[34] Controlling for IQ, VLBW children still showed low mathematics and reading comprehension scores. The duration of mechanical ventilation in the neonatal period was among the predictors of cognitive and educational outcome, as were full-scale IQ and motor skills scores at six years, head circumference at 12 years, maternal education, family size and income.

A knowledge of the Apgar score at one and five minutes after birth is useful, although this has come into question in recent years.[35]

The long-term developmental outcomes described in the above studies may engender some feeling of pessimism as regards neonatal care. While the knowledge of specific developmental difficulties helps in the provision of appropriate resources for the children, the fact remains that a vast number of survivors not experiencing hypoxic-encephalopathy in the neonatal period do as well as other individual children. Anticipatory guidance that builds on their strengths rather than focusing on 'deficits' is essential in helping the children to find their 'niche' in life.

Nutrition

Breastfeeding, besides being beneficial for nutritional, immunological and emotional developmental reasons, also facilitates cognitive development in the first four months.

This is related to the presence of docosahexaenoic acid (DHA), a long-chain polyunsaturated fatty acid present in breast milk, which facilitates synaptic transmission in the brain, as well as promoting visual development.[36]

Iron deficiency is now widely recognised as being associated with developmental delay in early childhood, although it is not clear if the relationship is causal.[37]

Atopy

Atopy may be a factor in recurrent upper respiratory tract inflammation, resulting in middle ear effusions. There has been recent interest in gluten sensitivity as a possible mechanism underlying autistic spectrum disorder, and there is sometimes parental pressure for a gluten free diet.

Family history

Apart from a family history of learning and mental health problems, an enquiry about the pattern of speech and language development in siblings and parents is useful. A familial pattern of language development may consist of delayed acquisition and rapid catching up.

Growth

Of particular importance is the child's head circumference. Microcephaly is associated with prenatal/perinatal insult and developmental delay and large head size is a recognised feature of Fragile X syndrome, and is also reported in autistic spectrum disorder.

Congenital malformation

Cleft lip/palate and other craniofacial abnormalities are discussed in Chapter 15.

Seizure disorder

Subclinical seizure disorder, particularly occurring at night, may be an aetiological factor in receptive developmental dysphasia.[38] Landau-Klefner syndrome presents in a previously normally developing child with an apparent loss of auditory verbal understanding and speech at around 3–8 years. EEG findings are typical with bitemporal repetitive spikes, and spikes and slow waves of high amplitude.[39]

ENT problems

Of significance is fluctuating hearing loss. A recent longitudinal study of a UK birth cohort described the link between early middle ear disease and behavioural, cognitive and language problems at five and 10 years.[40] There were some persistent adverse effects even at 10 years, especially with regard to language test data and behaviour problems. The effects were more marked at five years but the overall size of the effect was modest. This calls for continuing awareness of hearing problems in children who display communication difficulties.

General examination

An examination of fundi is necessary, though it is often difficult and largely unrewarding. An ophthalmologic opinion should be sought if significant abnormal findings are suspected.

Neurocutaneous syndromes are recognised by cutaneous findings, such as café-au-lait spots, white skin patches and shagreen patch. Wood's lamp examination is necessary for clarifying the presence of white patches of tuberous sclerosis.

Certain syndromes are associated with a specific speech and language pattern. For example, William's syndrome is associated with a pattern called 'cocktail party' speech with enhanced quantity and quality of vocabulary, auditory memory and social use of language, together with an IQ of 50–70, and characteristic dysmorphic features.[41]

Neurological assessment

Apart from the finding of cerebral palsy, spina bifida and any other previously recognised problems, the practitioner should also look for developmental co-ordination disorder (also called dyspraxia). This is a problem of higher motor control involving the planning of motor tasks.

Developmental review

A review of all the major aspects of development (*see* Box 4.4) based on parental reports, informal observations of the play and behaviour of the child and, ideally, his or her performance on screening tests, is essential. Normal developmental milestones at different ages are described elsewhere.[2]

Differential diagnosis/investigations

Investigations are necessary for the identification of a number of problems and for establishing if any contributory factors, e.g. nutritional, atopic etc, are present.

Audiology assessment

This is essential, even if the previous child health surveillance examinations have been reported to be normal. Further investigations/clinical actions depend on the finding and type of hearing loss.

Iron status

For the reasons described above, investigating the child's iron status (using ferritin as well as haemoglobin, MCV and MCH) is useful.

Atopy and food sensitivity

Specific IgE may be useful. Serum anti-gliadin antibodies, especially IgA antibodies, are highly sensitive indicators of gluten sensitivity and are therefore useful screening tests.

Metabolic screen (serum and urine samples)

S amino acid and organic acid are part of the 'metabolic screen' for inborn-errors of metabolism. Metabolic screening of urine for glycosaminoglycans (for mucopolysaccharidosis) and for amino acids and organic acids, is justified if there are clinical grounds.

Microbiology and Virology

TORCHS screening is no longer carried out routinely to investigate the cause of delayed communication development. It may, however, be necessary if the family has recently moved from a country with a different epidemiology of infectious diseases, and if there are specific findings on clinical examination which are suggestive of a congenital infection, e.g. CMV, Rubella etc.

HIV testing may be indicated in specific circumstances where there is a high risk of vertical transmission of this infection.

Chromosomes

Molecular genetic and cytogenetic studies are essential if autism is suspected. In other situations, the presence of clinical indicators (e.g. dysmorphic features), known behavioural phenotypes or specific problems (e.g. Angelman syndrome, Rubinstein-Taybi syndrome) necessitates this investigation.

EEG

A low threshold for an EEG examination is needed in view of the likely significance of sub-clinical seizures in children with communication difficulties. Nearly 30% of children with autism develop epilepsy in later childhood. Attentional difficulties may be present in children with atypical 'absences' for which EEG is very useful. Paediatric neurology advice in clarifying these issues is essential.

Neuroimaging

Apart from specific problems such as microcephaly (where neuronal migration defects, generalised cerebral atrophy and periventricular leucomalacia are likely) and macrocephaly (where hydraencephaly, hydrocephalus and Dandy-Walker malformation need to be excluded), neuroimaging studies are largely unhelpful. CT brain scans are gradually being replaced by MRI scans which require a general anaesthetic – an important consideration.

Functional imaging studies, such as a positron emission tomography (PET) scan, are not generally available in the UK outside research studies.

Clinical decision making/management

The process outlined above helps the clinician to obtain a broad range of information about the social and family context of the child and his or her physical, developmental and behavioural status. This enables the practitioner to decide if there is a 'significant' problem and if there are any factors causing it or associated with it. It is necessary to seek help from the professionals in other disciplines, most notably speech and language therapists and psychologists, as well as occupational therapists and physiotherapists, as appropriate. It may also be necessary to consult colleagues in tertiary specialities such as paediatric neurology and child psychiatry.

In a pre-school child the recognition of a significant communication difficulty has implications for education, and a prompt notification to the education psychology service is essential (and is a statutory responsibility for health professionals under successive Education Acts). In any case, interventions for communication difficulties are often based in the education setting, e.g. for Autistic Spectrum Disorder, and effective early collaboration is therefore called for.

The social dimension of children with communication difficulties is often the aspect requiring the highest level of intervention. Working with health visitors in their supportive role, as well as with social services and other local authority colleagues, e.g. the housing department, is essential in order to maximise the effectiveness of interventions for the child.

Parent groups and other voluntary organisations also play a significant role in supporting parents, and in promoting service developments.

Communication with parents

This is an aspect requiring careful thought. At the initial paediatric evaluation there is often uncertainty as to whether or not there is a significant problem. This uncertainty is likely to be most acute with the relatively milder presentations of pervasive problems such as Autistic Spectrum Disorder. Parents might already have had suspicions about such a problem, and they naturally seek a clear answer from the professionals as soon as possible. This is an area of professional practice requiring sensitivity and empathy, together with objectivity. It is important to highlight the child's areas of strength and to minimise the expectation of a diagnosis that explains all the problems. In fact, a specific physical condition is *only one* of the determinants of a child's health and development, and it does not necessarily preclude him or her from finding their 'niche' in society.

The process of giving bad news to parents requires consideration of the range of feelings such as shock, anger, denial, grief and sadness, guilt, despondency and helplessness that parents may experience, often simultaneously. While the expression of these feelings may seem hostile to the professional(s), the process of coming to terms with the situation often begins relatively quickly. It may take various forms and can include a vigorous determination to do their best (including learning new skills to help their child), searching for therapeutic advances (facilitated by the easier access to knowledge via electronic media), and getting organised to meet all the various logistic demands placed on them by the need to see a variety of professionals at different times and different places. Such an expression of resilience is part of the human spirit and clinicians need to support this process. They can do so by giving as much information as is sought; by objectively dealing with the sometimes unrealistic expectations generated by cures and 'therapies'; by organising services, especially the multidisciplinary teamwork, in as unobtrusive a way as possible; and, above all, by being empathetic and prepared to listen unhurriedly despite time-limited appointments.

Other medical contexts

The medical context in helping children with communication difficulties does not end with the individual clinical encounters described above. It continues into other medical roles such as management, professional and parental education, research, and other wider roles that clinicians undertake during their professional lifetime. By keeping the individual clinical context alive in those clinically less involved roles, clinicians may be able to achieve the much cherished goal of advocacy for children with communication difficulties.

Summary

- Children's language develops primarily for sharing and receiving feelings and ideas. Language development connects with physical health as well as other developmental domains of the child.
- The medical context in primary care provides an opportunity for promoting communication development and an early identification of any impediments to it.
- In the secondary care context, paediatricians can provide holistic assessment and management of communication difficulties through individual clinical and multi-disciplinary and multi-agency working.
- For complex and pervasive communication problems, tertiary level collaboration between paediatric neurologist, child psychiatrist, speech and language therapist and psychologist is essential.
- The medical context can potentially extend beyond the individual clinical encounters into research, management and educational roles.
- At all levels of the professional care of children with communication difficulties, medical practitioners need to remain responsive to the concerns and anxieties of parents, and as far as possible adapt their involvement to suit the needs of the child and family.

References

1   Bloom L (1998) Language acquisition in its developmental context. In: W Damon (ed) *Handbook of Child Psychology* (5th ed). Wiley, Chichester.

2   Tamhne R (expected 2000) *The Normal Child: a biopsychosocial approach in clinical practice.* Harcourt Brace/Churchill Livingstone, London.

3   Vygotsky LS (1962) *Thought and Language.* MIT Press, Cambridge, MA.

4   Santrock JW (1997) *Child Development* (8th ed). McGraw-Hill, New York.

5   Home Start UK, 2 Salisbury Road, Leicester LE1 7QR.

6   Hall DMB (ed) (1996) *Health for All Children* (3rd ed). Oxford University Press, Oxford.

7   Davis A (1995) Current thoughts on hearing screening. In: NJ Spencer (ed) *Progress in Community Child Health, Vol 1*. Churchill Livingstone, Edinburgh.

8   Davis A, Bamford J, Wilson I *et al.* (1997) A critical review of hearing screening in the detection of congenital hearing impairment. *Health Technology Assessment* **1**(10).

9   Baron-Cohen S, Allen J and Gilberg C (1992) Can autism be detected at 18 months? The needle, the haystack and the CHAT. *British Journal of Psychiatry* **161**: 839–43.

10   Bower H (1999) New research demolishes link between MMR vaccine and autism. *BMJ* **318**: 1643.

11   Nicoll A, Elliman D and Ross E (1998) MMR vaccination and autism. *BMJ* **316**: 715–16.

12   Moore JR (1999) A personal child health record for child with a disability. Personal communication.

13   Bishop DV and Edmundson A (1987) Language impaired 4 year olds: distinguishing transient from persistent impairment. *Journal of Speech and Language Disorders* **52**(2): 156–73.

14   Glascoe F (1991) Can clinical judgment detect children with speech-language problems? *Pediatrics* **87**: 317–22.

15   Hall DMB (1991) Shy, withdrawn or autistic? *BMJ* **302**: 125–6.

16   SDM Court (1976) *Fit for the Future*. HMSO, London.

17   Salt A (1998) *Child Development Centres: a directory*. RCPCH, London.

18   Illingworth RS (1987) *The Development of the Infant and Young Child* (9th ed). Churchill Livingstone, Edinburgh.

19   Bax M (1987) Paediatric assessment of the child with a speech and language disorder. In: W Yule and M Rutter (eds) *Language Development and Disorders*. Blackwells, Oxford.

20   Rutter M (1987) Assessment, objectives and principles. In: W Yule and M Rutter (eds) *Language Development and Disorders*. Blackwells, Oxford.

21   Rosenbloom L (1995) Communication disorder in recent advances in paediatrics. In: TJ David (ed) *Paediatrics*. Churchill Livingstone, Edinburgh.

22   Newton RW and Wraith JE (1995) Investigation of development delay. *Arch Disease Childhood* **72**(5): 460–5.

23   Waterstone T (1995) How can child health services contribute to a reduction in health inequalities in childhood? In: NJ Spencer (ed) *Progress in Community Child Health*. Churchill Livingstone, Edinburgh.

24   Murray L and Cooper J (1997) Effects of postnatal depression on infant development. *Arch Disease Childhood* **77**(2): 99–101.

25 Wallerstein JS (1991) The long-term effect of divorce on children: a review. *J Am Acad Child Adolescent Psychiatry* **30**: 349–60.

26 Harthup T (1996) Divorce and marital strife and their effects on children. *Arch Disease Childhood* **75**: 1–8.

27 Paul R and Rubin E (1999) Communication and its disorders. *Child and Adolescent Psychiatric Clinics* **8**(1): 11.

28 Naeye RL and Peters EC (1984) Mental development of children whose mothers smoked during pregnancy. *Obstetrics and Gynaecology* **64**(5): 601–7.

29 Hagberg B and Hagberg G (1993) The origins of cerebral palsy. In: TJ David (ed) *Recent Advances in Paediatrics*. Churchill Livingstone, Edinburgh.

30 Wolke D (1998) Psychological development of prematurely born children. *Arch Disease Childhood* **78**: 567–70.

31 Horwood LJ, Mogridge N and Darlow BA (1998) Cognitive behavioural and educational outcome at 7-8 years in a national very low birth weight cohort. *Arch Disease Childhood* **79**: F12–F20.

32 Luoma L, Herrgard A and Ahonen T (1998) Speech and language development of children born at $\leqslant 32$ weeks gestation: a 5-year prospective follow-up study. *Dev Med Child Neuro* **40**: 380–7.

33 Hutton JL, Pharoach PO, Cooke RW *et al.* (1998) Differential effect of pre-term birth and small gestational age on cognitive and motor development. *Arch Disease Childhood* **40**: 652–60.

34 Botting N, Pawls A, Cooke RW *et al.* (1998) Cognitive and educational outcome of very low birth weight children in early adolescence. *Dev Med Child Neuro* **40**: 652–60.

35 Marlow N (1992) Do we need an Apgar Score? *Arch Disease Childhood* **67**(7): 765–6.

36 Cockburn G (1995) Breast feeding and the infant human brain. In: DP Davies (ed) *Nutrition in Child Health*. RCP, London.

37 British Nutrition Foundation (1995) *Iron, Nutritional and Physiological Significance: the report of the British Nutrition Foundation Task Force*. Chapman & Hall, London.

38 Picavel A, Cheliyut Herayt F and Brauskraou M (1998) Sleep EEG and developmental dysphasis. *Dev Med Child Neuro* **40**: 595–9.

39 Appleton RE (1995) The Landau-Klefner syndrome. *Arch Disease Childhood* **42**: 386–7.

40 Bennett KE and Haggard MP (1999) Behaviour and cognitive outcomes from middle ear disease. *Arch Disease Childhood* **80**(1): 28–35.

41 Behrman RE and Kliegman RM (1995) *Nelson Textbook of Pediatrics*. WB Saunders, Philadelphia PA.

CHAPTER 5

Speech and language assessment

Alison Parkinson and Suzanne Pate

The aim of this chapter is to explain what underpins the process of speech and language assessment and how it works in practice. Parental views about their child's development play as central a part in this process as they do in surveillance, adding to the quality and accuracy of the assessment.

Describing the need

Surveillance and screening aim to identify children at risk of long-term difficulties. The process of identification attempts to involve parents and carers in describing their child, not only in terms of their development but also in terms of their well being. Once identified, children are referred onwards for specialist assessment. During this next phase speech and language clinicians who assess children's communication skills are generally looking to answer three questions, the first of which will also have been previously considered by members of the primary healthcare team during surveillance (*see* Chapters 3 and 4):

- Is there a problem?
- What is the nature of the problem?
- What can effectively be done about it?

This chapter will concentrate on the first two questions, the third is addressed in Chapter 7.

Figure 5.1 shows the process by which clinical decisions are made about the child's communication difficulties and future needs. There are three main sources of information:

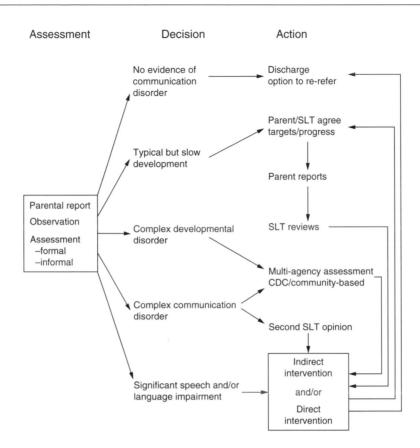

Assessment   Decision   Action

Figure 5.1   Describing the need.

- parental report
- observation
- formal and informal assessment.

These strands should not be seen as sequential. Observation, informal assessment and
parental report overlap both at the initial assessment and over time (Figure 5.2).

Parental report

The purpose of the initial contact with parents is to find out about their perceptions of
their child's current behaviour, early development and progress, through a detailed
case history. The aim is to establish whether they have any concerns themselves, in
part as a means of building rapport. Therapists are also interested in patterns of development and therefore parents are likely to be asked specifically about their child's

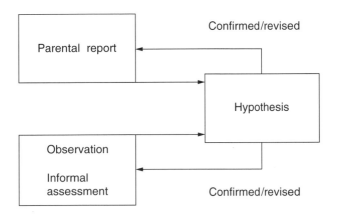

Figure 5.2 Strands of assessment.

strengths as well as those things they find hard. We know that parents make very good informants about their children's current behaviour (*see* Chapter 3). Personal Child Health Records may support their recollections of their child's early development. Discrepancies between the therapists' findings and parents' views probably reflect a different understanding of what is being discussed. The most typical example of this is parents expressing the opinion that their child understands everything said to them yet observation and assessment by the therapist indicating that this is not the case. In this situation the parent is probably talking about the way the child behaves at home in the presence of contextual cues, whereas the therapist is observing and assessing the child's response to spoken language without such contextual support.

In addition to case history information the therapist will seek specific information from other sources, including medical, educational and psychological advice, as appropriate. Subsequent contacts with parents and carers will particularly reflect on the child's progress, current areas of specific concern and strategies which have been particularly effective in supporting the child's development.

Observation

Over the past two decades, research has focused on the dynamic interactions between speaker and listener roles, the message to be conveyed and the context in which communication occurs. As evidence of the relationship between language and learning grows, so does the need to examine communication skills within the context of the child's home, school and daily living experiences. This shift in focus has led to an increase in the use of observation as the tool most appropriate to the assessment of children's functional language, i.e. the use and understanding of language within different settings and to meet specific requirements. Within such a model of functional language, the most critical purpose of assessment is to determine if communicative problems exist in the context of the child's experiences, and if they do, to determine the reasons for the lack of success. Observation of the child's communication skills within naturalistic contexts leads us to examine the degree to which any underlying linguistic impairment disables or handicaps the functions of everyday life. For young children, observations of them at home often provide clinicians with more information about their future potential than those in clinical settings. The clinical setting may limit the child's potential to use and understand language or may mask the child's difficulties as a result of the narrowness of the observations available. For logistic reasons, however, home- and school-based assessment are not always possible (*see also* curriculum-based assessment later in this chapter).

Equally, it is important to observe the parents' pattern of interaction.

Formal and informal assessment

Formal assessments have a predetermined procedure and structure; the majority of those most commonly used are standardised. Tests range from those which screen language skills to those which assess various aspects of communication in detail. The results of such assessments allow comparison with the population on which the assessment was originally standardised, and may be quoted in terms of an age-equivalence or more usually in terms of a standard score or percentile rank. Some tests will provide clinicians with a general view of the child's skills and point the way to other more specific assessments, others may lead to a diagnosis, or a description of the child's relative strengths and weaknesses. Informal assessments aim to investigate a particular area of skill but do not follow a given procedure. Clinicians describe behaviours or response patterns observed during the assessment, and take these into account when feeding back the results of the tests and formulating intervention plans. In some instances, how the child responded within the test situation can give information which is subjective yet more useful than the bottom line test score; information about processing skills, attention and listening, ability to scan, to self-correct, to rehearse overtly, etc. For further discussion regarding the use of informal and formal assessments see Chapter 6.

Analysing test findings

Standardised assessments are typically reported as standard scores, percentile scores or an age-equivalent score. Total or composite test scores are most often reported with a mean of 100 and a standard deviation of 15. Some measures report standard scores expressed as z-scores (mean = 0) or T-scores (mean = 50). Discrepancies between verbal and performance IQ are considered significant in the definition of primary language difficulties (*see* Chapter 1 for further discussion). Within some authorities it is not uncommon for agencies to use specific norm-referenced criteria to allow children to be given access to services, for example a differentiation between verbal and non-verbal IQ to enable access to a speech and language unit. This type of cognitive referencing can create problems because different tests can yield different recommendations for a single child at a single point in time. Within the UK, access to services is typically dependent more on an analysis of need made by various professionals than on the results of standardised assessments, with particular emphasis placed on progress over time (*see* the Code of Practice and curriculum-based assessment section of this chapter). A large number of standardised measures of language ability also provide information about age-equivalency. Age-equivalent scores simply represent the average score derived from a normative sample at a specific age. They do not take into account individual differences and tend to be misinterpreted by both lay and professional people. However, they may help parents understand what the test score implies. When using age-equivalence scores it is important that the therapist simultaneously describes other language parameters so that the parent understands precisely where the strengths and weaknesses lie. Any test represents a sampling of bits of behaviour to make a judgement regarding the larger picture. On those test instruments that look at more than one skill, it is recommended that attention is given to total or composite language scores because they represent a more valid estimate of global abilities.

Considerations associated with assessment

Certain factors affect the way in which children perform in a given situation and others may affect not only performance but also the way in which test results or observations are interpreted.

Speed

The speed of a child's ability to respond to tasks should be carefully monitored. Most formal measures of language ability provide an estimate of the amount of time typically required for test administration. Children who require longer than the average time may be at risk of failing to keep up with the pace of typical conversational interactions and classroom dialogue. Teachers report that these children are prone to daydream or engage in off-task behaviours. Slow information processing rate is one of the most common characteristics of children who have been diagnosed as having Attention Deficit Disorder (ADD) (*see* Chapter 10). The relationship between speed of processing and memory should also be kept in mind. Research indicates that language/learning disabled children and adolescents have been found to have consistent short-term memory deficits.[1-3]

Age

Young children tend to respond better to informal assessments than to those that are standardised because the more informal approach allows the tester to use various techniques including redirecting attention, repetition and praise to keep the child focused on the task. Older children generally do not require such devises, although older children with speech and language disorders may behave in similar ways to younger children in this respect. As children move through developmental stages their language needs vary greatly. Preschoolers, for example, need language to engage in imaginative and social play, whereas primary school children use language to strengthen peer relationships and learn how to present themselves well. By the time children reach adolescence, language has become a vital tool needed for self-exploration, self-definition and self-disclosure. The effectiveness with which a child is utilising language within each of these growth stages contributes valuable information to the assessment process. However, very few of these aspects of language functioning have norms against which we can compare an individual child's skills, and even fewer are tapped by formal testing measures.

Gender

A small number of formal assessments take gender into account to such a degree that they provide separate norms for girls and boys, the majority, however, do not. Research has shown that in general, girls develop a range of linguistic abilities earlier than boys, although there is a large degree of normal variation within any population.[4] Certainly speech and language impairments are more common among boys.

Ethnicity/bilingualism

Race and ethnicity influence the way in which one examines language development. It is fairly clear that tests based on standard English would not be appropriate for a child whose native language is not standard English. The same bias may apply when a child is learning a variation of English based on rules of a system such as Black Vernacular English (BEV) or other non-standard varieties of English. Furthermore, the learning of a second language before competency in the first language is fully developed may result in lower proficiency in each language. During the school years it can take up to seven years to become fully competent in English, so until then children cannot reliably be evaluated with standardised tests in English. Evaluating children from diverse cultures requires more than understanding the linguistic differences between the child's first language and standard English. For example, linguistic rules within a culture dictate styles that govern speaking and writing. *See* Chapter 6 for a more detailed discussion of multicultural/bilingual issues.

Case study

An example of the integration of parental report, observation and assessment

Ben is three years eight months of age. He was referred for speech and language therapy assessment following the three-year check by his health visitor. Although they had not brought any concerns to their GP or health visitor, Ben's parents had been aware that his speaking had been poor for some time.

Parental report

Case history

Ben is the elder of two children. His mum had herself been known to the paediatric therapy services and had attended a unit for children with moderate learning difficulties during primary school. She suggested that she found the children hard work and his parents described Ben as physical and boisterous. Both commented that they also felt he did not listen to what they said and did not concentrate well. He had a history of recurrent ear infections but had passed all hearing tests.

Communication and feeding

Ben had been late to start talking in comparison with other children his mum knew. At the time of his assessment his parents reported that he was using some words to ask for what he wanted, e.g. 'pop', 'biscuit', etc., and to name things he saw, such as 'bus' and 'train'. He was not putting any words together. He used pointing and taking his mum to show her if he could not tell her what he wanted. He often seemed frustrated and got angry if she did not understand him. His parents could understand the words he did use easily. Although his parents reported that he did not listen to them they felt that he did understand but was choosing not to do as he was told. Ben had never had any problems with sucking or chewing.

Play and interaction

Ben preferred physical play. Indoor play was mostly centred around watching TV and play with cars. He did not play for long periods with toys. He was said to get on well with his younger brother if they were outside or running around, but they did not find it easy to share toys. He did not have opportunites to play with other children. His mum reported that she did not get much chance to play with Ben.

Observation

Parent–child interaction

Observations of Ben, his younger brother and his mum in the playroom showed that she took the opportunity to allow them to play alone. She spoke to the two boys briefly, to control their behaviour. She used simple language when talking with the boys, neither of whom responded verbally to anything she said, but they did follow her instructions. Her speech was flat with little expression. She used few gestures to support what she said and she used a limited range of facial expressions. Within the assessment session she spoke to Ben mainly to direct his attention. When the boys' father came to pick them up he too spoke to them in simple, straightforward sentences, telling them what to do and explaining where they were going next. His speech was more highly intonated and louder than their mum's and he used gesture and facial expression to support his speech.

Play

In one-to-one play with an adult Ben showed that he was able to use objects to symbolise others. He related objects and showed by his actions that he understood their use. He copied many of the adult's ideas and incorporated them into his play, but was unable to extend them without further modelling. His own spontaneous play was based on toys 'crashing' and 'falling' rather than on construction. He handled the toys with assurance and dexterity but not very carefully.

Communication

Within the play setting Ben responded appropriately to the things said to him, for example he could pass a range of objects on request to the adult and carry out simple commands within the context of the situation. He was largely passive in his interactions with the adult, but often watched the speech and language therapist carefully and checked that he was being watched himself. He became more verbal as the play session progressed. He began to quietly imitate the things the therapist said and to comment on his play using single words and simple phrases such as 'It's gone', 'No horse', 'nother one, cow'. He began to show the therapist things, for example holding up two objects which were the same for inspection and comment. When attention was turned back to his mum he used both noisy actions with the toys and single words such as 'look' to regain the initiative and refocus attention back on to him. The words he used were easy for the listener to understand and showed no evidence of any speech sound difficulties.

Formal and informal assessment

Communication

Ben's understanding of spoken language was assessed using the Reynell Developmental Language Scales. His raw score converted to a standard score of −2.2. He concentrated well during the assessment and this was felt to be an accurate measurement of his general understanding.

Ben's use of spoken language was assessed informally. His vocabulary was measured through a picture-naming task which required him to label both objects and actions. It revealed significant gaps in his knowledge of verbs, with relatively good naming of objects from everyday categories. His grammar was assessed through analysis of a sample of spoken language taken from two play sessions, indicating Ben's predominant use of single words and holophrases with some two and three words linked to form phrases. Interpretation of the data suggested significant gaps in his use of grammar at both phrase and clause level. Ben's use of language to communicate functionally was assessed informally through a parent questionnaire, indicating that Ben mainly used spoken language to respond to things people said to him, to ask for what he wanted, to reject what he did not and to comment on what he could see and hear at the time.

Ben's speech was assessed initially through a phonological analysis of the data collected in the picture-naming task. This indicated that Ben had relatively good speech sound development in comparison with his language skills. Although the development of his speech sound system was not complete, for example his clusters of consonants were reduced to single phonemes, e.g. 'poon' for spoon, there was no evidence of a developmental delay or disorder of speech.

The three main branches of assessment – formal and informal, observation and parental report – can be used to investigate those abilities which underpin the communication and linguistic skills introduced in Chapter 1. However, some areas lend themselves more to one strategy than another, as indicated in the figures below. The assessment process may well begin before the clinician has seen the child or the family, dependent on referral details; on meeting them this is expanded to encompass initial information about the family and the physical characteristics and development of the child through a case history.

The assessment process
Underpinning abilities

Play

Watching children at play gives us an insight into the ways in which they are perceiving and thinking about the world, their social relationships, their motor devel-

Table 5.1   Play

Parental report	Observation	Assessment
Key questions	*Context*	*Formal assessment*
What are the opportunities for play?	Large or miniature toy play depending on age	The child is presented with a range of toys. The behaviours and language exhibited are recorded and compared with developmental norms
Where does the child like to play?		
With whom?	*Key questions*	
What does the child chose to play with?	Spontaneous play:	Standardised tests, e.g. the Symbolic Play Test, the Test of Pretend Play
	– Does the child show use of imagination and language in play?	
How long does the child stay with own choice of activity?	– Does the child sequence ideas?	
Does the child make up stories?	– Does the child involve adults?	*Informal assessment*
	– How?	Checklists of normal development, e.g. Living Language*
Does the child talk about what he/she is doing to comment on play?	– Play with adult support?	
	– Does the child take on adult suggestions?	

* Full references for the published formal and informal assessments can be found in the reference list. A summary of the quoted assessments can be found in Appendix 2.

opment and their cognitive skills. Clinicians want to know about the young child's interest in exploring his or her environment spontaneously, his or her curiosity (and later motivation, *see* Chapter 1), symbolic understanding, imitative skills and sociability with adults and other children. For older children the focus is on their imagination and social play with others. From a diagnostic viewpoint many children referred for assessment are likely to have a delay in the development of their play skills (*see* Part two for further details). The key issue is not only the presence or absence of early play, but the quality of it. As such it is important to look for what the child does, rather than what he does not do. The same is true for older children although here the focus is on their imagination rather than their play.

Interaction

Babies respond to humans, our faces and voices within the first days of life. He or she begins to communicate through cooing and screaming, with the parent interpreting the child's messages. The child gradually becomes a more active participant in the interactions, so that within the first weeks we see him or her acting as both speaker and listener; roles which will go on to form the foundation of 'real' conversations. The timing of these interactions, the child's active role in developing them and the parents responses are all crucial in maintaining this developing process. Even before young children develop the use of spoken language they are able to communicate their wants, needs and feelings to those around them, and respond to our attempts to

Table 5.2 Interaction

Parental report	Observation	Assessment
Key questions When did the child first show early interactions, e.g. smiling, joint attention, showing, pointing, giving and taking games, etc.? Did any early difficulties persist and for how long? Did any new difficulties emerge before three years? How does the child: get attention, anticipate, request an object, request repetition, comment, reject, express likes/dislikes, express happiness/enjoyment? Is the child able to: follow our pointing; follow who is speaking to whom; understand simple gestures, like an outstretched hand meaning 'give it to me' and body language, like a tap meaning 'turn to look at me'? Do the parents enjoy playing with and talking to the child?	*Context* Child interacting with parents, siblings, strangers, etc., in a range of settings *Key questions* Does the child distinguish between people and objects in his or her behaviours? Does the child show age-appropriate differential reactions to strangers and familiar adults? Does the child show joint attention, e.g. bringing things to show? Does the child use body language, eye gaze and gesture to regulate the timing of interactions? Does the child enjoy interacting? How do the parents respond to the child, following child's lead and topic, extending the interaction, etc.? Does the child use body language: proximity and movement, gesture, facial expression, eye gaze, pausing, vocalisations, volume of voice, intonation and words to express meaning? Does the child respond to the above in others to interpret meaning?	*Formal assessments* None *Informal assessment* Setting up scenarios which rely on the interpretation of non-verbal communication. Checklists of non-verbal communication, behaviours and gestures Checklists and diagnostic frameworks, e.g. for Autistic Spectrum Disorder

communicate with them. Moving on from the early interactions of the first few months of life children become increasingly sophisticated in their ability to manipulate their environment and the people in it. Over time the young child begins to be able to predict what is going to happen from a developing awareness of other people's behaviour and the routines in which humans engage. From these real-life and play situations children begin to find out about how humans communicate as well as what they communicate about. In the face of extreme communication and/or behavioural difficulties in their child, parents can themselves adopt some unlikely accommodating strategies so that they begin to look and sound as if they themselves have difficulties in interacting effectively. For further information about behavioural issues *see* Chapter 12.

From the perspective of assessment it is rare for young children to be referred to a speech and language therapist before two years of age in the UK unless there is known to be a congenital condition or the child is thought to be at specific risk of late onset of speaking (*see* Chapters 6 and 11).

Memory

There is a body of data from psychological research about memory, much of which has come from testing with adult subjects and from people following brain injury. From these and other sources, theories of memory processing have been developed, many of which have now become well established.[5] Three main processes make up a person's memory: encoding, storage and retrieval.[6] Theories of processing suggest two main memory systems, which, although not discrete, operate in different ways. Long-term memory is seen as the sum of knowledge acquired over the past. Its storage capacity is unlimited, although we may have difficulty in encoding information to be stored, storing it effectively, i.e. with a wide range of associations, or in information retrieval. Long-term memory itself is thought to have three component parts. Semantic memory has been described as a dictionary which stores information about concepts and meanings and knowledge of the world.[7] Although most of this information may be considered to be learned through language some comes from the input to other senses. Episodic memory is concerned with personal information, that

Table 5.3 Memory

Parental report	Observation	Assessment
Key questions Can the child remember events and talk about the past? Does the child learn and recall nursery rhymes? Can the child follow instructions? How does the child usually learn something new or remember something?	*Context* Interaction with parents and siblings and others, e.g. in play *Key questions* Does the child use memory strategies like overt rehearsal? Is the child helped by repetition of an instruction or question? Is the child helped to understand by visual cues like gesture pictures and demonstration? Does the child respond to verbal information quickly?	*Formal assessment* The child is asked to carry out a range of tasks, e.g. to follow instructions, repeat sentences, words and non-words Standardised tests: subtests of Clinical Evaluation of language Fundamentals Revised UK (CELFR UK), the Test of Non-Word Repetition *Informal assessment* For example digit span, sentence repetition, non-word repetition, reciting rhymes, retelling stories

gained from our 'experiencing self'.[8] Procedural memory is about 'knowing how', as opposed to the 'knowing that', which is semantic memory. It seems clear that information in long-term storage must be organised in some way, but it is not necessarily true that each person uses the same organisational system. There is likely to be a great deal of variation in the importance different people place on a shared event and different associations with it, which leads each person to encode and store this information in a unique way.

Items in short-term or working memory, are present for only as long as they are required for current mental operations to be carried out. Working memory has been compared to an internal diary of day-to-day events, which has a limited capacity and is subject both to interference and decay over time. Information within it is easily accessible but may need to be kept in a state of high activation if it is to be worked upon. A central executive is thought to plan and execute all work in short-term memory, supported by an articulatory loop which maintains activation levels and a visuo-spatial sketchpad where images can be temporarily stored and manipulated. Information can be shifted into long-term memory through the use of strategies like rehearsal and repetition. From what we know of the workings of memory it is apparent that difficulties in any of its functions or in either system may influence both a person's understanding and use of language. (For a discussion of the impact on literacy of memory deficits *see* Chapter 16).

Attention and listening

As with all other skills, the development of attention and listening follow a documented pattern, from single-channelled attention through to an ability to watch and listen and integrate information from different sources and speakers, and to do so within a group situation against a background of distractions. We usually see children moving smoothly through these stages to the point where they are ready for the demands placed on them by school-type environments at maybe four or five years old (*see* Box 5.1).

Box 5.1:   The developmental sequence of attention and listening skills[9]

Age
0–1	Can pay fleeting attention
1–2	Rigid attention to own choice of activity
2–3	Single-channel attention: can attend to adult's choice of activity but only under adult control
3–4	Single-channel attention: under child's own control
4–5	Integrated attention: for short spells
5–6	Integrated attention: well-controlled and sustained

Table 5.4 Attention and listening

Parental report	Observation	Testing
Key questions Does the child listen to what is being said? Do you have to raise your voice or say things lots of times to get the child's attention? In what situations is the child's attention best? Does the child enjoy listening to stories? Are there any reports from school or nursery that the child finds it hard to pay attention in a group situation?	*Context* Solitary play and with adults and children *Key questions* How long does the child spend with own choice of activity? How well does the child attend to adult choice of activity? If attention is lost what adult strategies help him/her return to task? Can the child be doing something and interpreting auditory information together? When interrupted from a task can the child pick up where he/ she left off?	*Formal assessment* None *Informal assessment* Developmental checklists of attention, *see* Box 5.1

For a child with suspected communication impairment there is the possibility that his or her skills in early auditory and visual discrimination (the ability to locate sound, to link it to what he or she sees, to perceive differences between sounds, and to sort out what is important for him or her to look at and listen to), may be limiting factors in the development of understanding, use of spoken language and of a complete sound system. The link between attention and communication is two-directional in that if a child is able to listen and look carefully he or she is more likely to understand the message being conveyed, and similarly, if he or she under-stands what is going on, and finds it interesting, he or she is more likely to attend to it. So children with delayed development of attention often miss out on opportunities to hear and learn from good models of language around them. The interactive nature of the development of attention, interaction, understanding and speaking means that clinically it is not easy to identify auditory perception as being the single cause of an individual child's difficulties (for further discussion *see* Chapter 13).

For some children the development of attention is an area of specific and significant difficulty. Such children's behaviour falls well outside typical parameters of development. Not all these children have problems in developing primary language skills, although they may go on to have problems in structured situations and may there-fore be in need of school-based assessment and support (*see* Chapter 10).

Table 5.5   Non-verbal understanding

Parental report	Observation	Assessment
Key questions Does the child pick up on things that are happening at home and respond to them appropriately, e.g. watching what is going on and joining in? Does the child copy things he/she sees others doing? Does the child know about family routines and predict what is going to happen next? Does the child understand any language about everyday events, e.g. 'it's bath time'?	*Context* Interaction with adults *Key questions* Does the child respond to non-verbal instructions like a chair pulled out to indicate where to sit? Does the child look for non-verbal cues to help him/her join in? Does the child look at the person who is talking?	*Formal/informal assessment* See section on interaction For children showing very delayed communication skills, detailed checklists of behaviours Non-standardised, e.g. the Pre-verbal Communication Skills Schedule

Non-verbal understanding

Young children begin to make sense of the world through integrating what they see and hear. The language spoken by the child's family is typically mapped on to familiar routines, the meaning of what people are saying becoming transparent in the context in which it is being said. Move the same phrase or word to a different context and the young child may struggle to understand. The child is effectively programmed to make sense of the whole message, not just the words, but the actions, tone of voice and facial expressions. This is what clinicians call non-verbal understanding. The development of non-verbal understanding has links with the development of interaction and pragmatic skills, as well as with verbal understanding. For parents, carers and professionals unfamiliar with early communication development the distinction between a child's ability to understand the gist of a message in context and his or her understanding of spoken language itself may seem artificial. For clinicians it is important to be positive about non-verbal understanding, however, for long-term progress in the acquisition of spoken language children need to be able to learn flexibly and to transfer their knowledge from one situation to another. This can only be done by learning the meanings of individual words.

Linguistic skills

The following section deals with the assessment of the understanding and use of spoken language. It is not always possible to separate out the various aspects, but clinicians typically look at receptive and expressive language skills. Once we begin to collect and analyse information at conversational level it is apparent that there is considerable overlap. For example, if a child has not understood a question it is likely that they will give an irrelevant response or one lacking in detail or fluency, a similar response to that seen in children with a specific expressive disorder. Where it has been possible to do so, this section has been subdivided into receptive and expressive skills.

Understanding

Understanding of non-literal language

By its very nature, idiomatic language is both language- and culture-specific. Standardised assessments are unlikely therefore to be useful across different populations, and because languages shift and develop possibly not even over time.

Although some attempts are being made to standardise assessment of non-literal understanding, much of this is currently carried out through contact with a therapist, testing out in therapy whether a child understands certain phrases and sayings, for example 'Keep it under your hat', 'I've run out of milk', etc., or the polite forms of various speech acts, such as requesting: 'Can you pass the salt?'; commanding: 'Would you like to sit on the carpet now'; requesting information: 'Could you tell me

Table 5.6 Receptive vocabulary measurement

Parental report	Observation	Assessment
Key questions Can the child match and sort and relate things in real life or in play by the way they go together, such as socks and shoes, cup and spoon etc.? Can the child fetch things on request? Has the child's school or nursery commented about the child's understanding?	*Context* Cognitive tasks, interaction with parents, etc. *Key questions* Can the child match similar objects/pictures? Does the child respond to simple requests to pass objects? In play does the child respond to simple requests to make objects act in specific ways? Can the child group objects by category?	*Formal/informal assessment* Object or picture recognition tasks in which the child is asked to look at a set of pictures or a selection of objects and choose by pointing or picking it up the one that goes best with the stimulus word spoken by the examiner Standardised, e.g. British Picture Vocabulary Scale (BPVS) and measures of conceptual relationships, e.g. subtests of CELFR UK Non-standardised, e.g. the Derbyshire Language Scheme Informal, e.g. responding to words about colour, size, number and shape*

*Beginning levels focus on basic nouns, verbs and concepts, while more advanced measures examine knowledge of multiple meaning words and word relationships.

Table 5.7 Word meanings and content

Parental report	Observation	Assessment
Key questions Does the child understand, e.g. instructions and questions at home? Do you need to rephrase or repeat things for the child to understand? Has the child's nursery or school commented about the child's understanding in group situations?	*Context* Interaction and conversation with others *Key questions* Does the child respond appropriately to simple instructions and descriptions? Does the child perform at a higher level with the support of visual cues like simple gestures?	*Formal assessment* Non-standardised, The Derbyshire Language Scheme uses the idea of word levels to measure understanding, information-carrying words* *Informal assessment* The child is asked to respond to utterances of differing word levels often in play-based tasks

*Information-carrying words (ICW)[10] which need to be understood in order to interpret the meaning of an utterance. A given utterance can be usefully measured by the number of ICWs until about a four-word level.

Table 5.8 Grammatical understanding

Parental report	Observation	Assessment
Key questions Do you ever feel that your child has not understood what you are saying? Does simplifying your sentences, making them shorter and using less complicated language help your child to understand?	*Context* Taped or videoed conversation with adults *Key questions* Does the child respond appropriately to utterances involving specific grammatical structures, for example negatives, adjectives, prepositions, wh- questions, embedded clauses, etc.?	*Formal assessment* The child is asked to select the one which best fits the target utterance from a series of different sets of pictures representing specific grammatical structures Standardised, e.g. the Test for Reception of Grammar (TROG), the Test for Auditory Comprehension of English, (TACL) *Informal assessment* A variety of tasks, e.g. judgements about the syntactical accuracy or anomaly of utterances

Table 5.9   Comprehension of oral commands

Parental report	Observation	Assessment
Key questions Is your child able to follow complicated instructions? Is he or she able to carry out these instructions in the order in which you gave them?	*Context* A formal setting *Key questions* Can the child follow a series of sequential instructions in order during play, drawing, etc.? Does the child respond appropriately to instructions involving 'first', 'lastly', 'before' and 'after'? Does the child use any strategies to help him or her remember?	*Formal assessment* The child is asked to follow oral commands of increasing length and grammatical complexity and/or in a specific order including words like first/last, before/after, instead/although, if/then, for example 'Before you do X do Y' Standardised, subtests of the CELFR UK, The Token Test

the way to...?' or 'Do you know the capital of...?', etc. Clearly this approach is time-consuming in that we are unable strictly to extrapolate from the child's response from one situation to another. However, it is important to make teachers and parents aware of a child's difficulty with literal interpretation because of the frequency with which adults use non-literal language like idioms and the impact not understanding may have on a child's behaviour and performance in class.

Table 5.10   Understanding of non-literal language

Parental report	Observation	Assessment
Key questions Does your child understand utterances which could have more than one meaning like: 'Can you pass me...', 'Pull your socks up', 'You're winding me up'?	*Context* Different settings over time responding to adult language *Key questions* Does the child understand typical family, classroom and playground language? Can the child explain the meanings of non-literal sayings?	*Formal assessment* The child is asked to choose which definition best fits the meaning of the target sentence Standardised, e.g. Understanding Ambiguities. An Assessment of Pragmatic Meaning Comprehension *Informal assessment* Researchers are currently devising ways to assess these skills through play-based acting out of stories containing non-literal language

Pragmatic skills

From the time they are able to utter single words and are beginning to put two words together, children can do other things with spoken language, such as argue, demand, seek information, deny, complain and much more. At the same time as they are developing these expressive skills they continue to learn how to recognise underlying meanings in the things people say to them. They process information from tone of voice, facial expression, gesture, body language and the words they hear to form a more complete picture of what it is people are 'saying' to them. As they experience and use more complex language functions children begin to find out more about how their language works. Some researchers have commented that from as young as two years old vocal children are able to think about their own language.[11] Certainly from about three years old children often make comments about things they have heard people say, about how words sound or about how difficult they find it to say a certain word. These metalinguistic skills continue to emerge in young childhood, so that by the time they go to school, children are often able, for example, to ask for the meanings of words, comment on rhyming words, tell people the first sound in a given word and, as they move towards literacy, talk about other aspects of written language and communication.

Table 5.11   Pragmatic skills

Parental report	Observation	Assessment
Key questions When and to whom does the child talk most? What does the child talk about? How does the child begin, maintain and finish a conversation? How does the child respond to an adult's language?	*Context* Taped or videoed spontaneous language sampling from play situations and conversation with peers and adults *Key questions* Does the child use a range of different sentence types? Does the child talk about range of different things? Is the child's language appropriate to the context? Does the child use language to meet nursery or classroom needs, discussions with pre-school or teaching staff*	*Formal assessment* Scenarios are acted out by the tester with prompts for the child to use target utterances Standardised, e.g. Test of Pragmatic Skills Non-standardised, Parent/ Teacher Interview Schedules, e.g. Pragmatics Profile of Early Communication Skills *Informal assessment* Conversational analyses

*In adult-directed environments it is difficult to gather data from children which will show their entire repertoire of potential language functions. In this type of situation children are likely to use spoken language to do certain things, such as ask or respond to questions, but may be less likely, for example, to make demands or give instructions; and this is as true of the clinic and surgery environments as it is of the classroom.

Spoken language grammar, content and use

Table 5.12   Expressive vocabulary measurement

Parental report	Observation	Assessment
Key questions How many words does your child know? What does your child like to talk about? Do you ever feel your child is searching for a word he or she knows but cannot remember? How quickly does your child learn to use new words?	*Context* Play- or conversation-based *Key questions* Is the child using words appropriate to the context? Does the child use words from a range of groups like verbs, nouns, adjectives, etc. Is the child able to talk about the functions and attributes of objects? Is the child showing evidence of word-finding difficulties by circumlocution or using non-specific filler words like 'this', 'it', 'thingy', etc.? Does the child show evidence of learning new words from adult language? Is the child able to correct his or her own errors?	*Formal assessment* The child is asked to name objects or pictures. Response times may be recorded Standardised, e.g. subtests of CELFR UK, tests of word-finding, e.g. Test of Adolescent/Adult Word Finding (TAWF), subtest of the Renfrew Action Picture Test (RAPT) Non-standardised, The 100 Pictures Naming Test *Informal assessment* The child is asked to perform a range of different tasks: − to name things from his/her environment or from pictures of objects, actions adjectives, etc. − to associate things, e.g. pencil and paper, socks and shoes, etc. − to categorise objects and to explain his/her choice by using category names, e.g. animals, clothes, etc. − to use words with multiple meanings, e.g. trunk, palm, etc., in sentences or to define their various meanings − to explain 'how to…', showing word usage in connected speech

Speech

From the first sounds a baby makes until he or she has acquired the complete sound system of his or her language, the process of speech development runs alongside that of language development. The underlying skills in auditory and visual perception, discrimination and memory, and the interest the child has in carers and their faces, are all significant for the development of speech. When looking at a child's speech development Grunwell[13] suggests the need to investigate four different dimensions:

- the anatomical and physiological dimension
- the phonetic dimension
- the phonological dimension
- the developmental dimension.

Table 5.13 Use of grammar

Parental report	Observation	Assessment
Key questions Is your child putting any words together? If so how many? Do your child's sentences sound the same as your own? If not how are they different? Does your child use word endings, e.g. -ing, -ed, -ly?	*Context* Sampling language in a range of settings *Key questions* What is the mean length of the child's utterances (MLU)?* Is the child using good word order? Is the child's grammar age appropriate?** Consider word endings, verb phrases, questions, negatives, expanded utterances	*Formal assessment* Formal analysis of sampled utterances, e.g. Language Assessment, Remediation and Screening Procedure (LARSP), indicating which structures are used routinely, or are emerging and highlighting significant gaps Grammatical analysis of elicited samples, e.g. South Tyneside Assessment of Syntax (STASS) North Western Syntax Screening Test (NSST)

*Up to a ceiling of about four or five words, the MLU is a gross but reasonably accurate index of grammatical development. It is a gross measure because it provides no information about the form or structure of the utterance.[12] Unfortunately, there is so much variability among children and conditions that an accurate prediction of which forms or structures should be expected at a given MLU age is difficult. The data from a young child can initially be analysed for length of utterance MLU, providing the child is producing some word combinations.

**Clinicians are often especially interested in verbs, verb phrases and verb-related structures such as tense markers, because of their complexity and apparent difficulty for children with problems in learning language.

Table 5.14 Language use

Parental report	Observation	Assessment
Key questions Can you have a conversation with your child? Does he or she respond to things you are talking about? Is he or she interested in your responses to things he or she is saying? Does the conversation flow?	*Context* Sampling of language in a range of settings *Key questions* How does the child initiate, maintain and close a conversation? Can the child sequence his or her ideas in a logical order? Can the child use narrative? Is there evidence of reciprocity? Does the child adapt his or her language to suit the audience?	*Formal assessment* *See* Pragmatics Non-standardised, checklists of linguistic behaviours, e.g. Pragmatics Profile for school-aged children, Evaluating Communicative Competence *Informal assessment* Analysis of conversations for fillers, pausing, interjections and repetitions and for fluency, coherence and effectiveness

In addition to these dimensions the child's skills in organising and planning across the levels of linguistic processing need to be considered, adding a further aspect to speech assessment which was introduced in Chapter 1 as praxis.

Anatomical and physiological dimension

The assessment looks at the structure and function of those parts of the body involved in speech production. Observation of the child at rest or in conversation will reveal any obvious anatomical problems with his or her head, face or neck. The GP may be advised to refer the child with suspected anomalies of hard or soft palate to the cleft palate team, or for further investigation of vocal fold functioning to the ENT consultant (*see* Chapters 15 and 17). The focus is particularly on lip, tongue and palate movement, and on breath control.

Phonetic dimension

Assessment at this level determines the range of speech sounds the child is able to use. Assessments may range from simple imitation of given sounds, looking particularly at consonant production, through picture-naming tests where all sound combinations in the language are represented, to analysis of a spontaneous speech sample. Omissions or differences in the sounds produced and any pattern to the difficulties the child may be experiencing are noted.

Phonological dimension

This level of assessment looks at the child's skill in using the speech sounds occurring in his or her phonetic inventory. This requires comparing the child's speech sound usage with that of the language he or she is hearing being spoken around him or her. The language sample needs to be large enough to look at any variability in the child's pronunciation patterns. Attention is paid to any patterns in the child's pronunciation of the language, and the differences between these patterns and those of the population speaking the child's language are described.

Developmental dimension

Speech sound systems are not static but develop through a child's life until the process is complete around five or six years of age. As with all other areas of communication development there is significant variation between children in their speech sound system development. At different stages in development certain typical patterns of development may be seen. Researchers have developed different types of phonological analysis to describe the processes the child uses throughout the various stages of development. A comparison is made between the child's pronunciation patterns with what might be expected at his or her age and stage of language development. A child

Table 5.15   Speech

Parental report	Observation	Assessment
Key questions Do you understand your child's speech? Do strangers understand him or her? Have you noticed anything about the sounds he or she can and cannot say? Does your child have any problems with feeding? Does your child dribble, mouth breathe, use a dummy for long periods in the day? Can your child imitate different facial expressions and movements of mouth, tongue, etc.?	*Context* Conversation and/or play. Phonological transcription of child's utterances contemporaneously or from taped sample *Key questions* Does the child have any oro-motor problems including dribbling? Can the child imitate different oro-facial movements including alternating patterns of movement? Can the child imitate speech sounds including alternating patterns at speed? What percentage of the child's speech is intelligible? Is the child's speech development age appropriate and/or in line with language development? Is there evidence of a speech delay or disorder?	*Informal/formal assessment* 1 Assessment of phonology. Data is collected through naming tasks, and/or continuous speech and is transcribed phonetically. Analyses are made of the data 2 Assessment of phonological awareness is carried out by, e.g. non-word repetition tasks, identification of sounds within words, sound blending and word segmentation 3 Assessment of auditory discrimination is carried out through the child listening out for specific sounds or sound differences in words Standardised, Phonological assessment (PACS); Edinburgh Articulation Test (EAT); Auditory discrimination assessment; Wepman Auditory Discrimination Test Non-standardised, Phonological Awareness Procedures, Nuffield Dyspraxia Assessment *Informal assessment* Oral examination

Note: Children with speech and language difficulties are at risk of later problems with literacy. Children with specific problems in learning to read share some of the same underlying difficulties as those with specific speech and language impairment; problems of short-term memory, of phonological awareness, i.e. with discriminating between speech sounds, with sound blending and word segmentation, for example. Assessment will include an investigation of these underlying skills. Further information about assessment for specific reading problems can be found in Chapter 16.

of two years old with a normally developing speech sound system is unlikely to be intelligible to strangers, a child of three is more likely to be able to make him- or herself understood. Information about normal developmental processes is also used to investigate whether a child's speech sound system development is simply delayed or whether atypical processes are apparent in his or her speech, suggesting a disordered pattern of development.

Praxis

Praxis is about the performance of an action, in this context an oro-motor or a verbal action. Speaking is an action which involves the temporal organisation and sequencing of speech sounds, and as such relies on a hierarchy of planning, execution and monitoring, from an ideational level through phonological, phonetic and motor programming levels to an articulatory level: a system which may break down at one or more levels. As with other groups of speech- and language-impaired children, the process of coming to a consensus about what constitutes verbal dyspraxia in terms of a set of symptoms or clusters of symptoms has been slow. Dyspraxia has variously been described as a motor programming deficit and a linguistic impairment, reflecting researchers' diverse opinions about the primary level of breakdown. The field has been further complicated by the use of a range of terminology: Developmental Verbal Dyspraxia, Developmental Articulatory Dyspraxia, Developmental Apraxia of Speech and Immature Articulatory Praxis. Focusing on Developmental Verbal Dyspraxia, Ozanne[14] describes it as a multideficit disorder with core deficits at the levels of phonological planning, phonetic programming and oro-motor and speech motor programme implementation. From a clinical perspective the key questions are about the level of severity and, related to this, the responsiveness to intervention. In terms of differential diagnosis it is also now becoming clear that the symptoms of dyspraxia merge at the margins with both those of dyslexia and phonological disorder.

Fluency

Children's speech, like that of adults, varies in fluency depending on the situation and what they are trying to say. At about 3–4 years of age the children typically pass through a period of non-fluency which reflects a time of explosive growth in their linguistic skills. This is called normal non-fluency, and the length of time for which it continues also shows considerable variation. Dysfluency refers to a wide range of presenting features in a person's speech which lead to a disruption to the flow of speaking and/or to covert aspects, such as anxiety about speaking and avoidance of certain words or situations. Differentiating between normal non-fluency and stammering is problematic and therefore any parental concern in this area should be taken seriously.

Table 5.16   Fluency

Parental report	Observation	Assessment
Discussion Describe your child's speaking. When is he or she most/least fluent? Discuss times, situations and people. How do you and other family members handle the most/least fluent times?	*Context* Child in play or conversation with parents *Key questions* Is there evidence of interjections of sounds, syllables, words or phrases? Is there evidence of repetitions of words, parts of words or phrases? Is there evidence of sound prolongation? How frequently do these occur in each utterance?	*Informal assessment* Checklists of fluency

Prosody

Information about what a word, phrase or sentence means comes from the interpretation of prosodic information as well as from a knowledge of word meanings and grammar and the interpretation of the context of the utterance. Prosody relates to information above the level of the syllable; stress, timing and intonation. Research has shown that it continues to develop, both expressively and receptively well into school years, with the development of intonation expected up to the age of 10

Table 5.17   Prosody

Parental report	Observation	Assessment
Key questions Does your child pick up on your tone of voice?	*Context* Conversation *Key questions* Is the child able to use intonation, stress and rhythm appropriately to convey a range of meaning and to maintain word and phrase boundaries? Does the child respond appropriately to different tones of voice?	*Formal assessment* None current in clinical practice, under development and used in research *Informal assessment* For example, matching tone of voice to photographs of emotion or to pictured/verbal scenarios

years.[15] It is an area that is often impaired in children with pragmatic difficulties, being clearly linked to the development of skills in interpreting ambiguous messages, as well as emotional tone of voice.[16] In this respect it has also been linked with the ability to process rapidly changing auditory information (*see* 'Attention and listening'). In terms of the use of intonation, children with Autism Spectrum Disorders are often identified as having specific deficits in this area. Prosody is also affected in some children with dyspraxia where timing and stress may be disrupted by difficulties in planning and co-ordinating the linguistic and articulatory levels of speech.

Curriculum-based assessment

For school children of all ages, clinicians and teachers use modifications to the educational curriculum as a basis for language assessment. This assessment is grounded in the various aspects of the curriculum which children are supposed to master in the UK.[17] Information is gathered from teacher assessment and Standardised Attainment Targets (SATs) about the level the child is reaching in each subject, the profile of achievement, especially across core subject areas, and about how the child is learning. For a child with identified special educational needs, The Code of Practice[18] provides a recommended protocol for the setting and monitoring of modified targets for the child. The critical dimension of this approach is that relevant content and contexts from the child's world guide the assessment process. The focus is not so much on whether the child is learning the course content but on whether the child is using language knowledge, skills and strategies effectively when attempting to learn. As part of the assessment the clinician is likely to work with teaching staff to examine the teacher's instructional style in the classroom setting, as it may relate to the student's performance; looking at the level of complexity of the language used, the pace at which the information is delivered, the time given for student reflection, and the teaching which precedes independent work. The therapist and teacher will also look at classroom layout, groupings of children and the visual transparency of the tasks the child has to follow in order to have access to learning opportunities. Essentially, the aim of this evaluation is to look at the potential barriers and facilitators to the child's learning within the environment.

Diagnosis

One of the outcomes of the assessment process is to provide parents and supporting professionals with a diagnosis of the child's condition. Increasingly, and possibly as a result of recent educational legislation, clinicians are focusing not so much on what the condition is called but on a description of the child's strengths, weaknesses and needs. It is true too that many children referred to speech and language therapists are presenting with complex communication disorders which cannot easily be classified, that is we are seeing very few instances of 'pure' speech or language impairments. Classification systems are available, but for a range of reasons they are not as widely used within speech and language therapy as they are within other disciplines, psychiatry and paediatrics for example. (Chapter 1 outlines the differential diagnosis for speech and language disorders from DSM-IV.) Rather a series of clinical decisions are made based on the needs of the child (*see* the Decision and Action columns in Figure 5.1). In practice, parents and carers vary in their need for a diagnosis. For some, having a name for their child's disorder helps to explain what is going on and facilitate the search for a possible cause, for other parents a diagnosis may be a pigeonhole from which their child will never escape despite progress, advances in medicine and education and changes in thinking: labelled for life. In some situations a diagnosis provides access to specific health or educational resources. Certainly a diagnosis will help in putting parents and families in touch with support organisations, a statutory duty for healthcare professionals in the UK, and may alert other health and non-health professionals to the need for specific assessments and interventions in their fields of expertise. Clearly, professionals need to be sensitive to the needs and wishes of the child's family in deciding whether to (i) describe his or her needs, (ii) make a diagnosis, or both. Being in the position of knowing more than one is sharing with the parents is uncomfortable. Parents need to be given the authority to decide how much they wish to know and when they wish to be informed.

Summary

- Speech and language therapy assessment uses theories, processes and practices from both educational and medical models.
- The assessment aims to investigate whether there is a problem and if so how significant it is. Judgements are made in comparison with what is known about normal development.
- Parental report and observation are used in conjunction with informal/formal assessment approaches.
- Typically an assessment is a snapshot of the child's sampled skills at any one time. It begins with areas of communication about which the parents are concerned.
- Clinical decisions are made on the basis of extrapolation from the sampled skills.
- The process of assessment is never complete. The skills outlined in this chapter may all be sampled over time for an individual child. More likely the assessment will focus on key areas of development at any given time.
- Flexibility in the process accommodates the divergent requirements of education to provide a needs-based description of the child, and medicine to follow a system of referral–assessment–diagnosis–treatment.
- The best indication of a positive, long-term prognosis is the child's level of development and rate of progress until the time of assessment.

References

1   Gathercole SE and Baddeley AD (1990) Phonological memory deficits in language disordered children: Is there a causal connection? *Journal of Memory and Language* **29**: 336–60.

2   Haynes C and Naidoo S (1991) *Children with Specific Speech and Language Impairment.* MacKeith Press, Oxford.

3   Johnston JR (1992) Cognitive abilities of language impaired children. In: P Fletcher and D Hall (eds) *Specific Speech and Language Disorders in Children.* Whurr, London.

4   Bornstein MH, Haynes MO and Painter KM (1998) Sources of child vocabulary competence: a multivariate model. *Journal of Child Language* **25**: 367–93.

5   Baddeley AD and Hitch GJ (1974) Working memory. In: G Bower (ed) *Recent Advances in Learning and Motivation.* Academic Press, New York.

6   Stelmach GE (1982) Information-processing framework for understanding human motor behaviour. In: J Scott Kelso (ed) *Human Motor Behaviour.* Erlbaum, Hillsdale, NJ.

7   Baddeley AD (1990) *Human Memory: theory and practice.* Erlbaum, Hove, Sussex, and Hillsdale, NJ, p. 354.

8   Tulving E (1983) *Elements of Episodic Memory.* Oxford University Press, Oxford, p. 28.

9   Cooper J, Moodley M and Reynell J (1978) *Helping Language Development.* Arnold, London.

10 Masidlover M and Knowles W (1982) *The Derbyshire Language Scheme.* Ambervalley and Erewash Education Authority, Derby.

11 Hakes DT (1980) *The Development of Metalinguistic Abilities in Children.* Springer-Verlag, Berlin, New York.

12 Bernstein DK and Tiegerman E (1992) *Language and Communication Disorders in Children.* (3rd edn). Macmillan, New York.

13 Grunwell P (1981) *The Nature of Phonological Disability in Children.* Academic Press, London.

14 Ozanne A (1995) The search for developmental verbal dyspraxia. In: B Dodd (ed) *Differential Diagnosis and Treatment of Children with Speech Disorders.* Whurr, London.

15 Wells B and Peppe S (1998) *The development of intonation in the preschool years.* Child Language Seminar, 4–6 September 1998, Sheffield.

16 Courtright JA and Courtright IC (1983) The perception of nonverbal vocal cues of emotional meaning by language-disordered and normal children. *Journal of Speech and Hearing Research* **26**: 412–17.

17 DfEE (1995) *National Curriculum.* HMSO, London.

18 DfEE (1994) *Code of Practice on the Identification and Assessment of Special Educational Need.* HMSO, London.

CHAPTER 6

Communication difficulties in a multicultural context

Deirdre Martin

Bilingualism is a linguistic, sociocultural and cognitive phenomenon and it is not a language pathology. There is no longer substantial evidence that becoming bilingual is disadvantageous for children (see ref. 1 for an overview of these studies). The growing understanding is that being bilingual is not like being monolingual twice over. The languages are not completely separate but are inter-related and bilingual speakers and listeners draw on both. Indeed, being bilingual is the child's language. Further, it is a recognised human right that bilinguals have the opportunity to maintain their languages.

This chapter looks at the issues involved with linguistic minority children who have difficulties learning language, similar to other cases discussed in this book. However, in the case of children developing two or more languages, there are two immediate challenges facing the professionals involved. First, to clarify whether or not the language delay or difficulty solely concerns the later developing language, which will be English in most English speaking-countries, or whether it concerns both (all) the child's languages. That is, is the child's difficulty a second language problem or a problem developing language itself? Each type of difficulty has different implications for managing the child's support. The second important challenge and concern is underdetection, explored in Chapter 3. It is easier for professionals to detect, and intervene with, severe difficulties in children when they do not share their language. However, it is more difficult to detect and support problems at higher levels of language functioning when professionals and particularly speech and language therapists do not share the child's or young person's language.

The chapter explores these challenges and other areas which concern appreciating the size of the bilingual population and the potential caseload, the assessment, intervention and support of bilingual children with speech and language difficulties, and the professional issues involved in meeting the needs of this client group. First of all, it is important to understand what we mean by bilingualism.

Bilingual, English as an additional language and linguistic minority

The term 'bilingual' or 'emergent bilingual' is often used to refer to children developing two or more languages. For some children they may have acquired their home language and English at about the same time and be 'simultaneous bilinguals'. Referring to this group of children only by their skills in developing English is misleading. For example, they may not be developing English as a second language (ESL) but rather as a third or fourth language, consequently, English as an additional language (EAL) is more accurate. In the USA emergent bilingual children may be referred to as having 'limited English proficiency' (LEP), which labels what they do not have linguistically rather than what they do have. It is important that practitioners involved with this group are alert to the fact these children are constantly communicating and learning and being communicated to through two languages. The term 'linguistic minority' is often used to describe children from bilingual communities. In many countries there are substantial communities which are distinguished by their languages, cultures and heritage countries. They are often in lower socioeconomic groups. Many communities are established for two or more generations and chose to maintain their language and culture as part of their identity. There are also other, newer, linguistic minority communities and refugee groups. Many linguistic minority children enter school speaking languages other than English as well as some English, and English develops after their home language, which is 'sequential bilingualism'. They comprise the majority of linguistic minority learners in most primary schools in the UK. They are potentially linguistically richer than their monolingual peers and teachers.[2] Many preschool children are monolingual in their home language.

Being bilingual

Being bilingual is a complex achievement at both societal and individual levels. There are linguistic skills involved, which include both spoken and written forms, cognitive skills, where language is used for learning, and there are issues of culture and identity, which are mediated by language and the language community. Bilingual speakers often have a preferred language, one which they feel they are more fluent in, which is the dominant one.[3] Practitioners need to consider all these aspects and looking at only one will be insufficient for the needs of children with language difficulties who are in constant contact with two languages.

The aim for practitioners working with potentially bilingual children is not necessarily to work towards developing a 'balanced' bilingual: 'someone who is equally fluent in two languages across various contexts' (ref 1: 8). Language skills develop to different levels to meet communicative need and most bilinguals will have different communicative demands for their languages. The practitioner needs to consider supporting potentially bilingual children with language difficulties to develop language skills to meet the language demands from both their different environments, such as home, school, park and temple.

When neither language is thought to be fluent then the term 'semilingual' is sometimes used:

> *A semilingual is considered to exhibit the following profile*
> *in both their languages: displays a small vocabulary and*
> *incorrect grammar, consciously thinks about production, is*
> *stilted and uncreative with each language, and finds it*
> *difficult to think and express emotions in either language. (ref 1: 9)*

Semilingual is a controversial term because it is usually used disparagingly, associated with low expectations and underachievement, and suggests that poor language development may be due to within-child factors rather than being due to social factors. It overlooks the fact that languages may be competent in certain contexts. Further, quantitative assessment of language skills may not give the full picture of a bilingual child's abilities in both languages. Moreover, comparisons are made with monolingual speakers' language skills rather than more appropriately with other bilinguals' performance.[1] The term 'semilingualism', rather than being a descriptor of language difficulties, serves to remind practitioners of the need to be rigorous about assessment purposes and practices with bilingual children.

Considering language skills only limits understanding the needs of emerging bilinguals. The important issue for teachers and others involved with bilingual learners with potential special needs is to distinguish and assess the relationship between social factors and within-child factors which contribute to the language needs of bilingual learners who have substantial difficulties.

Gathering information about your area and your potential clients

The equality of service to linguistic and ethnic minority clients may present a challenge to service providers in terms of access and provision. Consequently, in a district where there are ethnic and linguistic minorities it is important that health and educational services gather demographic information about the minority groups in order to develop resources. This information should include the number of languages and whether they are both spoken and written, how long the communities are established, and some account of the size of each minority community or group of speakers. For service provision to potential clients who are bilingual, this kind of demographic information is important because it should enable some forecast to be made about potential referral numbers and the resources needed to support them. Estimating the size of the problem has been discussed in Chapter 1, which summarises that up to 7% of children may have difficulties which warrant attention. We may anticipate that a similar estimate can be made for bilingual children. The estimate for the bilingual child population in England is between 7 and 8% of the total population, which suggests that the number of linguistic minority children with potentially significant language problems will be small. Yet, a survey of the speech and language therapy departments in England shows that under 60% of speech and language therapists working with children have bilingual children on their caseload.[4] There are implications from these figures that we need to organise minority language resources appropriately.

Other aspects of the bilingual client's community which have direct implications on case management concern the family structure of the child's community, linguistic information and naming systems. In the family structure it is important to know whether the family is extended or nuclear, the adjustments made as a consequence of living in the new country, the isolation of any members of the family, such as a young mother, who are the primary caregivers to the client, parents or others. Awareness of different child-rearing practices across the communities, in particular the role of play and the pattern of child–adult communication, is essential.[5]

It is important to know something of the language of your clients and how it is used. This may include knowing how and whom to greet, non-verbal politeness forms and what is appropriate to ask to whom. Speech and language therapists would need to know in some detail the linguistic aspects of the child's mother tongue for the purposes of assessment.

Understanding the naming system in a linguistic minority community is essential if important administrative confusions are to be avoided. In many cultures, parents and children may share the same names. In other cultures, religious names may be part of the child's name or there may be gender forms, for example in the Sikh religion boys are given the name 'singh' and girls the name 'kaur'. In some cultures a family name has less importance than the clan or village name. It is important not only to document the child's official name, but also to note the personal name that the child is most frequently referred to by, as well as the name by which the child wishes to be called.[6]

It is fundamentally important to see the individual client and family within their cultural perspective and to challenge stereotyping. Generalisations are easily made when working in cross-cultural contexts. It is important to bear in mind that groups originating from the same country will vary considerably. While remaining aware of general patterns of behaviour, each client and family needs to be considered individually.

Resources

Resources need to be directed at facilitating clients' access and to providing a service which clients are able to make use of. These resources may include language and cultural support for the practitioners and clients where they do not share the same language, such as a bilingual paraprofessional or co-worker. They may include assessment and intervention materials. They may extend to support groups across different language and cultural communities.

Since resources are finite, effective planning and management are necessary. For example, in a district with large linguistic minority communities, investing in recruiting and training professionals and paraprofessionals or co-workers may be considered. In the case of small numbers of linguistic minority clients, sharing bilingual resources across disciplines, services and districts may be an efficient support strategy for the clients and practitioners involved.

Referral patterns

In an overzealous attempt to prevent any child with possible difficulties from 'slipping through the net' it may become practice to refer many linguistic minority children for speech and language assessment. Some health workers may place these children on an 'at-risk' register so that they are continually monitored. This is an expensive and unnecessary approach, which may also alarm parents if they were made aware of it. Health workers need to consider how they can refine their screening procedures to develop sensitive indicators for referring linguistic minority children for speech and language assessment. In this respect, working with speech and language therapists can be rewarding. For example, making linguistically appropriate some of the early language development indicators, such as babbling, first words, combining words and using grammatical markers such as verb tenses, gender and plural marking in the home language.

Case history taking

The initial interview is a sensitive and important part of the contractual relationship between the client and the practitioner. On the basis of the information exchanged the practitioner decides whether or not the child has a difficulty and how this might be supported, and the child and family decide whether they wish to collaborate with the practitioner.[7] It is essential to this relationship that the child and family develop a satisfactory understanding of the process of assessment and intervention.[8] Central to this are feelings of trust and empathy between the child and family and the practitioner. In the case of an initial interview with a bilingual family there may be several factors which may complicate the situation.

Language

The practitioner and the child and family may not share a language. Alternatively, they may share a language but at differing levels of ability.

Cultural perceptions

The practitioner and client may not share a mutual cultural background. Perceptions of the client/practitioner relationship may differ substantially concerning power, authority and equality, which has implications for working together and counselling. There may be differing perceptions of disability as well as intervention and 'cure', which would influence the nature of a support programme.[9]

Priority of language difficulties alongside other difficulties

It is important that the practitioner is sensitive to the priorities the family may place on the child's difficulties. For example, if the family has housing difficulties, or political asylum problems or family breakdown, then the child's speech and language difficulties may not be prioritised by the family.

Predisposing factors in the practitioner

Practitioners need to be aware of their own attitudes towards working with linguistic minority clients. For example, practitioners need to ask themselves whether they feel that they have received adequate and appropriate training for working with this client group? Do they have views about assimilation, speaking the majority language, racial prejudice? Antipathetic views made by the practitioner towards the linguistic minority client group are likely to have a negative influence on any working relationship with this group. Practitioners and their managers need to be sensitive to these factors and respond appropriately.

Developmental information

The same principles in gathering a case history in the majority culture apply to children from linguistic minority communities. Information about the child's birth and development are the focus, across the parameters of medical, social, emotional, motor and cognitive development.

The practitioner needs to be aware that in some cultures, women may be sensitive to talking about pregnancy and birth particularly in the presence of a man or even an older child. The gender of the practitioner and co-worker will be an important consideration. In some societies, marriage within the extended family, known as 'consanguinity', is a social practice. Studies[10] have shown that this may cause genetically based difficulties, which commonly affect physical and sensory development, giving rise to, for example, skin disorders, learning difficulties and hearing impairment.

When assessing the account of the child's development, the practitioner needs to balance what may be 'universals' of development and what may be cultural expectations. Often what are thought to be 'universals' of development are based on research findings from white, Western societies and may not generalise to other societies. For example, hearing and vision may be objectively measured, while height and weight at certain ages, the amount and nature of socialising with adults, familiarity with toys and play are all relative to the community. The guidance offered in Chapter 2, about aspects of development associated with language, such as attention, memory, motor skills and co-ordination, needs to be contextually embedded in the child's environment and interpreted through what parents say about the child's experiences. In this respect, the practitioner may need to rely more than usual on the views and advice from the family and co-worker to make an informed opinion about the child's development.

Two important difficulties for practitioners who refer linguistic minority children with alleged speech and language difficulties are highlighted in the summary of Chapter 3, on surveillance. Although practitioners may have good observation skills, in the case of the development of other languages, they are likely to have limited frameworks for interrogating and interpreting what they see. For example, there is a lack of knowledge about developmental expectations for language in most languages other than English. Furthermore, they may not have elaborated 'effective trigger questions to tap the observation skills of parents' in the preferred language of the parents. More research needs to be done in these areas to build up a body of knowledge. Working with speech and language therapists specialising in this area and trained bilingual personnel can be rewarding.

Context, setting and patterns of language use

In most cases, the case history interview takes place in the health or school clinic. There are a growing number of practitioners who believe that seeing the linguistic minority child in the home environment may be the best place to begin to gather assessment information. There are also other reasons for visiting the child's home, such as the family's non-attendance, when the practitioner may need to consider obtaining the case history information elsewhere, such as in the family's home. This may require sensitivity regarding the appropriateness of the visitor in terms of language, background, gender and status.

Language use among bilingual families will depend on the context, the speakers and the topic. It is essential that the practitioner explores the patterns of language use in the bilingual child's family and notes who speaks what language to whom and about what topic. This information promotes understanding of the bilingual environment of the child, and informs assessment, management and advice on language support.

Assessment process

There are four main issues involved in the assessment of language and communication in bilingual children. They concern assessment in both languages, language and culture sensitivity, the assessment procedures and who is involved in the assessment process.

The practitioner needs to be clear about the purpose of the assessment. Is it for screening, for educational placement, or for identifying the nature or severity of difficulty, and in the case of bilingual children for comparing the language skills of both languages? Assessments may aim to draw a profile of the child's strengths and weaknesses across a variety of language and communication skills. It is increasingly acknowledged that assessments do not measure ability but rather achievement in the test. Moreover, low achievement is not necessarily synonymous with low ability. The points raised in Chapter 3 about evaluating the appropriateness of screening tests is possibly more pertinent with this population group.

Assessing both languages

The linguistic minority child may present as a monolingual speaker of the home language or as an emerging bilingual speaker. In both cases the practitioner needs to assess the full language repertoire of the child, that is, assess both languages, as the following case study illustrates.

Case study

Hasan, a four-year-old child of Turkish Cypriot parents, was assessed on a standardised monolingual English comprehension test. The practitioner scored his age equivalent language level as being at a level of one year seven months. This was relayed to the parents as evidence of Hasan's severe language delay. No assessment was attempted of the child's first and most familiar language, Turkish. Important decisions about the child's educational provision were made on the basis of the speech/language therapy report which stated that the child was delayed in his language ability by over two years. No reference was made in the report to the fact that the child had only been assessed in English, his less developed language.[11]

Language and culture sensitivity

Language and culture are inextricably linked. Halliday[12] sees language as the vehicle for culture. Others see 'culture' as the structure and 'communication' as the process (Birdwhistle, cited in ref. 12: 183). The implications for the assessment of language and communication skills are that assessment needs to be culturally embedded. In many cases, practitioners aim to find assessment approaches and materials which are acultural and beyond cultural influence. It would be more rewarding to aim for language assessments which are embedded in the culture of the child and thus are more likely to encourage the child's optimum achievement. This would necessarily involve developing assessments which were sensitive to language and culture specifics. This would have resource implications.

One strategy is to adapt assessment procedures. Tests and assessment procedures may be modified successfully from one language to another.[14] However, a great deal of preparation needs to be invested in this adaptation. Cultural and linguistic appropriateness needs to be taken into account. *Simple translation of the test is not recommended*, particularly in language and communication assessments. For example, vocabulary items may not be directly translatable or there may be aspects of grammar which are language specific. Moreover, there are ways of asking for information which vary across languages and would need to be taken into account in the test procedure.

Assessment procedures

'Another approach to non-discriminatory assessment is to use standardised tests in a non-standard manner'.[13] The bilingual child can be allowed to perform on a test without the testing constraints. For example, the stimuli may be selected based on familiarity or unfamiliarity to the child, instructions may be reworded, longer response time may be allowed, ceilings and baselines may be ignored, all the responses made by the child are recorded in whatever language or dialect the child uses. Practice items should always be developed and available to the child to make clear what is required. Of course, the decision to use a standardised procedure in a non-standardised manner means that the test norms cannot be applied.

Assessments may be standardised or they may be criteria-referenced. Standardised tests compare peers' performance across a set of tasks, where the performance of the majority is called the standard or the 'norm'. The norms can only be used for comparison among children of the same population group. Hence, norms for first-language English speakers cannot be used for second-language or bilingual speakers of English. When using criteria-referenced assessments, caution needs to be exercised in the appropriateness of 'age-stage' information, and interpreted through the developmental history and sociocultural background of the bilingual child.

In many cases the experienced practitioner may prefer to use informal assessment procedures, such as observing bilingual children with alleged language difficulties at play and in interaction with objects and people familiar to them. They may set the criteria by the toys or objects set out for the child, such as fine or gross motor activities, sequencing games or doll play. Alternatively, they may observe the child selecting who and what they choose to play with. Furthermore, they may rely on others, such as the parent or teacher, to collect this information in a variety of settings, such as home, the classroom, nursery, the playground, the park. It is important that the practitioner has a recording format for the observations. In this way a degree of detailed consistency can be maintained across the settings and the observers. One such inventory is the Bilingual Oral Language Development (BOLD) inventory of communication skills for bilingual children. It concerns noting the child's communicative behaviour in both languages, such as 'comments on own actions, describes events sequentially, follows directions, expresses imagination'.[15] Interestingly, children with substantial speech and language difficulties are identified more accurately by teachers according to language use criteria rather than by grammatical accuracy criteria.[16] Another assessment procedure, which is based on interviewing the caregiver about the child's communication, is the Pragmatics Profile,[17] which has been trialed successfully with linguistic minority communities. It offers a profile of the child's communicative behaviour across both languages, whether the child is preverbal or verbal.

The interpretation of the information from these observations needs to be modified by the language and cultural practices of the bilingual child's speech community. In some communities children are not encouraged to ask adults questions or to initiate conversation and the absence of these pragmatic features of language use might not necessarily indicate disability.

One of the issues raised at the beginning of this chapter concerned the importance of differentiating between second language difficulties and more profound language delay because of the implications for supporting the child's language needs. If the home language is developing satisfactorily according to parental report and home language assessment, but there seem to be difficulties in the development of the second language, then further assessment, monitoring and support would be indicated in the second language. Usually this is the province of specialist language teachers. If the child has difficulties in the development of both languages then it is likely that the child has problems processing aspects of language, whatever the language. These children need to be referred to speech and language therapists. There are implications concerning which language support and intervention should be offered.

Assessment team

Assessment is ideally done in a team and in the case of the bilingual child with alleged language difficulties the team needs to comprise a speaker of both the child's and the practitioner's languages who will be able to influence the presentation of a case profile which is as linguistically and culturally balanced as possible.

The practitioner who shares the languages and culture of the bilingual child with identified language and communication difficulties is in an optimal position for assessing bilingual children. However, such practitioners are in short supply and it is important that they are not professionally 'ghetto-ised' into working exclusively with one population group. In terms of equal opportunities, they are entitled to a similar range of options in career development as their colleagues.

In cases where practitioners do not share the language(s) of the child, there are several possibilities for language support. One of the best options is trained bilingual paraprofessionals or co-workers who work alongside the practitioner and the child and family. Their role is multifold and includes interpretation, advocacy for the client, language and cultural advice, advising on materials, case history and assessment support, counselling and intervention programme support.[18]

It is possible to recruit non-trained personnel, and community centres in the linguistic minority community are good sources of potential recruitment of untrained bilingual support personnel. There are professional issues, such as confidentiality, which would need to be well established first. In all these cases, consideration needs to be given to briefing time before the assessment or intervention session, seating arrangements in the session, materials and the management of communication in the session between the child, family, co-worker and practitioner.[19] It may be possible to make a video or audio cassette recording of the child functioning in both languages and at a later time to analyse it with a bilingual speaker in a professional capacity. When parents or family are involved in the assessment process, practitioners need to be aware that there are issues surrounding training and objectivity which compromise the assessment and influence the outcomes.

Range of difficulties

Bilingual children with communication and language difficulties may manifest difficulties at all levels of language, speech sounds, vocabulary and meaning, grammar and sentence formulation, and using language in a variety of ways, such as in conversation, to problem solve and tell stories. Bilingual children may also show some interaction between the two languages. For example, some speech sounds from one language may appear in the other language. Similarly, some words or word endings and even the formulation of phrases and sentences may show an interaction between the two languages. Language-mixing is a normal aspect of bilingual development and it precedes the languages separating and functioning independently. Code-switching is an essential form of a bilingual's repertoire, where bilingual speakers move between their two languages without difficulty because it is part of their use of language (pragmatic skills). It is important that the practitioner differentiates between these features of bilingual children's language skills.

There is a small percentage of children who present with difficulties only in the area of language, while many more children have language difficulties together with other difficulties, such as difficulties with learning, hearing or physical development. In the case of bilingual children, differentiating between difficulties in learning and language is a substantial challenge to most practitioners. The assessment procedures for assessing cognitive and intellectual functioning are as fraught with cultural and linguistic bias as are the language assessments. The practitioner needs to be aware of these issues and try to bring to bear effective strategies for appropriate assessment of the linguistic minority child's cognitive skills.

The second issue which was raised at the beginning of the chapter was identifying higher-level language difficulties in linguistic minority children. It is clear that the non-verbal preschool child or the child with unintelligible speech will be referred for further language assessment. The risk is that the less severe difficulties will go unassessed and consequently unsupported, with implications for the education and employment of that young person. For example, assessing phonological difficulties, such as dyspraxia, word-finding difficulties, conversational skills and certain pragmatic skills, and related literacy difficulties. Identifying and supporting higher-level language difficulties in emerging bilingual children is very challenging. There are obstacles at each stage in the process. There are few resources and few people who are able to assess and identify higher-level language difficulties across both languages. Those children with severe language difficulties who have specialist language support or attend language units, are usually offered intervention only in English. There are implications for the families of these children, their understanding of their child's difficulties and their inclusion in intervention and support. More research is needed to develop our understanding of the relationship between languages in higher-level language difficulty in bilingual children.

Parental involvement

As with every child, parental involvement is essential and it is important that parents from differing linguistic and cultural communities understand and appreciate the opportunities open to them to be involved in the assessment and intervention process of their child's language and communication difficulty. They must be encouraged and enabled to do this and a counselling/consultative framework offers parents and families these opportunities. It is highly likely that the parents from ethnic minority communities have perceptions of difficulty and disability which are different from the practitioners'.[20] Parental involvement and support depends upon practitioners and parents having some mutual understanding of each other's views and some shared agreement about each other's role in the support of the child's difficulty. Practitioners and parents need to spend time together developing this understanding. What is to be avoided is the situation where the parents and practitioners are following separate and different approaches to the child's language difficulty and developing different expectations about the communication need and abilities of the child.

Intervention and support: which language(s)?

The central issue here is in which language intervention and support for bilingual children with communication and language difficulties should occur. In principle, both languages of the linguistic minority child need to be supported so that the child is not alienated from accessing either community. The practitioner needs to consider that it is likely to be the minority community, in the minority language and culture, which cares for the disabled child and adult. Linguistically, developing the mother tongue builds on the child's communication strengths, which can help the child develop additional languages. However, there may be resourcing constraints which obscure principled decisions and these need to be recognised and managed to enable the preferred line of intervention and support.

Case study

Sidrar is a four-year-old girl with moderate–severe learning difficulties. Her mother speaks no English and the only language spoken at home is Urdu. Sidrar is attending a school nursery and will be going into mainstream school. The educational psychologist and the speech and language therapist involved agree that working on Sidrar's strengths would be the preferred approach, in particular enhancing her Urdu and using this language as a means of enabling her to access English. Sidrar's mother is unable to help her at home with language and learning support, so a bilingual Urdu/English nursery assistant would be the most appropriate support for Sidrar.[21]

This case study exemplifies one of several possible scenarios for intervening and supporting bilingual children with communication and language difficulties. Bilingual parents and co-workers need to be involved, as well as bilingual teachers and classroom assistants. Advising linguistic minority families to speak English-only to the child, when English plays only a partial or possibly no role in the family's communication, is not appropriate advice. It can be harmful because it can result in the child being excluded from home language interaction and being spoken to infrequently.

As in the case of assessments, commercial intervention programmes for monolingual English children with developmental difficulties need to be appraised for appropriateness of material and linguistic aims. Caution is needed in the translation of any aspects of it. Ways of saying things in one language are rarely the same in another. The linguistic structures elicited and practised in one language through materials and activities may be different in another language. In addition, programmes may be based on developmental information which is language-specific and may not be the same across languages.

Conclusion

In the case of the linguistic minority child with alleged speech and language difficulties, understanding the nature and extent of a child's bilingualism will allow the practitioner to assess and advise sensitively. Appreciating the role and importance of the child's and family's mother tongue and culture are important in offering management and support for language difficulties. The practitioner needs to involve the parents and family in supporting the development of the mother tongue and the additional language where possible. Finally, practitioners are advised to monitor their own skills and limitations in this area, in terms of language and cultural diversity, and to seek appropriate resources, such as bilingual paraprofessionals and further professional development.

References

1   Baker C (1993) *Key Issues in Bilingualism and Bilingual Education*. Multilingual Matters, Avon.

2   Gregory E (ed) (1997) *One Child, Many Worlds*. David Fulton, London.

3   Fishman J (ed) (1971) *Advances in the Sociology of Language*. Mouton, The Hague.

4   Winter K (1999) Speech and language therapy provision for bilingual children: aspects of the current service. *International Journal of Language and Communication Disorders* **34**(10): 85–99.

5   Ara F and Thompson C (1989) Intervention with bilingual pre-school children. In: D Duncan (ed) *Working with Bilingual Language Disability*. Chapman and Hall, London.

6   Duncan D (1991) Communication. In: AJ Squires (ed) *Multicultural Health Care and Rehabilitation*, pp. 78–85. Edward Arnold and Age Concern, London.

7   Miller N (1979) The bilingual child in the speech therapy clinic. *British Journal of Disorders of Communication* **13**(1): 17–30.

8   Cunningham C and Davis H (1985) *Working with Parents: frameworks for collaboration*. Open University Press, Milton Keynes.

9   Harry B and Kalyanpur M (1994) Cultural underpinnings of special education: implications for professional interactions with culturally diverse families. *Disability and Society* **9**(2): 145–65.

10 Bundey S and Allam H (1993) A five year prospective study of the health of children in different ethnic groups with particular reference to the effects of in-breeding. *European Journal of Human Genetics* **1**: 206–19.

11   Stokes J and Duncan D (1989) Linguistic assessment procedures for bilingual children. In: D Duncan (ed) *Working with Bilingual Language Disability*. Chapman and Hall, London.

12   Halliday MAK (1975) *Learning How to Mean: explorations in the development of language*. Edward Arnold, London.

13   Taylor OL (1986) *Nature of Communication Disorders in Culturally and Linguistically Diverse Populations*. College-Hill Press, San Diego.

14   Duncan D (ed) (1989) *Working with Bilingual Language Disability*. Chapman and Hall, London.

15   Mattes LJ and Omark DR (1984) *Speech and Language Assessment for the Bilingual Handicapped*. College-Hill Press, San Diego.

16   Damico J and Oller JW Jnr (1980) Pragmatic versus morphological/syntactic criteria for language referrals. *Language, Speech and Hearing Services in Schools* 11: 85–94.

17   Dewart H and Summers S (1995) *The Pragmatics Profile of Everyday Communication Skills*. NFER-Nelson, Windsor.

18   Martin D (ed) (1993) *Services to Bilingual Children with Speech and Language Difficulties*. AFASIC, London.

19   Barnett S (1989) Working with interpreters. In: D Duncan (ed) *Working with Bilingual Language Disability*. Chapman and Hall, London.

20   Harry B (1992) *Cultural Diversity, Families and the Special Education System: communication and empowerment*. Teachers College Press, New York.

21   Gadhok K (1994) Languages for intervention. In: D Martin (ed) *Services to Bilingual Children with Speech and Language Difficulties*. AFASIC, London.

CHAPTER 7

Intervention for children with communication difficulties

James Law

The potential size of the population of children with communication difficulties and the range of the problems which present through the language system were discussed in Chapters 1 and 2. Such difficulties may be significant in their own right and warrant specific remedial language support, but they may also be flags for other conditions and point to other interventions. But it is of little value picking out difficulties in a population unless something can be done to improve them. Remedial services offer one solution here, but given the large numbers involved there are likely to be issues which need to be dealt with at a wider, population level.

There are many approaches to promoting speech and language skills in young children with communication difficulties. The way in which such a service is offered depends on a great many contextual factors. Clearly the difficulties experienced by the child constitute one dimension. But it is also necessary to take into consideration the experience of the clinician or teacher, the extent to which family or carers are involved in the intervention and also what is available at the point at which the service is delivered. This chapter presents a broad overview of the type of interventions available for the child with speech and/or language difficulties. It does not focus on children with complex communication needs – for example those needing augmentative and alternative means of communication. Many aspects of intervention are impairment- or disability-specific and these are covered in more detail in Part Two of this book. The evidence for the value of different approaches will be presented in each section. The main effects of intervention will be summarised at the end of the chapter. The chapter ends with a discussion of the economic evaluation of intervention for communication difficulties.

Who receives help for speech and language delay?

The intervention literature suggests that it is broadly possible to pick out three groups of children with communication difficulties:

- Children with language delays secondary to other conditions, such as developmental disabilities, mental handicap, autism and the like.
- Socially disadvantaged children who have poor speech and language development concomitant to their other developmental skills but are considered to be experiencing environmental deprivation.
- Children with speech and/or language delays in the absence of other handicapping conditions. These are the primary language delays described in Chapter 1.

To a great extent these are service-orientated classifications. What is actually offered to the child and the family may be similar in each of the three categories. Many different professional groups may be involved with supporting these children. At the centre must be the education/social care system but, depending on the nature of the problem and the age at which the child is identified, there will also be speech and language therapists, clinical psychologists, psychiatrists and the primary care professionals, such as health visitors and general practitioners who often play such an important role in responding to parental anxiety regarding the child's communication skills. The range of interested parties is hardly surprising given the interdependence of the different aspects of development and well being which are reflected in communication, but it can be bewildering for parents trying to establish who might offer the best for their child.

The reader wishing more detail should look at one of the many narrative reviews in this area.[1–5] A full review of the literature related to intervention for handicap and social disadvantage is provided by Farran.[6]

A word on the nature of the evidence

It is sometimes difficult for those familiar with trials methodology to feel confident when examining the intervention literature related to communication difficulties. Few studies present with the kind of statistical power that is routine in studies associated with the introduction of new drug technologies, and both the nature of the cases and the interventions are often not as well described as they might be. Thus a study may describe the children as being 'language disordered' but there may be little data on the children apart from the specific measures used to indicate change. It may not be clear, for example, whether they had a history of hearing loss or whether they presented with any associated behaviour problems. Another central issue is the extent to which the child is able to generalise newly taught skills. The impact of an intervention is much more powerful if the child is able to take a skill taught in treatment and generalise it to other contexts both within the language system and to other environments. For example, a child may be taught to use subject-verb-object constructions with a set of four action verbs. The child, who is able to generalise this newly acquired structure to other verbs and use them in the playground or at home as well as in the clinical context is clearly at an advantage relative to the child who is not.

These are all areas of concern because they make it difficult to interpret the evidence. Nevertheless a substantial body of intervention literature is now available and it is appropriate to consider it as a hierarchy of experimental evidence. Randomised control trials (RCTs), where they exist, do still offer the best protection against bias when addressing the question of whether an intervention works relative to nothing. But other sources of evidence such as quasi-experimental designs and experimental single-case designs are widely used in this field and are able to offer some solid confirmatory evidence. Indeed the experimental single-case studies may be particularly useful in allowing us to get some feel for the level at which the intervention generalises across contexts, a feature often lacking in the RCT design but crucial to the understanding of intervention in this area. Much of the literature to date has been of a descriptive, non-experimental nature. Although this limits the extent to which it is possible to find commonalities and draw inferences from the findings, it often provides the texture which aids interpretation of the data. Of course the same is true of more traditional medical interventions, many of which have not been evaluated.

Even when there is a body of evidence that intervention can be shown to be useful, there is no guarantee that it is being offered in the same format as that in the intervention study. To a certain extent this is a problem inherent in the interpretation of any literature related to effectiveness, whether it be behavioural or chemical in nature. The difference is that at least the drug is held constant. While a behavioural intervention can be said to be of the same type across studies, the nature of the needs of the client will alter the way in which it is administered. We can show that such intervention *can* work but cannot guarantee that it *will* work in all cases and even if they do it is not clear by what mechanism it is happening. The therapeutic process is, by its nature, iterative in that the therapist may start out with a broad schema of what is intended but will modify strategies according to the response of the individual. The individual reacts to these modifications and so on. It is very hard to factor out the context in which the intervention takes place. Nonetheless there is now a substantial body of literature which has attempted to do just that.

The bottom line – do interventions for communication difficulties work?

At one level it is possible to synthesise the intervention literature to answer the question 'does the intervention work?' The technique most commonly used to determine whether intervention in a given area works is the combination or meta-analysis of effect sizes from all the available intervention studies. This process results in an average effect size. Understandably, number crunching in this way can be treated with suspicion because, combining the effects of studies without due consideration for the differences between them may lead to inappropriate conclusions. Equally, confining attention to a small number of studies meeting specific design criteria may appear to oversimplify the process of intervention and thus detract from clinically valid conclusions. For example it may be common practice for the best-quality studies, and thus the ones that are included in the meta-analysis, to use outcomes which do not reflect those commonly used by clinicians. Nevertheless, meta-analysis does provide a bottom line and does allow those commissioning health services to answer the question 'is there reasonable evidence that referral to such and such a service will result in gains for this client?'.

The extent of the evidence regarding intervention for communication difficulties in children does not compare with that for many medical interventions, at least in terms of the number of studies. Although the extent of the literature in this area remains narrow relative to that for many medical conditions, it is increasing and bears consideration.[6,7]

The most comprehensive meta-analysis of the literature related to intervention for primary speech and language delay comes from the systematic review carried out for the NHS in the UK by Law et al.[5] Only the best-quality studies were synthesised in this review. They include randomised and quasi-experimental designs, but studies were only included if the designs incorporated a no-treatment control group. The studies were grouped into four main clinical areas based on the literature available, namely expressive language, receptive language or comprehension, articulation/phonology and auditory discrimination. Effect sizes from studies with RCT/quasi-experimental designs were averaged across language areas, as in Table 7.1, to allow a comparison between the data from children with primary speech and language delay and those from meta-analyses of studies involving children with secondary delay. Note that an effect size of $+1.00$ corresponds to a level of progress equivalent to that from the 5th to the 25th percentile on a norm-referenced test, representing a considerable degree of improvement and indeed normalisation in the sense that the child's performance approaches what would be considered normal given the age of the child and the assessment in question.

Table 7.1   Summary of effect sizes (d) by language area

Area of language	No. of effect sizes	Average d	95% confidence interval
Articulation/phonology	29	$+0.35^*$	$+0.10/+0.60$
Expressive language	57	$+1.07^*$	$+0.85/+1.29$
Receptive language	7	$+1.09^*$	$+0.44/+1.74$
Auditory discrimination	14	$+0.23$	$-0.10/+0.56$

*Indicates statistically significant results; $p < 0.05$.

The data then suggest consistently high effect sizes for expressive and receptive language but much lower effects for auditory discrimination and articulation. It is possible to conclude that intervention does not affect these areas. In fact these lower overall effects are partly a function of the process of combining studies and they mask the differential effects of direct and indirect work. The relative value of direct and indirect work will be discussed further below.

The results from this analysis are comparable to the only other synthesis of intervention studies focusing on speech and language data.[4] Analysing data across a wider range and a larger number of studies, Nye and colleagues found an average effect size of $+1.42$ from 23 effect sizes for outcomes in syntax, and an average effect size of $+0.65$ from 13 effect sizes for comprehension. The effect size for syntax ($+1.42$), although higher, corresponds relatively closely to the $+1.07$ for expressive language in Table 7.1 although the constructs do no overlap completely. The figure for comprehension ($+0.65$) is rather lower than the figure for receptive language quoted in Table 7.1 ($+1.09$). It is not easy to explain these differences except to say that effect sizes may be higher for children with more discrete problems and that those with expressive difficulties are likely to be just such a group. By contrast, children with low receptive language skills are more likely to be more delayed in other aspects of their development and therefore more resistant to intervention. The figure for receptive language skills may have been higher[5] because the synthesis only included studies with participants with *primary* speech and language delays and thus the more broadly developmentally delayed child would have been excluded.

Although the discussion above has tended to focus on speech and language measures it is evident that many children with speech and language delay have difficulties that are not confined to speech and language and many of the interventions focus on other developmental skills. For example, early communication difficulties are clearly linked into literacy and there has now been an extensive literature developed in this area suggesting that a wide range of interventions can be successful but that many depend on the level of early adult/child interaction in the classroom and at home.[8] Such early intervention programmes have been subjected to considerable attention. Shonkoff and Hauser-Cram[9] reported an average effect size of $+1.17$ for language outcomes from 31 studies. This analysis included non-controlled studies and this may explain the fact that these results are rather higher than other meta-analyses of the literature related to general developmental disabilities. For example, Casto and Mastropieri[10] report an average effect size of $+0.67$ for language in a meta-analysis of the outcomes from 37 early intervention programmes for a broad range of handicapped preschool children and Arnold *et al.*[11] report an average effect size of $+0.59$ from 30 studies. However, these latter results are difficult to interpret as: (i) effect sizes are based upon a wide range of measures, including IQ; and (ii) factors such as severity of the handicapping condition are confounded with the type of intervention programme and other factors, such as the age of the child.

In summary, there is good evidence that interventions in this area can be shown to work. Indeed the effect sizes appear to be higher for children with primary speech and language delays than they are for interventions for children with more disabling conditions and those from adverse social environments. This would rather suggest that speech and language delays are relatively amenable to intervention, although there are issues here relating to the long-term effects of such interventions. As already indicated there is a concern that syntheses of this kind may not pick up areas where intervention is available but which have yet to be subjected to appropriately controlled trials. For example, the issue of pragmatics is discussed in Chapter 1 and again in Chapter 5. Many children with communication difficulties find it very difficult to communicate effectively even when they have sufficient grammatical skills to do so. This has considerable implications for the level of disability experienced by the children, yet intervention in this area of communication has, to date, rarely been the subject of empirical investigation. Thus although this may be the focus of much clinical activity it is not reflected in such meta-analyses. Reducing the data in this way, while providing convincing evidence of an effect of intervention relative to no intervention, fails to cover many of the issues facing the clinician. It is to this broader discussion that we turn next.

Types of intervention

Intervention is sometimes construed as a single phenomenon. Does speech and language therapy work? Such simplification is not helpful because it masks a considerable degree of variability in the practice and in the clients themselves. Of course, if it is genuinely possible to say that children respond to intervention irrespective of type, then there might be a case for saying that any contact of a therapeutic nature would be beneficial. In fact, there is considerable debate about which treatments work more effectively with different groups of client. But first it is helpful to look at some of the sources of variation. It is possible to differentiate between treatments on the basis of length and intensity, on the basis of the professional group with prime responsibility for carrying out the intervention, and on the basis of what is actually carried out in the intervention programme. These axes reflect what the professional does to the child and the family. But it is now widely recognised that the child and the family do not respond in a passive fashion but rather have a decisive role to play in the uptake of intervention.

   The length and intensity of intervention can be divided into three types: inoculation, dosage or nutritional. The inoculation approach provides a highly circumscribed level of input (perhaps two hours) in which advice may be given and recommendations made. This level of intervention is most often used at the level of identifying whether the child has a problem or not and of addressing parental anxiety. This sort of intervention might be construed as a form of primary prevention in that it may prevent children who might have subsequent difficulties going on to do so. Such provision, although undoubtedly recognised by many primary healthcare workers, is poorly specified in the UK. The only exception to this is the WILSTAAR programme for children identified at ten months as having poor listening skills.[12] The intervention is made up of an average of four sessions in total provided within the context of the home. This type of intervention is of considerable interest because of the substantial effect sizes obtained in the original study.

If the child does have a recognisable communication difficulty at that point the child may be taken on for a period of treatment or what is sometimes known within the UK context as a 'package of care'. These 'dosage' treatments may be of up to ten weeks' duration and may be renewable according to the needs of the child concerned. This approach suggests that a relatively short burst of help can redress imbalances within the child or between the parent and child which can then result in self-sustaining modifications to the interaction and may lead to a level of normalisation in the child. It is this type of intervention which has been for the most part the focus of the efficacy literature in this area.

Even the term 'dosage' suggests a model derived from medicine, with children being referred to practitioners because of an identified or a suspected need. For many children their first contact with an interested professional may well be in nursery or even in school. In such cases the children may be referred to outside agencies but it is as likely that they will be monitored in the classroom using existing assessment procedures within the school. This process may mean that the child receives additional help within the classroom. This may be of a specific nature aimed at the impairment experienced by the child but is more likely to be support for work that is expected within the classroom. For example, the teacher would determine the target area of the curriculum for the child in question, and the speech and language therapists or specialist teacher would support them in developing a programme which incorporated the area designated and the remediation for the particular difficulties concerned. Thus the teacher might specify mathematics as the area in question and the therapist develop ways of training specific skills related to sequencing number experiments into sentences and narratives. Alternatively the teacher might specify a concern with behaviour and the therapist might indicate that the behaviour difficulties were closely associated with the child's lack of comprehension. Intervention would then comprise modifying the teacher's spoken language levels to maximise the child's understanding of instructions by using visual re-enforcers. This is rather different from the therapeutic model which aims to modify the way the child approaches materials, to provide the child with a framework rather than provide more of what the class is already doing. It is possible that there is therapeutic involvement at this level in the school or nursery. This may take the form of the therapist working directly with the child but will be more likely to mean that the therapist will work in collaboration with the teacher.

Such interventions are monitored at regular intervals. The professionals, in collaboration with parents, make a decision as to whether further intervention is needed or whether the child can cope without further support. If more help is needed and a more nutritional model is indicated a decision has to be made as to how this can best be provided. The existing support services may not be able to provide sufficient input if long-term needs are identified. Usually this would involve the child being identified as being in need of special educational help. The child would then be closely monitored with different levels of support at different stages of the process, where necessary leading to a statement of special educational need, committing the educational authority to long-term support. It is increasingly recognised that while many communication difficulties may be amenable to dosage treatments, for many children there are likely to be long-term implications for the difficulties experienced.

Who provides the intervention?

At one level everyone who speaks with the child potentially modifies the child's language environment. This may be family, primary care professionals or therapists and specialist teachers. But at the point at which the child is identified as needing professional help a decision has to be made as to who should be 'doing the work'. Traditionally the locus of control rested squarely with the professional. The child was brought to the clinic or taken to school and the parents' responsibility was restricted to transporting the child to the clinic or carrying out discrete tasks to promote carry-over. The implicit understanding in such a model is that communication skills reside in the child and that these skills can be treated in isolation from the environment in which the child is developing. This model may have advantages as far as the parent is concerned in that someone else is taking responsibility for what is done and the problem is seen to be within the child. The professional may effectively collude with this because it may be more convenient for the child to be seen on their own or in a group with other children. However, there has been an increasing awareness in recent years that speech and language are not independent from the linguistic environment to which the child is exposed. The communication difficulty is not just between the ears of the individual child but between speakers. This recognition immediately suggests a change in emphasis in the way that intervention is offered. The role of the therapist shifts from one of taking responsibility for training the child to one of fostering the role of significant others – most notably parents and teachers – in that child's environment to do so. Effects are more likely to be both sustained and generalised if the communication environment around the child can be changed. This is too big a job for the child to do on his or her own. So modifying the significant others can do the job as well.

A number of studies have drawn comparisons in this way and in the review quoted above it was possible to synthesise the results accordingly (*see* Table 7.2).

These findings suggest that there is a differential effect of direct or indirect models of intervention according to the difficulties experienced by the child. The data suggest that the child with an articulation or phonological difficulty would, at face value, be better provided for using a direct model of service delivery, whereas the indirect model appears to be rather more effective than the direct model for intervening to promote expressive and receptive language skills. Thus the average effect size for articulation across all studies is $+0.35$ but the equivalent figures for direct and

Table 7.2 Summary of effect sizes by language area and by direct/indirect treatment

	N	Direct	N	Indirect
		Norm-referenced measures (and 95% confidence intervals)		
Articulation/phonology	2	+1.11* (+0.46/+1.77)	2	+0.20 (−0.44/+0.83)
Expressive	5	+0.65* (+0.23/+1.10)	9	+1.08* (+0.83/+1.34)
Receptive	2	−0.02 (−0.66/+0.63)	5	+1.43* (+1.09/+1.77)

N refers to the number of studies which contributed an effect size.
*Indicates statistically significant results; $p < 0.05$.

indirect intervention are $+1.11$ and $+0.20$ respectively. This suggests that in terms of articulation, direct intervention is much more promising. Of course, care needs to be taken in not overextrapolating from such data, especially given the relatively small number of studies involved.

The indirect interventions discussed above refer to the work being carried out by parents. Care has to be taken not to assume that all parents are equally willing to take on the responsibility for supporting their children's communication skills in this way. One of the immediately appealing aspects of the indirect model is that it should be cheaper as far as those providing health or educational services are concerned. There is the cost of the initial training but if the parent then continues with the same activities at other times, the skills will continue to be taught but not by the therapist. But, of course, this means that it is correspondingly more expensive for the parent who has to give time to the intervention. Because this is not a cost covered by the health service it may prove an attractive option for health managers. It seems likely that placing demands of this nature on parents may be ideal for those who are highly motivated to learn how to optimise their child's communication skills. It is less clear whether it would be universally applicable. Some parents may feel that they are not able to take on this additional responsibility and this may indeed result in non-compliance and in children being referred back to the services if the intervention proves not to be successful.

Parents are not the only intermediaries. Indeed for the older child it is far more likely that the teacher will play a central role. For example, the teacher might identify the needs of a child and request assistance. The speech and language therapist might then visit the school and discuss the child with the teacher and the special needs co-ordinator in the school. The result might be a programme of intervention which is administered by the class teacher and his or her assistant and which is then monitored every half-term by the speech and language therapist. Indeed this consultative pattern is one adopted by many services offering support to schools. However, it is unclear how well it works overall. There are no intervention studies that examine the role of the therapist and teacher in helping the child's communication skills in this way. This is not to say that it could not be as effective, simply that at this stage we do not know what that effect is nor how consistent it could be. In practice, much of the support work for children with communication difficulties comes from within the school setting.

The direct/didactic approach

This takes as its starting point the training of specific communication skills in the child. The child's performance is assessed and specific communication behaviours targeted. For example, it might be established that the child of four is still not combining words. The target might be to increase the overall vocabulary by 20 words and to introduce the use of verbs as a way of triggering the child's use of syntax. The vocabulary would be identified and the child exposed to a variety of stimuli associated with those words. He or she might be required to repeat the words in the first instance in conjunction with the stimuli and alongside a model presented by an adult. The stimuli and the modelling would gradually be withdrawn and the child's production of the target words monitored within the clinical context and extended into the context of the home and the classroom to identify whether generalisation had occurred.

Strictly behavioural methods are more commonly applied to the communication difficulties of children with more general learning difficulties. Results suggest that there is a range of positive effects, with changes occurring more commonly with the way the child uses a particular grammatical construction than in the dramatic increase in tested language performance.[13] In some cases outcomes have focused on reducing inappropriate linguistic behaviours, most notably echolalia, rather than specifically training the acquisition of new language skills. Promising results have been shown using sustained intensive interventions with autistic children[14] (see Chapter 11). These studies have received considerable critical attention but the results remain impressive for both the relatively crude language outcomes used and for educational placement. However, more didactic behaviour modification techniques have also been used to some effect with children with primary speech and language delays and those with stammers.[15,16]

The indirect/interactionist approach

In practice, many educationalists and speech and language practitioners use behaviour modification techniques routinely in their work but do not adhere to strict behavioural procedures in the sense of introducing specific vocabulary items in a controlled fashion through imitation and modelling. Rather they take a view that the most important factor for the child and the parent is that interaction is meaningful. Where communication breaks down it is often because the parent and the child cannot find a way of communication in a satisfactory and reinforcing way. The child finds the process difficult and the parent cannot identify and respond to communication attempts effectively. This can lead to a stalemate between carer and child where they function together 'in parallel'.[17] This need not be due to a conscious withdrawal, but the cumulative effect of not interacting effectively may be fewer and fewer attempts at communication on the part of both parties. The result is a very limited set of communication strategies which can discourage the child from making effective use of other communication partners, teachers, nursery staff, other family members and the like. The other side to this coin is the well-substantiated evidence that children who do have these communication strategies are best suited to taking advantage of the educational environment.

The emphasis in the interactionist approach then shifts from changing the child's specific skills to optimising the opportunities for communication. And the targets shift from performance within the setting of a specific communication environment such as a clinic to performance wherever the child communicates. Sometimes such interventions are described as 'ecological' in the sense that they aim to modify the child's whole environment not just target specific language skills. There are many such programmes available. One of the most clearly described and the one which is most widely used is the Hanen Early Language Parent Programme.[18] In the first instance practitioners have to be explicitly trained in the rationale and techniques associated with the approach. They then have to abide by explicit rules as to how the approach should be delivered to ensure integrity of the programme. Distinctive characteristics of the programme are the emphasis on teaching the parent to 'Observe, Wait and Listen' and to follow what they term the three As: Allow your child to lead, Adapt to meet the needs of the child and Add language at a level appropriate for the child. This approach is normally seen as 'naturalistic' in the sense that it reflects what normally happens when children learn language. This may seem slightly misconceived because it is clear that whatever normally happens when children learn language has not been sufficient for the child in question. In fact, such approaches probably make the link between the environment and the communication used that much more explicit than parents routinely do when they talk with their children and it is this level of explicitness that makes the difference. They also provide parents with specific practical techniques for getting back into the interaction.

The interactionist approach can be used in more formal educational settings such as classrooms but, more commonly, the targets in such settings are bound by curriculum and the teaching tends to be correspondingly formal. Consequently the carer and all other adults in the child's immediate environment will play a central role in the intervention, particularly with the younger child. Groups are set up and parents encouraged to attend. In some cases the children are involved. In others it is made clear from the start that the focus of the intervention is the promotion of the parents' communication skills. Indeed the extension of such interactionist approaches is the improvement of the overall communication environment for all children, not just that of the child with an 'identifiable' problem. Thus parents may modify the way they speak to other children in the same family once they have been involved in such a programme.

Which is most effective – the behavioural approach or the interactionist approach?

It would seem that the more naturalistic approach best reflects the way children normally learn language and should be more effective as a means of promoting speech and language. However, it is not possible to make this call at this stage simply because the evidence is not there. There have been some attempts to establish whether more formal didactic measures are more effective than interactive approaches for children with and without developmental delays. Some authors have argued that children with developmental delays respond more effectively to the interactionist approach. Others have suggested the reverse. There has also been some discussion as to whether more didactic approaches have a differential effect on the response of the child to training for specific types of syntactic skills. The results suggest that more didactic methods may be more effective for syntactic forms which do not require a context, such as gerunds (swimming, walking), whereas naturalistic techniques may be more useful for syntactic forms which are context bound, such as passives. Thus it is necessary to know the context to interpret fully 'it was hit', i.e. who hit what? It has also been suggested that didactic methods may be more useful for first introducing a communication skill but that naturalistic methods are more useful for ensuring that the skills are generalised.[19]

In the final analysis the choice between the more formal behavioural techniques and the more context-sensitive interactionist techniques may reflect a difference in learning styles in the children themselves. Any effective intervention will incorporate aspects of both of these approaches. Over the years this is indeed what has happened. There has now been extensive examination of the effectiveness of what in the USA is known as 'milieu teaching'. The characteristics of this technique are:

- teaching occurs following the child's lead or interest
- multiple, naturally occurring examples are used to teach simple, elaborated language forms
- child production of language is explicitly prompted
- to varying extents, the teaching episode is embedded in ongoing interactions between the milieu teacher and the student
- naturalistic techniques are often supplemented by adult-directed techniques such as 'mand modelling' and 'time delay', and child-directed techniques such as 'incidental learning'.

The same tendency to combine the two general approaches has been observed in modifications proposed to the Hanen Programme described above. Initial evidence suggested that this primarily interactionist technique was more effective in changing the parents' interaction skills than in increasing the child's language skills. This may have been appropriate for the more obviously handicapped children, but for children who had some language but remained very delayed modifications were clearly necessary. The resulting changes included what has become known as the 'focused stimulation' approach. As before, the interaction skills were emphasised but more specific linguistic targets were added to the intervention package. Again the results showed that this identification of specific linguistic targets had a dramatic effect on language outcomes for the children concerned.[20]

The timing of intervention

Many of the decisions regarding intervention depend on the stage of the child's development at which they are referred. Some would argue that the earlier the children can be identified the better, on the grounds that more can be done in the first two or three years than can be done when the child is entering secondary school. The concept of sensitive periods, and in particular the idea that if you do not provide intervention at a specific (early) point in the child's development the window of opportunity will close and there is little more that can be done, is one which is extremely complex. At one level it is clearly advantageous to all concerned to provide intervention at an early stage such that the child no longer has need of supporting services in the years to come.

However, it is important that the process of identifying such children needs to be clearly defined and accurate. If too low an age threshold is set, it is likely that more children will be referred than need to be with a resulting increase in over-referrals. These are clearly expensive for the services to which they are referred but there may also be a psychological cost to the individual. We know from other screening programmes that false positives have costs in terms of increased anxiety. This is one effect, but there is also the potential risk of lowered expectations resulting from inappropriate identification. On the other side of the equation there may be costs of not referring children whose parents construe that the child has a difficulty. There is likely to be anxiety associated with the frustration of trying to have something done in the face of inappropriate reassurance from professionals.

The economics of intervention

There are many social and moral reasons for providing intervention to children with communication difficulties because they are at risk of poor outcomes and because intervention can be effective. However, as with any intervention the issue of the costs relative to the benefits needs to be considered. The study of economic evaluation in this area is still in its infancy. The costs of time and space are relatively easy to assess but this is not sufficient to address this question. There needs to be a measurement of whether the costs outweigh the benefits to the individual, to the families and ultimately to the services which may subsequently be needed for those children. Only two studies have examined economic issues in this level of detail.[21,22] The first of these compared home-based, parent-delivered intervention with centre-based intervention, with a combination of the two and with a no-treatment control group. Costs included those for staff, facilities and transport, and also parent time. The results suggested not only that the home-based programme was more effective but also that it was considerably cheaper – in the region of half the price. The second of these two studies addressed the same issue and concluded that the outcome was equivalent rather than distinctly weighted in favour of the home-based intervention. The interpretation of these findings depends on how parental time is interpreted. If parents are willing to put in the time, the home-based programme is likely to be more efficient. But it is important to recognise that in both these studies the mothers did not work outside the home and were well-educated.

Long-term outcomes

Finally, it is desirable that the long-term implications of intervention are monitored. The best documented long-term follow-up studies of intervention come from the large-scale HeadStart and HomeStart programmes which have been offered in the USA since the 1960s as a result of government policy aimed at reducing social deprivation. Initial interpretation was clouded by problems of design but in recent years a much clearer picture has emerged of long-term effects of early intervention programmes in terms of socially significant outcomes, such as a reduction in the number of those imprisoned, reduced teenage pregnancy, etc. Although speech and language are likely to have been contributory factors in the early development of such children, this sort of measure is rarely used in the later assessment of such children. Evidence which would provide a sound test of the extent to which one or other model of speech or language intervention had been effective would include reduction in the prevalence of literacy problems, reduced difficulties in socialisation, etc.

The long-term outcomes of interventions devised for children with general or specific communication difficulties have yet to be properly evaluated. There has been a range of prospective studies of children who have been through specialist 'language unit' provision, but they do not generally provide enough control to influence clinical judgement at a case management level. Long-term outcomes are discussed in greater detail in Chapter 8. In general the evidence suggests that children who have difficulties that extend into the early school years are likely to be in need of support for a substantial part of their school careers and may go on to be vulnerable young adults.[23] There is also evidence from retrospective studies that young adults with histories of communication difficulties are disproportionately represented in prison populations. This presents something of a dilemma. On the one hand intervention appears to be effective, at least in short-term circumscribed studies. On the other hand these effects do not appear to be translated into long-term effects. Such a conclusion would be premature at this stage. In fact, the children who go on to have poor outcomes are often those with the greatest levels of impairment in the first instance. It is unclear whether the ones who benefit from the intervention would be the same ones who attend specialist intensive help later on. It seems more likely that there is a group with severe problems who would not obviously stand to gain from dosage intervention in the same way as a group who had a much more uncertain outcome, for whom intervention may prove critical.

Summary

- There is now a reasonable body of evidence to suggest that intervention for communication difficulties can be effective. It is possible that speech and language difficulties, particularly for children with primary difficulties, may be more amenable to modification than other areas of developmental skill and more amenable to change than the same type of difficulties occurring in children with secondary communication difficulties.
- To date most interventions have focused on changing the child's communication behaviours rather than altering the environment in which the child communicates.
- This does not mean that all intervention works everywhere. It will always depend on the abilities of the therapist and teacher, on the difficulties experienced by the child, on the extent to which parents choose to be involved and on the extent to which the programme of intervention mirrors those that have been evaluated. There is also the problem of extrapolating from studies to clinical practice – the relation between efficacy and effectiveness. Intervention studies often down-play the role of crucial features of the clinical intervention which are not captured by outcome measures. For example, the role of parental counselling is rarely mentioned in the intervention studies but this will be a feature of most interactions between parent and therapist or teacher.
- The issue of the long-term implications has yet to be addressed. Progress has been shown in the early years (up to five years). This period has been the focus of intervention studies to date. The long-term evidence of children with more entrenched difficulties suggests that secondary prevention may be less likely and that interventions will be more focused on tertiary prevention – preventing associated difficulties – than normalisation.
- Interventions are likely to be sensitive to the interactions between child characteristics, the context and the skills of the therapist/teacher. This introduces a level of

variability which make research in this area difficult.

- The cost implications have yet to be fully explored but there is preliminary evidence of differential effects for different types of intervention.
- The intervention evidence allows us to conclude that there is a good case for identifying children who are at risk for speech and language delays. These difficulties can prove problematic in their own right. They can lead to a wide range of associated difficulties in school, whether in the acquisition of literacy skills, in socialisation or self-esteem and because it is possible to do something about them.
- Appropriate information needs to be made available to parents to allow them to make reasonable decisions about their child's language skills and whether intervention is likely to be beneficial. This should include evidence about the potential effects of intervention.
- However, there remain many gaps in the literature, most notably in terms of long-term outcomes. Absence of documented evidence is not the same as negative evidence.

References

1 Enderby P and Emerson J (eds) (1995) *Does Speech and Language Therapy Work?* Whurr, London.

2 McClean LK and Woods Cripe JW (1997) The effectiveness of early intervention for children with communication disorders. In: MJ Guralnick (ed) *The Effectiveness of Early Intervention*. Paul H Brookes, Baltimore.

3 Law J (1997) Evaluating early intervention for language impaired children: a review of the literature. *European Journal of Disorders of Communication* **32**: 1–14.

4 Nye C, Foster S and Seaman D (1987) Effectiveness of language intervention with language/learning disabled. *Journal of Speech and Hearing Disorders* **52**: 348–57.

5 Law J, Boyle J, Harris F and Harkness A (1998) Child Health Surveillance: screening for speech and language delay. *Health Technology Assessment* **2**(9).

6 Farran DC (1990) Effects of intervention with disadvantaged and disabled children: a decade review. In: SJ Meisels, JP Shonkoff (eds) *Handbook of Early Childhood Intervention*. Cambridge University Press, Cambridge

7 White K and Casto G (1985) An integrative review of early intervention efficacy studies with at-risk children: implications for the handicapped. *Analysis and Intervention in Developmental Disabilities* **5**: 7–31.

8 Fraser H (1998) *Early Intervention: key issues from research*. The Scottish Office Education and Industry Department, Edinburgh.

9 Shonkoff JP and Hauser-Cram P (1987) Early intervention for disabled infants and their families: a quantitative analysis. *Pediatrics* **80**(5): 650–8.

10 Casto G and Mastropieri MA (1986) The efficacy of early intervention programs: a meta-analysis. *Exceptional Children* **52**: 417–24.

11 Arnold KS, Myette BM and Casto G (1986) Relationships of language intervention efficacy to certain subject characteristics in mentally retarded pre-school children: a meta-analysis. *Education and Training of the Mentally Retarded*. June: 108–16.

12 Ward S (1994) Validation of a treatment method. 2nd Conference of the Comite Permanente de Liaison des Othophonistes-Logopedes del'UE [CPLOL], Antwerp.

13 Howlin P (1987) Behavioural approaches to language. In: M Rutter, W Yule (eds) *Language Development and Disorders*. MacKeith Press, Oxford.

14 Lovaas OI (1987) Behavioural treatment and normal educational and intellectual functioning in young autistic children. *Journal of Counselling and Clinical Psychology* **55**(1): 3–9.

15 Connell PJ (1987) An effect of modeling and imitation teaching procedures on children with and without specific language impairment. *Journal of Speech and Hearing Research* **30**(1): 105–13.

16 Conture EG (1996) Treatment efficacy: stuttering. *Journal of Speech and Hearing Research* **39**: 518–26.

17 Wulbert M, Inglis S, Kriegsman C and Mills B (1975) Language delay and associated mother–child interaction. *Developmental Psychology* **11**, 61–70.

18 Manolsen HA (1992) *It Takes Two to Talk*. Hanen Centre Publications, Toronto.

19 Camarata SM and Nelson KE (1992) Treatment efficiency as a function of target selection in the remediation of child language disorders. *Clinical Linguistics and Phonetics* **6**(3): 167–78.

20 Girolametto L, Pearce PS and Weitzman E (1996) Interactive focused stimulation for toddlers with expressive vocabulary delays. *Journal of Speech and Hearing Research* **39**(6): 1274–83.

21 Barnett WS, Escobar CM and Ravsten MT (1988) Parent and clinic early intervention for children with language handicaps: a cost-effectiveness analysis. *Journal of the Division of Early Childhood* **12**: 290–8.

22 Eiserman WD, McCoun M and Escobar CM (1990) A costs effectiveness analysis of two alternative program models for serving speech-disordered pre-schoolers. *Journal of Early Intervention* **14**: 297–317.

23 Haynes C and Naidoo S (1991) *Children with Specific Speech and Language Impairment*. Blackwell Scientific, Oxford.

CHAPTER 8

The outcome of speech and language impairment

Corinne Haynes

Much of this book has focused on the concepts of identification, description and treatment of communication difficulties and, given our state of knowledge about the subject, this is as it should be. Yet many of the resulting decisions rest on our knowledge of the natural history of the communication disorders themselves. What happens to these children once they come into contact with health and educational services? What sort of outcomes can be anticipated? After all, if the outcomes are good if a child has received little or no intervention, is intervention warranted at all?

However, the concept of natural history assumes that these children do not receive any special help, that they are somehow exposed to education in a way that children without such difficulties experience it. This makes little sense because these children affect the services to which they are exposed from the moment they come into contact with them and this relationship is reciprocal. We are then faced with something of a dilemma when attempting to evaluate therapeutic outcomes. If natural history includes whatever intervention the children would naturally be exposed to, it will prove very difficult to disentangle specific effects of different therapies.

Notwithstanding these difficulties a number of attempts have been made to examine the outcomes for these children. The earliest studies followed up children who attended specialist educational facilities,[1] but more recently attempts have been made to examine clinical populations who may not have received such extensive specialist provision[2–5] or in normal populations.[6,7] The extent to which children continue to be affected in school and beyond depends on the severity of their difficulties at outset. The more severely affected are likely to have a worse prognosis, although a significant proportion of children with language scores below, for example the fifth centile, go on to be at risk for associated educational, social and behavioural problems even if the language difficulties may have receded somewhat. In general, IQ, level of co-morbidity and the range of linguistic domains affected provide the most effective predictors.

There is a difference too, depending on the period over which outcomes are measured. The shorter the time-frame the more specific the predictors can be but the impact of many of these predictors may wash out over time. While these shorter-term gains may be clinically interesting and may indeed help the children concerned to get a sound overall picture, it is necessary to follow up children over their entire childhood and to cover areas of development beyond those confined to linguistic skills. This chapter looks in detail at the outcome for the group of children with primary or specific speech and language disorders, that is children for whom the communication handicap does not emerge secondary to some other cause, such as hearing impairment or physical disability. This population (primary or specific speech and language disorder) provides insight into outcomes without the wide range of additional associated problems experienced by children with less specific difficulties. That is not to say that the difficulties many of them experience are confined to language development, merely that we are seeing development here with less interference than we might in broader conditions such as autism (Chapter 11) or cerebral palsy (Chapter 14). However, although there may be condition-specific implications for disabilities with readily recognisable causes, such as cranio-facial abnormalities (Chapter 15) or traumatic brain injury (Chapter 23), there will be factors inherent in impaired communication skills which affect educational and social outcomes.

The study

The specific outcomes described are taken from a study of 156 children diagnosed as having a specific language impairment (SLI) attending a special school for language impaired children between 1974 and 1987.[8] In that study, possible causative or associated factors – birth history, familial factors, middle-ear problems, social environment, motor development, auditory processing, cognitive ability and neurological correlates – were extracted from the school records and these were compared for nine subgroups of SLI children. The subgroups of this nominally homogeneous group of children were based on the degree and balance of their disabilities in the three linguistic areas of comprehension, expression and speech. The final achievements (at school-leaving age 13) were considered in the light of the factors listed above, and the nature of their language profile. An additional follow-up study of 34 ex-pupils who had reached the age of 18–22 years was included to allow some consideration of their continuing language status and also of the effects of early language handicap on career and social life.

Outcomes will be considered under three headings:

- language and communication
- education and career
- personal and social skills.

In each section the problems will be briefly outlined with an indication of the changes that can be expected with appropriate intervention. Finally the outcomes for a subsample of the children are reported when they became young adults.

In the majority of cases language disabilities reflect a brain organisation which does not favour the development of good linguistic function. Brain organisation does not greatly change in non-traumatic conditions and children with very poor language skills generally become adults with very poor language skills. The difference between the skills of children and adults is one of degree and style. Clinicians and teachers who seek to help language-impaired children are essentially seeking to reinforce useful strengths, to compensate for weaknesses, to find useful alternative processes and to instil feelings of confidence and self-esteem in the child as a whole.

Complete eradication or 'cure' of severe SLI is no longer recognised as a meaningful concept. The good outcome that is the goal of intervention is the development of an aware and self-appreciative adult, able to communicate with and relate to others, able to minimise the adverse effect of language impairment as the result of therapy, education and the acquisition of well-practised strategy, and able to pursue realistic goals in career and social life through a knowledge of his/her strengths and weaknesses.

Language and communication

A number of specific aspects of communication were measured throughout the children's career in the school. Each is reported in turn.

Auditory processing

Auditory processing encompasses auditory discrimination of speech (ADS) – the ability to differentiate between minimal essential differences in speech sounds – and auditory short-term memory (ASTM) – the capacity to retain phonologically based material in a primary store while processing takes place. Poor auditory processing is found in the majority of SLI children and this pattern was repeated in the population discussed here; a marked difficulty in speech discrimination was found in 62% of the children and 75% had limited auditory sequential memory.

Comprehension

Objective test results do not support the view frequently expressed by the parents of SLI children that comprehension is intact. Two-thirds of children, including those referred with expressive language or speech problems, were found to have significant problems in the area of comprehension of both vocabulary and language structure. The parental belief may be an indicator of the unconscious accommodations made by parents to their child's linguistic abilities.

Expressive language

This is the classic area of difficulty in children with communication disorders very few of whom, even with a known primary cause not related to language production *per se*, have an expressive language level comparable with unimpaired peers.

Speech

Deficits of speech production are more discrete than other language areas, inasmuch as a child can have impaired comprehension or expressive language but a normal phonological system. Rarer are children with impaired speech and no other language problems, since the opportunities for using and developing good language skills are reduced when there is a bar to intelligibility. Over 95% of the SLI children in the study had phonological problems varying from a slightly immature system to complete lack of intelligibility.

What changes can be made?

Changes in auditory processing

The nature of the relationship between improved auditory discrimination and improved speech and reading is unclear. Children can have good speech and poor discrimination and vice versa. Learning to discriminate speech sounds is an inherent part of most programmes to improve speaking and reading undertaken by therapists and teachers. But it has been suggested that improved speech discrimination is secondary to improved speech production or they may improve *pari passu*.[9] Children in the study all took part in programmes to improve their discrimination skills and as a group they made significant gains in test scores[10] and also made gains in speaking and reading, but there was no evidence of causal correlation in either direction, and improvements in some children occurred in one area and not another. The conclusion reached in the present study was that it is hard to justify spending valuable time on programmes aimed at the general stimulation of speech discrimination and ADS, but the available evidence supports training which is specifically geared to those sound contrasts which are the current focus of therapy or teaching. There is no such justification for training in the area of auditory short-term memory, a point argued by Rees nearly 30 years ago but still ignored by some teachers and therapists who, being appalled at the deficiencies of SLI children in this area, feel they must intervene.[11] Limited ASTM is strongly associated with impaired speech and language. The poorest ASTM is associated with the greatest degree of language impairment and reading difficulty, and was found to be a highly significant predictor of outcome in the Haynes and Naidoo study.[8] This same study also found that trained or untrained, there was very little change in ASTM but actually a deterioration if compared with normal age levels. Instead of attempting to train something that is merely an indicator of one aspect of linguistic function, time can be better spent teaching coping strategies (such as use of visual imagery), awareness of the problem and the confidence to ask for necessary repetition.

Changes in receptive language

Vocabulary gains are very slow for SLI children, who continue to have difficulties of phonological analysis and who are almost invariably poor readers. Thus the vocabulary age gap grows compared to normal peers. However, the important fact is that vocabulary continues to increase and reaches a level which, although poor for age, is adequate for most practical purposes. Two-thirds of the 13-year-old school leavers in the study were found to have adequate (i.e. better than −1 standard deviation on testing) comprehension of vocabulary. Comprehension of grammatical structure responds well to intervention. Most SLI children will have been swamped at the normal language acquisition age by the need to decode the rules of grammar while having to cope with unknown vocabulary, too fast a rate of input and the semantic and psychological demands of the situation. Teachers and therapists who can structure a classroom interaction so that the context is known to the child but the target grammatical rule is new, and who can provide activities and visual aids to support comprehension of the situation, are able to effect reasonable, if slow, progress in their charges. Seventy-nine percent of the study children were felt to have adequate comprehension (better than −1 standard deviation on testing) at age 13.

Changes in expressive language

Similar strictures affect the improvement in expressive language as those affecting the understanding of language. Phonological difficulties in analysis and synthesis make the production of new words slow, but vocabulary reaches a level of functional adequacy. Grammatical structure can be acquired, again to a level of day-to-day adequacy, when the learning load is consciously reduced. Around 95% of study children reached a good functional level. Although they will never shine as orators in the cut and thrust of debate, SLI children will be able to communicate effectively if they are well taught. Tests did not exist at the time of the study to assess the more subtle skills of expressive language – persuasion, humour, reasoned argument, etc. It is highly likely that such skills remain poorly developed for many.

Speech

In the absence of physical causes, the prognosis for speech improvement *per se* is good. There is indubitably a degree of improvement that occurs with maturation, and good improvement can be expected with appropriate therapy for deviant as well as delayed speech. The effects of a dysfunctional phonological system on reading and spelling are longer lasting and cogent reasons in themselves for beginning therapy for speech difficulties as early as possible. Of the 95% of children entering the study between the ages of 5;2 and 12;11 with poor intelligibility, 38% of leavers between the ages of 6;10 and 13;10 after a mean stay of three years nine months, still had problems. Of these 15% were considered disabling. Many of those children who scored well on final testing still had some problems with polysyllabic words and it is interesting that this problem is one which featured in the awareness of their own difficulties reported by 20-year-olds (*see below*).

Education and career

Those who support special segregated education for SLI children point out that the pervasive nature of this condition makes it very difficult for such children to excel or even to hold their own in any educational area. Academic subjects rely increasingly over the school age range upon a good vocabulary and understanding of language, in conjunction with the ability to read. For most, but not all SLI children, difficulties with mathematics are legion.[12] Poor motor co-ordination also renders achievements on the playing field hard to attain and can affect pencil control, drawing ability and skill in using tools. Auditory sequential memory problems are closely associated with the attention deficits commonly experienced by these children and necessarily make the retention of instructions difficult.

The best attainments, and occasionally very good attainments, are made in science subjects but difficulties with symbolism, vocabulary and sequential reasoning adversely affect most pupils in this area. It is hardly necessary to point out the difficulties that will be experienced with second languages for pupils still not in control of a first. In every class and in every subject these children are likely to compare poorly with normal peers. Add to this an emotional immaturity and an inability to appreciate schoolchild humour (based often on puns) and an increasing spiral of failure can safely be predicted in comparison with a non-impaired group.

What changes can be made?

The normal precepts of good education – making topics meaningful and relevant, instilling an active desire to learn rather than be taught passively, proceeding at a pace appropriate to the child with change of subject when appropriate, giving choice and encouraging participation – all apply, rather more so, to language-impaired children. Since progress must be slow and hard won, the allocation of time must be well-planned. Success can be produced by changing and slowing the pace, paying attention to teacher language, using graded motor programmes, and always supporting the weak aural–oral channel with visual and tactile aids. It is important to set realistic goals and achieve them, rather than aiming too high and failing. This does not mean that there should be a general lowering of expectations and ready acceptance of less than the child can achieve, but that educational programmes should be founded in a real understanding of the child's abilities and disabilities.

Even when attention is paid to all these things, and class sizes are reduced, problems will remain, in particular problems with reading and spelling may continue into adult life.

Changes in reading ability

These are reported, since the data are available, not because this is the only or necessarily the major area of educational handicap. Around 90% of the study children entering school were non-readers or retarded readers on a test of word-recognition which did not require a spoken response. Most of the non-readers were aged five or six years, but among the seven-year-olds only 3–4% could read at age level. Observation of children without speech and language difficulties as they read suggests that, at around a reading age of seven years, an incipient ability to work from letters to sounds, the beginnings of phonological awareness, emerges. Around 60% of seven-year-olds in the study had not reached this stage. A comparison with other language skills found that reading ability was more significantly related to a low level of expressive language structure, expressive vocabulary and auditory sequential memory than to limited comprehension, poor speech or weak auditory discrimination. The ability gap between normal and poor readers, in mainstream as well as special education, is likely to increase with time.[13] This was generally true of the study children, although a few did reach a reading ability commensurate with their age. The reading skills of all children improved while at school, but relative to peers without speech and language difficulties their skills were falling further behind. Most had severe difficulties and 77% left the special school with a reading age more than two years behind chronological age and considerable ongoing problems both in word-recognition and reading for meaning, in spite of the intensive and specialised help they had received. Final reading ability correlated with measures of comprehension of spoken language as well as with expressive ability.

Personal and social skills

Behaviour problems and disorders have been shown in many studies to occur more frequently than expected in children with speech and language disorders.[14] It has been suggested that in the population under discussion, the behaviour problems stem directly or indirectly from the language difficulties themselves[15] and it is easy to understand the confusion, frustration and humiliation experienced by SLI children which may cause or exacerbate problems such as poor peer relationships, solitariness, uncontrolled temper, aggression, anxiety, inhibition and emotional lability. When language cannot be used effectively to mediate these feelings and consequently to deal with the resulting behaviours – by the child needing either to follow an explanation or express his or her own feelings – then the situation may easily deteriorate.

The group of children studied exhibited, in order of frequency, the following behaviours after entry to the special school: lack of confidence, easily evoked distress, poor attention, poor peer relationships, aggression, frustration and solitariness. These are descriptive terms applied to the behaviour of the children and do not necessarily constitute clinical levels of behavioural difficulty (see Chapter 12). They are derived from staff and parental reports and not from an objective measure. Some children attended the school as boarders and others as day pupils. Behaviours in these two groups were found to be the same, with the exception of better peer relationships and better attention among the boarders, possibly supporting the suggestion of Siegel et al.[16] that playmates of a similar age and communication level aid the development of peer relationships. Children with problems of comprehension were, unsurprisingly, more likely to be solitary.

What changes can be made?

At the time discussed in the study there was no focused management of particular behaviours in the school, although individual children with a particularly severe difficulty could receive help from the school's educational psychologist. Some support was offered to develop social skills and there was a generally caring environment with small class and residential groups, and therapists, teachers and care workers who were always ready to listen and were skilled in communicating by whatever system the child found most accessible, including a manual sign system.

School leaving age at this period was 13, the beginning of the adolescent years, which are often marked by an increase in emotional upheaval and disturbed behaviours. The study children were facing an additional hurdle in the need to change school. Behaviours of the leavers were again measured by subjective report and so cannot be directly compared with behaviour at school entry, but some general observations can be made. Aggression had reduced and was a continuing problem for only a few pupils. Most had formed satisfactory peer relationships. Poor attention was a problem for about 25% as opposed to 50% at entry. However, in this final year, lack of confidence and poor coping strategies – including being easily upset and an ongoing need for adult approval – were common, affecting about 75% of the pupils.

The outcome for this group of children with severe language impairment who were given intensive speech and language therapy and special education for one to seven years can be summarised as:

- Communication: comprehension and expression of language both improved, normally to a level considered adequate for functional purposes and accepted as unproblematic by many interlocuters. However, problems did remain which were more covert but would almost certainly adversely affect education and career prospects, and social life. In most cases speech was intelligible but the range of speech ability varied from complete lack of intelligibility to faultless pronunciation.
- Education: some children were able to cope in mainstream education (62% of the study children) but almost all continued to have marked educational problems, particularly in the areas of language, reading and spelling.
- Social: most children learned to cope with feelings of anger and aggression, and had some skills in making friends. Friends were sometimes younger or disadvantaged in a different way – therefore perhaps less threatening – and sometimes older and protective. Generally these relationships were fragile. Self-image was generally poor. This was more likely to be related to educational failure than to communication failure.

Young adults

To assess the effects of language impairment in the longer term, telephone interviews were conducted with 34 young people between the ages of 18 and 22 who had been subjects in the study, and/or their parents. The decision as to who was to be interviewed was taken by the families concerned. For the majority of young men and women, language impairment continued to affect their lives in some way, but the extent of the ongoing effect varied considerably.

Language and communication in adults

Only three of the 34 considered there were no residual language problems and the interviewers – the special school headmistress, who was an educational psychologist, and the author, a speech and language therapist – had doubts about the accuracy of this report in two cases. Problems with written language are included in this count. The breakdown of reported residual problems is shown in Table 8.1. Many of the problems described seemed trivial – problems using polysyllabic words, following films or using the telephone – but these were not necessarily minor problems for the young people experiencing them. The interviewers were sometimes aware of more communication problems than were being reported, and other studies have indicated that communicatively handicapped young people are likely to play down the extent of their disability.[3]

Table 8.1 Residual language problems reported by 34 young adults

Problem	Number
Comprehension	14(16)*
Expressive language	19
Speech	22(24)*
Reading	12(13)*
Writing	17
Spelling	21

*Numbers in brackets indicate differing reports from subjects (first figure) and parents.

Difficulty with written language remained but was considered more of a problem by parents than by the young people who, to a certain extent, could choose to ignore it. Although reading difficulties were reported as a problem by only 14, only four listed reading as a hobby, and in all four cases the reading was of hobby magazines not books or newspapers.

Education and career

There was a very wide span of educational attainments between the ages of 13 and 18. Thirteen pupils leaving their final school took no externally moderated examinations. Twenty-one pupils passed between one and seven subjects in the Certificate of Secondary Education (CSE). Five pupils passed between one and 12 subjects in the General Certificate of Education. The three advanced level pupils all went on to university, where they graduated in economics, chemistry and aeronautical engineering. These were exceptions to the rule, however, and the majority of examination subject successes were in practical subjects or the sciences.

Education was prolonged and students in tertiary education were often rather older than their group. Often the only courses available in colleges of further education were those designed for slow learners and these were disappointing to SLI students whose difficulty in communication masked a better learning potential. Some reported

Table 8.2 Educational attainments of 34 young adults in final school placement

Examinations	Number	Range
No public examinations	13	
Certificate of Secondary Education (CSE)	21	1–7
General Certificate of Education (Ordinary)	5	1–12
General Certificate of Education (Advanced)	3	2–4

Table 8.3 Socioeconomic status of 34 young adults and their families

Groups	Families	Subjects
Top professional	4	0
Managerial	3	1
Skilled non-manual	3	2
Skilled manual	17	5
Partly skilled	6	9
Unskilled	1	8
Unemployed	0	4
(Students)	0	4
Total	34	34

the frustration they experienced when tutors and careers officers failed to understand the nature of their problems – a finding also reported by Baginsky.[17] Of the 34 young people interviewed, five were currently not working or were still students. Two had become unemployed in the previous month and were expecting to be back in work shortly. Two had only ever had intermittent casual work and one who was severely depressed had never worked. This represents a high level of employment for the period in which the study was carried out, although many of the jobs were not skilled and poorly paid (for details see ref. 8). Significantly, the jobs obtained failed to reflect the socioeconomic status of the families (Table 8.3).

Social life

The interviewers asked questions about leisure activities, friendships and outings. There was a predictably varied response but the general picture was one of continuing dependence on their families for a social life at the age (18 to 22) when most young adults are branching out on their own. The young people lived with family (29), relatives or family friends (2) or in student accommodation (3). For two-thirds, hobbies were home-based and solitary or involved only other family members, but a similar number did go out for some sort of social activity with friends at least once a week. This included groups of work mates and also family friends. Of the 26 young men and eight young women questioned, it was the young women who seemed to be finding involvement in social life easier, possibly because at that time a more passive role for women was common. Four of the eight young women had boyfriends while only three of the 26 young men had girlfriends. Few of either sex had a lively and independent social life. Parents who were interviewed expressed their greatest concerns not with career prospects or language skills, but with the lack of social activity outside the family circle. It is perhaps not surprising that late physical and emotional maturation compounded by the specific difficulty of communication handicap should at least delay social confidence and competence. However, these skills are essential for personal fulfilment and to gain more insight into the variation in achievement, early behaviours at school were compared for those pupils who achieved the greatest social success or failure.

The results of this comparison showed, predictably, that the most severely handicapped communicatively were the most unfulfilled socially, but this applied to language rather than speech handicaps. There was no social advantage or disadvantage in having been a boarder rather than living with family while attending school. When earlier behaviour patterns were considered, the one that best separated the social achievers from the non-achievers was their attitude to communication. Thus although in both groups there were people with marked problems of intelligibility, those who in their schooldays had felt positive about their ability to communicate were now coping better than those with better communication skills who had a more negative image.

Summary

- Children with communication difficulties severe enough to warrant special educational provision are likely to become adults with communication difficulties, although these vary from communicative near isolation to minor difficulties with written language or pronunciation of polysyllabic words.
- The impairments adversely affect communication, education, career and social life.
- All aspects of the handicap improve if given appropriate intervention, but language handicaps are more disabling than speech handicaps, and within language handicap, difficulties with comprehension are more pervasive than expressive problems.
- Help at an early age is essential to enable the children to cope with their difficulties and to allow them to be supported through the school system.
- Impaired communicative skills can affect social relationships, career prospects and – crucially – self-image. While specifically focused therapy for aspects of the language handicap are fruitful and essential, equal importance and time should be devoted to promoting a positive self-image as an effective communicator.

References

1   Griffiths C (1969) A following study of children with disorders of speech. *British Journal of Disorders of Communication* 4(1): 446–56.

2   Renfrew CE and Geary L (1973) Prediction of persisting speech deficit. *British Journal of Disorders of Communication* 8(1): 37–41.

3   King RR, Jones C and Lasky E (1982) In retrospect: a fifteen year follow-up report of speech-language disordered children. *Language, Speech and Hearing Services in Schools* **13**: 24–32.

4   Schery T (1985) Correlates of language development in language-disordered children. *Journal of Speech and Hearing Disorders* **50**: 73–83.

5   Stothard SE, Snowling MJ, Bishop DVM, Chipchase BB and Kaplan CA (1998) Language impaired pre-schoolers: a follow-up into adolescence. *Journal of Speech, Language and Hearing Disorders* **41**: 407–18.

6   Silva PA, Williams SM and McGee R (1987) A longitudinal study of children with developmental language delay at age three: later intelligence, reading and behaviour problems. *Developmental Medicine and Child Neurology* **29**: 630–40.

7   Drillien CM, Pickering RM and Drummond MB (1988) Predictive value of screening for different areas of development. *Developmental Medicine and Child Neurology* **30**: 294–305.

8   Haynes C and Naidoo S (1991) *Children with Speech and Language Impairment: clinics in developmental medicine No. 119.* Blackwell Scientific Publications, Oxford.

9   Prins TD (1963) Relations among specific articulatory deviations and responses to a clinical measure of sound discrimination ability. *Journal of Speech and Hearing Disorders* **18**: 382–8.

10   Wepman JM (1958) *Auditory Discrimination Test.* Language Research Associates, Chicago.

11   Rees N (1973) Auditory processing factors in language disorders: the view from Procrustes' bed. *Journal of Speech and Hearing Disorders* **38**: 304–15.

12   Grauberg E (1999) *Early Mathematics and Language Difficulties.* Whurr, London.

13   Share DL and Silva PA (1986) Classification of reading retardation. *British Journal of Educational Psychology* **56**: 32–9.

14   Butler NR and Golding J (1986) *From Birth to Five.* Pergamon Press, Oxford.

15   Baker L and Cantwell DP (1982) Language acquisition, cognitive development and emotional disorder in childhood. In: KE Nelson (ed) *Children's Language*, vol. 3. Lawrence Erlbaum, Hillsdale, NJ.

16   Siegel LS, Cunningham CE and van der Spuy HIJ (1985) Interactions of language delayed and normal preschool boys with their peers. *Journal of Child Psychology and Psychiatry* **26**: 77–83.

17   Baginsky MR (1990) *Vocational Educational Opportunities for Students with Specific Speech and Language Impairment.* NFER, Slough.

PART TWO

CHAPTER 9

Maltreated children

Maureen Sanger

Case study

Steven was four years old when he was referred for psychological evaluation due to concerns regarding his psychosocial adjustment. By his preschool teacher's report, Steven exhibited mild cognitive delay and had an articulation problem that hindered his interaction with peers. He was observed to be an anxious and fearful child, who was often aggressive, at times for no apparent reason. His behaviour, according to his mother, seemed to deteriorate following contacts with his father. A detailed social and developmental history revealed that prior to his parent's divorce, at the age of two years, Steven had been subjected to harsh physical punishment, to the point of bruising, and emotional rejection by his father. He had also witnessed multiple episodes of marital violence. At the time of his parents' separation, Steven was non-verbal and failing to thrive. In the first month following his parents' separation, Steven's appetite increased and he gained six pounds. His language also began developing rapidly. Despite these gains, Steven continued to exhibit communicative and behaviour problems, and it was evident that ongoing parental conflict continued to impede his psychological development. During the course of the evaluation, when asked to sketch a picture of his family, Steven drew his father shooting his mother with a gun and explained, 'Daddy's killing mamma cause she divorced him'.

Definitions

There are a number of categories of maltreatment. While each category may be theoretically defined in practice there is likely to be a considerable degree of overlap across categories.

- Maltreatment: an action or failure to act by a parent, caretaker or other person defined by law as a perpetrator of abuse or neglect, that resulted in death; physical, sexual, or emotional harm; or risk of harm to a child.

- Neglect: a type of maltreatment that refers to the failure to provide needed, age-appropriate care.
- Physical abuse: a type of maltreatment that refers to physical acts that cause or could have caused physical injury to a child.
- Sexual abuse: a type of maltreatment that refers to the involvement of the child in sexual activities to provide sexual gratification or financial benefit to the perpetrator, including contacts for sexual purposes: prostitution, pornography, exposure or other sexually exploitative activities.
- Psychological or emotional maltreatment: a type of maltreatment that refers to acts or omissions that cause, or could have caused conduct, cognitive, affective or other mental disorders, such as emotional neglect, psychological abuse or mental injury.

Aetiology

The level of child maltreatment is of epidemic proportions. Data compiled in annual surveys by the National Committee For Prevention of Child Abuse in the USA and by the National Society for the Prevention of Cruelty to Children in the UK have documented a gradual but steady increase in the number of reported cases of child abuse and neglect since 1985. In the USA at least there was an increase in reported cases of the order of 50% in the eight years between 1985 and 1993.[1]

A growing body of empirical research supports widespread clinical evidence that maltreatment negatively impacts on children's development across multiple domains of functioning and there is some suggestion that speech and language may be particularly sensitive to adverse environments.[2] Child abuse and neglect may result in insecure attachments, negative self-representations, difficulty regulating emotions and behaviour, impaired social development and intellectual deficits.[3] Abused and neglected children also appear to be at risk for difficulties with language and communication skills. Although epidemiological data are lacking, Taitz and King[4] reported that in a sample of 260 consecutively referred children with histories of physical abuse or neglect, 33% evidenced speech and language or other developmental delays.

It is not clear whether communication problems in children contribute to maltreatment or are a consequence of living in an environment marked by abuse or neglect. Many researchers and clinicians believe, however, that maltreatment may well play a causative role in the development of children's speech and language problems. Studies of normal child language suggest that a consistent, warm, sensitive and contingent parent–child interaction style is optimal for early communication development.[3] These are the very factors that seem to be impaired in the dysfunctional relationships between maltreated children and their caregivers. Researchers examining the social communicative environment of maltreated infants indicate that, for some, their caregiver interactions appear to be less stimulating, less active, less positive and more negative than interactions observed in non-maltreated infants.[5]

Several possible mechanisms by which maltreatment may result in speech and language difficulties have been hypothesised. Some posit that environmental stressors acting on maltreated children limit lexical learning.[6] Others believe that maltreated children may not be exposed to the variety of experiences and interactions necessary for the learning of new words and that the paucity of language stimulation contributes to the development of communication problems. Another explanation is that abused children may be afraid to risk talking and therefore suffer language delay due to restricted practice.[7]

In one of the few empirically rigorous studies to examine the relationship between child maltreatment and language problems, Allen and Oliver[8] compared performance on the Preschool Language Scale for four groups of children: abused only, neglected only, abused and neglected, and a non-maltreatment group. They found that neglected children scored significantly lower on measures of expressive and receptive language than children in the other groups. Abuse did not appear to correlate with language performance in this study. It was hypothesised that a lack of stimulation in the environment of neglected children hindered language development. Fox and colleagues[9] similarly found in their study of abused, severely neglected and generally neglected children that the severely neglected children earned the lowest scores in all three areas of language comprehension examined and that these children had significantly greater difficulties with language comprehension tasks compared to non-abused peers. These studies suggest that psychological rather than physical maltreatment could be the critical factor associated with language disability. Further research is needed to examine whether maltreatment of a certain type or severity can cause specific speech and language impairment, or whether the speech and language impairments linked to maltreatment are long-lasting.[10]

Identification

Given that child abuse and neglect is not associated with a specific pattern of speech or language impairment, nor with a unique constellation of behavioural symptoms, identifying maltreatment as a factor contributing to communication difficulties in children is difficult. However, the prevalence of child abuse and neglect warrants that maltreatment be considered whenever a child presents with speech or language concerns.[11] While the psychological and developmental effects of maltreatment vary considerably from child to child, the impact of abuse and neglect often impacts on children in many domains of functioning. Thus, assessing children's development and adaptation in areas beyond speech and language may clarify the diagnostic picture.

In the physical domain, examining children for signs of injury (e.g. dislocations, fractures, bruising and scarring) and eliciting reports of how the injuries were obtained, may identify physical maltreatment in some children. Whenever an injury is inconsistent with the history given, physical abuse should be suspected. Physical indicators of sexual abuse include complaints of pain, itching or irritation in the genital area, evidence of trauma to the anus, external genitalia or vaginal area, and presence of sexually transmitted disease. Another physical parameter to consider is the child's growth. As Skuse points out,[6] both physical growth and the development of language in children is critically dependent on the provision of appropriate attention and stimulation by a caretaker. The physical consequences of persistent neglect of preschool children, according to Skuse, often includes poor growth, not only in height and weight, but also in head circumference. The important issue here is that medical practitioners need to monitor the growth trajectory of the child not simply the birth weight.

Assessing a child's behavioural status may provide further clues as to the possibility of abuse and neglect. Children who are unusually aggressive and destructive or shy and withdrawn, who exhibit sophisticated or atypical sexual knowledge or behaviour, who demonstrate frequent and severe mood changes, who appear fearful or depressed, who exhibit sleep disturbance, who have extremely poor self-esteem or who regress from age-appropriate behaviours may be exhibiting the effects of maltreatment. As Berliner notes,[11] all of these behaviours may have alternative explanations that are not related to maltreatment, but they provide clear evidence of a disturbance that should be further assessed.

While parents may be the best and most convenient source of data regarding a child's behaviour, questioning a child's school or daycare teacher may provide further evidence of a problem. School personnel can provide information regarding the perceived extent and impact of a child's developmental and behavioural difficulties, as well as observations of the child's family relationships. Teachers who report a child to be withdrawn or listless, to relate poorly with peers, to be frequently absent or chronically tardy, or to show a consistent tendency to stay at school after the other children have been sent home, may be observing the effects of maltreatment. School reporting may well conflict with reports from the family or other sources and these inconsistencies need to be followed up. There may also be cases where parents deliberately mislead professionals by giving false accounts.

Directly observing interactions between a parent and child during the course of a paediatric visit may raise suspicion about the presence of abuse and neglect. Parents who use inappropriately harsh discipline, make disparaging remarks or fail to respond to their child's attempts to gain assistance, guidance or support may have a dysfunctional relationship with their child. Approaching parents in a non-threatening, non-accusatory manner to explore these observations and to elicit information about issues such as discipline, the extent to which they find parenting rewarding and enjoyable, their resources for child-rearing assistance and stresses in the home may provide further clues as to the status of family relationships.

While reports and observations of a child's behaviour and development may raise concerns about abuse and neglect, child maltreatment is most accurately learned about by statements from and observations of the child. Professionals need to recognise the obstacles to effective reporting experienced by children with communication difficulties. Children may, during interactions with their healthcare provider, reveal that they are being abused, or they may make spontaneous statements during physical examination that should be pursued by gentle questioning. That children offer information about their own abuse, unprompted, is often the exception rather than the rule, however. Indeed the questioning of young children with communication difficulties may be problematic because, by definition, they are less able to express themselves. In a study of children referred to a psychiatric outpatient clinic, sexual abuse was discovered in four times as many cases when children were directly asked by clinicians whether they had been molested.[12] Asking children whether their bodies have been touched in a hurtful or inappropriate way may result in substantially increased identification of child abuse. Professionals also need to be mindful of the underlying level of development required to lie or mislead when seeking to determine the accuracy of children's reporting (see Chapter 1).

Implication for service delivery

Intervening in cases of child maltreatment must occur at two levels: the level of the social system and the level of the family system. Involvement of the social services system is necessary to protect children from immediate harm and to ensure that families comply with needed rehabilitative services. In the UK, every local authority has designated responsibility under the Children Act (1994) to produce local child protection procedures in conjunction with police and health authorities. Similarly in the USA, every state has enacted a child abuse reporting law and, as in the UK, it is incumbent upon professionals working with children that they are knowledgeable and respectful of their legal and ethical duty to recognise possible abuse and to report it to the appropriate authority as the law requires. Professionals do not have to be certain that a child has been abused before making a report to their local social services department; they must only have a reasonable suspicion that child maltreatment has occurred. A report is simply a request for an investigation so that concerns can be explored and ameliorative services provided as warranted.

At the level of the family system, multimodal intervention is essential for promoting positive, long-lasting outcomes in maltreated children. One key to intervention is securing services for caregivers of abused and neglected children. These may include individual and family psychotherapy, education in child development and parenting skills, and assistance in meeting physical and social needs, such as adequate food and shelter, job assistance, childcare and social support. The importance of family-based intervention was underlined by Webster and colleagues[13] who documented unexpectedly little improvement among children with communication difficulties who had received regularly scheduled individual language tutoring to accelerate their communication skills. The factor consistently identified as contributing to the lack of improvement was the absence of familial support, and raised the obvious question

'How can children be helped when they're living in homes where they're consistently hurt, neglected, or ignored?'.

In addition to intervention with caregivers, children who have been maltreated need special services to address the social, emotional and behavioural consequences of their abuse or neglect. Individual and/or group counselling may facilitate children's psychosocial adaptation and provide a safe environment in which they can express their thoughts and feelings. Many communities have therapeutic preschool programmes for maltreated children that can address children's emotional needs in an intensive manner.

For abused and neglected children who exhibit speech and language disabilities, language intervention is required. Historically, therapeutic programmes for maltreated children have not included speech and language therapy or intensive language stimulation. Rather, they have focused on emotional issues with the assumption that when these are resolved, language will improve. However, as Blager and Martin observed,[7] these children are likely to need specific language intervention to correct the effects of abuse on their communication skills.

References

1   Lewit EM (1994) Reported child abuse and neglect. *The Future of Children* **4**(2): 233–42.

2   Law J and Conway J (1991) *Child Abuse and Neglect: the effect on communication development – a review of the literature*. Available from the Association for All Speech Impaired Children, 347 Central Markets, Smithfield, London EC1A 9NH, UK.

3   Coster W and Cicchetti D (1993) Research on the communicative development of maltreated children: clinical implications. *Topics in Language Disorders* **13**(4): 25–38.

4   Taitz LS and King JM (1988) A profile of abuse. *Archives of Disease in Childhood* **63**(9): 1026–31.

5   Katz KB (1992) Communication problems in maltreated children: a tutorial. *Journal of Childhood Communication Disorders* **14**(2): 147–63.

6   Skuse D (1992) The relationship between deprivation, physical growth and the impaired development of language. In: P Fletcher and D Hall (eds) *Specific Speech and Language Disorders in Children: correlates, characteristics, and outcomes*, pp. 29–50. Singular Publishing Group, San Diego.

7   Blager F and Martin HP (1976) Speech and language of abused children. In: HP Martin (ed) *The Abused Child: a multidisciplinary approach to developmental issues and treatment*, pp. 83–92. Ballinger, Cambridge.

8   Allen RE and Oliver JM (1982) The effects of child maltreatment on language development. *Child Abuse and Neglect* **6**: 299–305.

9   Fox L, Long SH and Langlois A (1988) Patterns of language comprehension deficit in abused and neglected children. *Journal of Speech and Hearing Disorders* **53**: 239–44.

10   McCauley RJ and Swisher L (1987) Are maltreated children at risk for speech or language impairment? An unanswered question. *Journal of Speech and Hearing Disorders* **52**: 301–3.

11   Berliner L (1993) Identifying and reporting suspected child abuse and neglect. *Topics in Language Disorders* **13**(4): 15–24.

12   Lanktree C, Briere J and Zaidi L (1991) Incidence and impact of sexual abuse in a child outpatient sample: the role of direct inquiry. *Child Abuse and Neglect* **15**: 447–53.

13   Webster L, Wood RW, Eicher C and Hoag CL (1989) A preschool language tutoring project: family support– the essential factor. *Early Childhood Research Quarterly* **4**: 217–24.

CHAPTER 10

Attention Deficit Disorder

Anna Baumgaertel

Developmental impairments, be they physical, mental or social, create increased potential for the emergence of psychiatric disturbance. As clinicians we tend to focus on specific dysfunctions and diagnoses, and frequently forget that even narrowly circumscribed problems have repercussions for the whole individual in his or her context. We also tend to think of 'psychiatric disturbance' as implying classic psychiatric diagnoses, such as major affective disorders or schizophrenia. Attention Deficit/ Hyperactivity Disorders and Oppositional/Conduct Disorders, while making up the majority of childhood psychiatric diagnoses, are often not considered psychiatric problems of the first order. This may indeed be related to problems of syndrome definition, and also to the fact that these behavioural disorders occur on a continuum of severity and co-morbidity,[1] only the most severe of which are consigned to the territory of the psychiatrist.

Language plays such a central role in human development as the dominant vehicle of communication, socialisation and cognition that it is not surprising to find that language dysfunction is highly associated with behavioural and affective disorders as well as cognitive difficulties, even though the directionalities and causalities are not as obvious as they may first appear. To illustrate, one need only imagine existing in an environment in which everyone else converses in a foreign language only poorly mastered by one's self to get a flavour of the limitations and strain placed not only on one's linguistic abilities, but also on all levels of cognitive, social and emotional functioning. On the one hand, intense mental effort is required to attend, remember, learn, conceptualise and organise. On the other hand, initiating and maintaining communication, feeling 'connected' to others, in control, competent, flexible and secure are as much emotional as linguistic challenges that will be met in a highly individualistic way depending on the context and one's previous experience as well as one's temperamental make-up.

To illustrate the complexity of the relationships that interact in language impairment, let us examine the case of JL, a young boy presenting in our clinic for developmental evaluation.

Case study

JL is a five-year five-month-old Caucasian boy with a prior diagnosis of Attention Deficit Hyperactivity Disorder (ADHD), who has been on stimulant medication for the past year, which apparently has improved his hyperactivity and impulsivity but has not had an impact on his poor attentional control or his social interactions, which are getting worse. He has been referred for evaluation because of his increasingly disruptive behaviour in his kindergarten class.

He was the full-term product of a normal pregnancy of a 21-year-old, born by normal spontaneous vaginal delivery with a weight of 8 lb 13 oz. There were no medical developmental risk factors except that his mother smoked one pack of cigarettes per day throughout the pregnancy and his father was an early-onset severe alcoholic who engaged in substance abuse. JL's medical history is otherwise unremarkable.

JL was described as an 'easy', undemanding infant, who showed normal motor but delayed language milestones. A developmental evaluation at two years revealed significant delays in communication and social development with low average cognitive abilities. He was enrolled in an early intervention programme until the age of three years, but did not meet eligibility criteria for further interventions on subsequent testing.

At three years six months increasingly hyperactive-disruptive behaviour led to the establishment of an ADHD diagnosis and initial good therapeutic response to stimulant therapy (methylphenidate). In his kindergarten placement he was described by his teacher as having a short attention span, and an inability to follow directions, to stay focused and to retain information. He was loud, overly talkative, hyperactive and frequently 'out of control'. He was very moody and experienced peer rejection because of his overbearing intensity and bossiness in his attempts at relating to them. However, his teacher also saw him as eager to please, compliant and affectionate.

JL's family history was significant for 'slowness' of his father and maternal half-brother as well as alcoholism in several members of the paternal family. The psychosocial history is significant for multiple stressors, including low income, limited maternal education, two closely spaced younger siblings in the same household and two older half-siblings in their father's household. In addition, JL's father abandoned the family three years ago. However, a good deal of social support was available from the maternal extended family.

JL's medical examination was normal except for mild immaturity of his neurological 'soft signs', but no generalised or focal neurological findings. The psychological evaluation confirmed a low-average IQ (full-scale 85, verbal 86 [WIPPSI-R] see Appendix 2). The language evaluation (CELF; see Appendix 1)[2] showed a severe generalised receptive-expressive language disorder. Specific difficulties in receptive language included difficulties interpreting oral directions requiring logical operations, understanding complex sentence structure and following complex directions. In expressive language he showed a limited ability to plan, organise, produce or imitate compound or complex sentences. He also had significant problems in auditory word discrimination.

This case illustrates the complexity and heterogeneity of the components of dysfunction which together are much more than the sum of their parts. This young boy has a speech-language disorder and ADHD, a common combination which is probably associated with as yet unidentified biological and environmental mechanisms. Individually and together these disorders confer significant risk for adverse psychosocial development. As is the case more often than not, there are other major risk factors for neurodevelopmental as well as psychiatric morbidity in JL's life: poverty, poor maternal education, single parent household, multiple siblings to name some of the environmental factors. Biological risk factors are:

- paternal and sibling 'slowness' as a probable genetic indicator of cognitive impairment
- maternal smoking during the pregnancy as a teratotoxic factor implicated in language and behavioural morbidity[3]
- long-standing paternal alcoholism, which also is associated with independent vulnerability towards language and attentional/behavioural dysfunction, although the pathologic mechanisms remain obscure.[4]

Last, JL's low average IQ places him academically and vocationally at risk and makes it more difficult for him to rationally approach the world and its complexities, find healthy compensations for his ADHD as well as language difficulties, and deal with his own emotions constructively. In conjunction with his speech and language problems, his low average intelligence and ADHD increase his risk for specific learning disabilities, which are strong independent risk factors for psychiatric disturbance. However, not all the cards are stacked against him, as he has a supportive extended family and also does not have aggressive or oppositional behaviour. On the contrary he is compliant and eager to please, at least in school, even if his peer interactions are intense and unmodulated.

Speech-language difficulties and psychiatric morbidity

Speech and language difficulties commonly co-occur with behaviour problems as they do with other environmental or individual risk factors. However, even if these other contextual adversities are controlled for or eliminated, speech-language impairments in and of themselves continue to be associated with increased psychosocial and behavioural morbidity. Rutter and Martin[5] had found that children with brain damage and psychiatric disorders had a higher rate of speech-language disorders than children with brain damage but without psychiatric disorders. Cantwell and

Baker,[6] studying 600 children with diagnosed speech-language disorders found that 50% had identifiable psychiatric disorders. Conversely, Cohen et al.[7] and Love et al.[8] found that 28% and 66% respectively of children seen in psychiatric clinics had previously undiagnosed significant speech and language difficulties. Beitchman et al.,[9,10] in a representative population of non-referred children, searched for a correlation of specific language profiles with specific clinical psychiatric syndromes, and was one of the first to identify statistically distinct psychosocial differences among children:

- pure articulation (speech) problems
- poor auditory comprehension
- children who had low overall scores on multiple measures of speech-language development.

The latter group differed most significantly from the normal group in social/environmental factors, cognitive measures and medical risk factors by being more likely to come from lower income, single-parent families and having lower (though still normal) scores on verbal and non-verbal measures of IQ, and higher (25%) failure rates on audiometry than the other groups. The pure articulation group was most similar to a normal group with respect to these non-linguistic variables. In this population, 75% of a random sample of the low overall group had psychiatric disorders compared to 33% in the poor articulation, 38% in the poor auditory comprehension group and only one child in the normal group. ADHD was the prevalent diagnosis for both low overall (59%) and poor auditory comprehension (38%) groups, and these children also tended to have higher levels of aggression, while emotional disorders were more common in the articulation group. Cantwell and Baker also found socioenvironmental stressors to be significantly associated with psychiatric morbidity in their large cohort of children with speech-language disorders, but the most significant factor was the severity and type of linguistic impairment itself, specifically in the areas of language comprehension and auditory processing, with the psychiatrically ill group (50% of the cohort) having higher and more severe rates of combined speech-language disorders and pure language disorder and lower rates of pure speech disorder. A subgroup of children with coexisting specific learning disorders had especially high prevalence (68%) of psychiatric disorders. ADHDs were the predominant psychiatric diagnoses in this study (19% ADHDs, 7% Oppositional-Defiant/Conduct Disorders and 20% emotional disorders) as in the other cited studies.

These investigations substantiate the findings of other researchers and the experience of clinicians of the high prevalence of language problems in children with psychiatric disturbance and of the high prevalence of psychiatric disturbance in children with language problems. They demonstrate further that socioenvironmental factors and male gender are strongly associated with language impairment as well as with psychiatric comorbidity, but that the severity and type of language disorder is the most significant variable for psychiatric vulnerability in children with speech-language disorders. Although there is a significant proportion of children with affective and emotional problems Disruptive Behaviour Disorders, primarily ADHDs are the most common psychiatric diagnoses in this group.

Definitions and criteria for Attention Deficit Hyperactivity Disorders

Despite ongoing controversies regarding the symptomatology, nosology and aetiology of Attention Deficit Hyperactivity Disorder, ADHDs are the most common neurodevelopmental syndrome diagnosed in children. Depending on the source, 3–18% show the 'core symptoms' of dysfunctions of attention and cognitive organisation (doesn't listen, distractible, forgetful, disorganised, does not complete tasks, etc.), and/or developmentally abnormal degrees of impulsivity and motor activity. ADHDs are more common in boys by a ratio of between 3 and 5:1 and show strong co-morbidity with oppositional and conduct disorder as well as learning and language disorders. The diagnostic criteria predominantly utilised in the USA are based on DSM classifications which have undergone a series of revisions from an Attention Deficit Disorder with Hyperactivity/without Hyperactivity (1980), to an Attention Deficit Hyperactivity Disorder (1986) requiring the presence of all three core symptoms for the diagnosis, to a return to a 'monothetic' model in 1994. Current criteria are listed in the Appendix to this chapter. Based on the factor analytic identification of two distinct behavioural factors designating hyperactivity and impulsivity on the one hand, and inattention and cognitive disorganisation on the other, three distinct diagnostic subtypes of ADHDs have been formulated in DSM-IV:[11] a predominantly inattentive type, a predominantly hyperactive-impulsive type, and a combined type. Field trials of the new DSM-IV criteria in Germany and the USA have found that the predominantly inattentive type represents a clinically distinct group that is associated with a high degree of academic failure whereas the hyperactive-impulsive type appears to be associated with at least average academic performance, although these children are at risk of academic and social difficulties due to disruptive, usually non-aggressive, behaviour. The combined type has the worst of both worlds with academic problems as well as disruptive and oppositional-aggressive co-morbidity. In the European, ICD-based nomenclature (ICD 10 WHO), ADHD has been classified as the Hyperkinetic syndrome, which does not specify the role of attention and cognitive disorganisation, but otherwise is conceptually compatible with the DSM classification and criteria. According to the latter, the core symptoms are required to have been present for at least six months beginning before the seventh year of life, manifest in several different settings (i.e. at home as well as in school), associated with impairment of academic, behavioural and social-emotional functioning, and not part of an autism spectrum, major affective or thought disorder. Because of the pervasive nature of the symptoms and frequent co-morbidities with other developmental dysfunction and disorders, children with ADHDs continue to be at considerable social, academic and vocational risk as adults.

Aetiologically, ADHDs appear to be clinically related symptoms of multiple and heterogeneous influences on the developing brain: children with close relatives with ADHDs, with conditions of pre- or perinatal morbidity and adversity, and with postnatal insults to the developing brain are at risk for ADHDs (as for speech-language impairments). The underlying mechanisms appear to be associated with neurotransmitter system inadequacy as well as disturbance of frontal lobe, basal ganglia and brainstem functions. The evidence for the neurophysiological aetiology thus far remains indirect at best but is further supported by the response of most children with ADHDs to stimulant medication (methylphenidate, dextroampheta-mines, etc.) which inhibit dopamine uptake. As with all chronic impairments, the context given by psychosocial circumstances, temperament and intelligence will affect the mode and degree to which the underlying symptoms are expressed and lead to impairment. Whether these adversities develop into aggressive conduct-disordered behaviour appears to depend heavily on the 'goodness of fit' between these difficult children and their home and school environment.

Cognitive and behavioural features of individuals with ADHD are often reflected in language development and linguistic 'style':[12] language milestones are frequently delayed, and articulation problems and stuttering are also often clinically observed. Impulsivity and hyperactivity may be manifested in a number of ways. For example there may be an inability to wait, a tendency to constant interrupting, in a driven, hyperverbal, compulsive speech quality, or difficulty in listening and engaging in the 'give and take' of normal conversation.[12] They may also be characterised by impulsive, uncontrolled and unmodulated content, i.e. in inappropriately direct, crass, rude (but sometimes also wonderfully insightful or original) statements without an awareness of their effect. Attentional and organisational dysfunction may be evident in that verbal interactions may be initiated in pursuit of a train of thought but then with difficulty responding coherently to questions, and problems with semantic and grammatical organisation may occur (Milne's 'Pooh Bear' giving wonderful examples of these difficulties!).

SLDs and ADHDs: some connections

The nature of the relationship of ADHDs and speech and language difficulties remains largely speculative, but it would appear that they should become clearer as research into ADHD better defines the syndrome and as speech and language difficulties become more differentiated clinically and conceptually. One of the pieces of this puzzle may well be found in dysfunctions of Central Auditory Processing Deficit (CAPD) (*see* Chapter 13), which is described as a deficit in the processing of auditory signals, not due to impairments in hearing or intelligence. CAPD appears to lie at the intersection of language development and attention. Some investigators speculate that CAPD disorder is the mechanism responsible for the high co-morbidity of ADHD behaviours and language disorders since abnormal CAPD has been found in a high proportion of children with ADHDs. However, investigators searching for consistent relationships between CAPD disorders, speech and language impairments and ADHD subtypes have found high overall co-morbidities, but have not been able to demonstrate patterns that would yield satisfactory causal explanations.[13] It is feasible that the co-occurrence of language impairment and ADHD may arise as a result of inhibited language learning because of attentional dysfunction during critical periods of language acquisition from early childhood. On the other hand, ADHD symptoms may represent a behavioural/emotional response to impaired language processing (as indeed receptive language impairment was more prevalent in children with ADHD in the Los Angeles study[6]), and inability to manipulate one's environment through communication of one's needs is certainly a powerful force in the development of negative behaviours. Then again, neurophysiologic, individual and environmental factors may interact in a dynamic process whose individual components will only gradually become disentangled as our methods become more sophisticated.

In summary, population studies as well as studies of clinic-referred children demonstrate a high co-morbidity of language with psychiatric disorders, primarily ADHDs, and of psychiatric disorders in children with language disorders. The reasons for the co-morbidities remain speculative but appear to involve neurophysiological vulnerabilities in interaction with individual and socio-environmental risk factors.

Implications for service delivery

For paediatricians and other clinicians working with children there is a clear mandate that speech and language difficulties should be considered and ruled out as a standard part of the evaluation of children with psychiatric diagnoses, especially of the disruptive behaviour disorders. On the other hand, evaluation and treatment of children with suspected speech and language impairment should include a psychosocial component, in the hope that early addressing of these vulnerabilities may prevent or ameliorate the development of serious psychopathology.

References

1   Epstein MA, Shaywitz SE, Shaywitz BA and Woolston JL (1991) The boundaries of attention deficit disorder. *Journal of Learning Disabilities* **24**(2): 78–86.

2   Semel E, Wiig EH and Secord W (1991) *The Clinical Evaluation of Language Fundamentals – Revised (CELF-UK)*. Psychological Corporation, Sidcup.

3   Ferguson DM, Horwood LJ and Lynskey MT (1993) Maternal smoking before and after pregnancy: effects on behavioral outcomes in middle childhood. *Pediatrics* **92**(6): 815–22.

4   Tarter RE, Jacob T and Bremer D (1989) Specific cognitive impairment in sons of early onset alcoholics. *Alcoholism: Clinical and Experimental Research* **13**: 786–9.

5   Rutter M and Martin JAM (1972) *The Child with Delayed Speech*. Heinemann, London.

6   Cantwell DP and Baker L (1991) *Psychiatric & Developmental Disorders in Children with Communication Disorders*. American Psychological Press, Washington DC.

7   Cohen CJ, Davine M and Meloche-Kelly M (1989) Prevalence of unsuspected language disorders in a child psychiatric population. *Journal of the American Academy of Child Adolescent Psychiatry* **28**(1): 107–11.

8   Love AJ and Thompson MG (1988) Language disorders and attention deficit disorders in young children referred for psychiatric services: analysis of prevalence and a conceptual synthesis. *American Journal of Orthopsychiatry* **58**(1): 52–64.

9   Beitchman JH, Hood J, Rochon J and Peterson M (1989) Empirical classification of speech/language impairment in children I. Identification of speech/language categories. *Journal of the American Academy of Child and Adolescent Psychiatry* **28**(1): 112–17.

10 Beitchman JH, Hood J, Rochon J, Peterson M, Mantinti T and Majumdar S (1989) Empirical classification of speech/language impairment in children II. Behavioral characteristics. *Journal of the American Academy of Child and Adolescent Psychiatry* **28**(1): 118–23.

11 *Diagnostic and Statistical Manual of Mental Disorders* (4th edn) (1994) American Psychiatric Association, Washington DC.

12 Humphries T, Hadley K, Malone M and Roberts W (1994) Teacher-identified oral language difficulties among boys with attention problems. *Journal of Developmental and Behavioural Pediatrics.* **15**: 92–8.

13 Riccio CA, Hynd GW, Cohen MJ, Hall J and Molt L (1994) Comorbidity of central auditory processing disorder and attention-deficit hyperactivity disorder. *Journal of the American Academy of Child and Adolescent Psychiatry* **33**(6): 849–57.

Appendix

Diagnostic criteria for Attention-Deficit/Hyperactivity Disorder (DSM-IV)
A1
Six or more of the following symptoms of inattention have persisted for at least six months to a degree that is maladaptive and inconsistent with developmental level:
(Check all that apply)
Inattention
—   (a) often fails to give close attention to details or makes careless mistakes in schoolwork, work or other activities
—   (b) often has difficulty sustaining attention in tasks or play activities
—   (c) often does not seem to listen when spoken to directly
—   (d) often does not follow through on instructions and fails to finish schoolwork,

chores or duties in the workplace (not due to oppositional behaviour or failure to understand instructions)
— (e) often has difficulty organising tasks and activities
— (f) often avoids, dislikes, or is reluctant to engage in tasks that require sustained mental effort (such as schoolwork or homework)
— (g) often loses things necessary for tasks or activities (e.g. toys, school assignments, pencils, books or tools)
— (h) is often easily distracted by extraneous stimuli
— (i) is often forgetful in daily activities

A2
Six or more of the following symptoms of hyperactivity-impulsivity have persisted for at least six months to a degree that is maladaptive and inconsistent with developmental level: (Check all that apply)

Hyperactivity
— (a) often fidgets with hands or feet or squirms in seat
— (b) often leaves seat in classroom or in other situations in which remaining seated is expected
— (c) often runs about or climbs excessively in situations in which it is inappropriate (in adolescents or adults, may be limited to subjective feelings of restlessness)
— (d) often has difficulty playing or engaging in leisure activities quietly
— (e) is often 'on the go' or often acts as if 'driven by motor'
— (f) often talks excessively

Impulsivity
— (g) often blurts out answers before questions have been completed
— (h) often has difficulty awaiting turn
— (i) often interrupts or intrudes on others (e.g. butts into conversations or games)

Check all that apply:
B — some hyperactive-impulsive or inattentive symptoms that caused impairment were present before age seven years
C — some impairment from the symptoms is present in two or more settings (e.g. at school (or work) and at home)
D — there is clear evidence of clinically significant impairment in social, academic, or occupational functioning
E — The symptoms do not occur exclusively during the course of a Pervasive Developmental Disorder, Schizophrenia or other Psychotic Disorder and are not better accounted for by another mental disorder (e.g. Mood Disorder, Anxiety Disorder, Dissociative Disorder, or a Personality Disorder

Diagnosis

Check the appropriate diagnostic code below based on the above information:
— 314.01 Attention-Deficit/Hyperactivity Disorder, combined type: if both criteria **A1** and **A2** are met for the past six months and **B–E** are checked.
— 314.01 Attention-Deficit/Hyperactivity Disorder, predominantly inattentive type: if criterion **A1** is met but criterion **A2** is not met for the past six months, and **B–E** are checked.
— 314.01 Attention-Deficit/Hyperactivity Disorder, predominantly hyperactive-impulsive type: if criterion **A2** is met but criterion **A1** is not met for the past six months, and **B–E** are checked.
Coding note: For individuals (especially adolescents and adults) who currently have symptoms that no longer meet full criteria, 'In Partial Remission' should be specified.
— 314.9 Attention-Deficit/Hyperactivity Disorder, not otherwise specified: this category is for disorders with prominent symptoms of inattention or hyperactivity-impulsivity that do not meet criteria for Attention-Deficit/Hyperactivity Disorder.

Treatment needed

_____ further evaluation through the schools to determine presence of language impairment____ learning disabilities _____ intellectual skills _____ emotional/ behavioural status _____
____ behaviour management programme at school
____ parent training through schools
____ family counselling
____ individual counselling
____ resource classroom services through schools to assist in building school skills
____ after-school tutoring
____ summer school
____ trial of medication type_____ dosage_____
____ medication administered at school _____
____ speech-language therapy/evaluation

_____   _____
Date   Signature of Physician

_____
Address

_____
Telephone

CHAPTER 11

Autism

Wendy L Stone and Opal Y Ousley

Case study

Jesse was the product of an uncomplicated labour and delivery. He was described as an easy baby who rarely cried. His motor milestones developed within normal limits. At his two-year well-child visit, his mother expressed concern about his lack of speech. She reported that he rarely babbled like his older brother had and that he often did not respond when she called his name. His physical examination at two years was normal. However, the paediatrician noted difficulty engaging Jesse's attention through conversation or toy play. Jesse was most responsive during a tickling game; he laughed heartily when tickled, yet did not look at the paediatrician to communicate his enjoyment or request that the activity be continued. Upon further questioning, the paediatrician learned that Jesse never tried to communicate by pointing at things, and he usually attempted to obtain objects on his own rather than ask his parents. Occasionally when he needed help with something, such as unscrewing a jar lid, he would take his parent's hand and place it on the lid to indicate what he wanted. When asked, Jesse's mother reported that Jesse usually played by himself at home, showing little interest in his older brother's activities. His favourite activities were described as lining up his toy cars and opening and closing the kitchen cabinets, and he was reported to entertain himself with these activities for hours at a time. Based on this information, the paediatrician recognised a pattern of limited social interactions, delayed development of non-verbal communication as well as speech, and restricted play interests. She referred Jesse for a multi-disciplinary evaluation to rule out autism.

Jesse received a comprehensive evaluation at the age of two years six months through a clinic specialising in the early diagnosis of autism. The evaluation included formal cognitive/developmental and speech and language testing, as well as assessment of Jesse's play, motor imitation and spontaneous communication skills. An extensive parental interview was also conducted. Jesse was found to be functioning at the 16-month level cognitively, and his receptive and expressive language skills both were at the 12-month level. His play was repetitive, consisting mostly of opening and closing the doors on a toy schoolbus and rolling the bus on a table at eye level as he watched the wheels intently. He failed to imitate actions modelled by the examiner, such as drinking out of a toy teacup or clapping his hands. Jesse did not use any words, and his communicative gestures were limited to reaching for desired objects or placing the examiner's hand on toys he needed help operating. Based on clinical observations as well as parental report, the evaluation team concluded that Jesse demonstrated a triad of deficits in social interactions, verbal and non-verbal communication, and play skills that were consistent with a diagnosis of autism. Jesse was referred to an early intervention programme specialising in the treatment of children with autism.

Autism is a developmental disorder characterised by a triad of symptoms: impaired social relating and reciprocity, abnormal language and communication development, and impairment of imagination resulting in a restricted behavioural repertoire including stereotypies and unusual sensory responses. The prevalence of core autism is estimated to range from 4–5 children per 10 000[1] to 10–13 children per 10 000.[2] The figures for the more common Asperger's syndrome may be as high as 20–25 per 10 000.[3] Autism occurs more commonly in males than females, with sex ratios ranging from two to four males : one female.[4,5] The majority of children with autism (i.e. 70–80%) have a range of learning disabilities. Many children with autism demonstrate an uneven pattern of abilities, with relative strengths in visual-motor skills and auditory memory and relative weaknesses in language and abstract thinking.

Aetiology

Despite early views of autism that emphasised psychological or emotional causes, autism is now conceptualised as a biological disorder with diverse organic aetiologies. Neurobiological investigations have examined genetic influences, structural abnormalities, and neurophysiological and neurochemical factors. Genetic studies have revealed higher concordance rates for autism in monozygotic versus dizygotic twins, high familial rates of cognitive, social and language impairments, and an association of autism with several known genetic disorders, including Fragile X syndrome, phenylketonuria, tuberous sclerosis and neurofibromatosis.[6] Structural brain abnormalities have been found in some individuals with autism, with affected areas including the left temporal horn, cerebellum and forebrain. Some neurochemical investigations have reported abnormal levels of serotonin or endogenous opioids. In addition, seizure disorders have been found to occur in 11–42% of autistic individuals.[7] Despite evidence that central nervous system abnormalities play a role in the aetiology of autism, no single neurobiological factor has been shown to be uniquely and universally associated with autism.[8] Rather, there appear to be a variety of organic aetiologies which may contribute to the development of autism in individual cases.

Identification

At present there are no biological markers or medical tests that can detect the presence of autism; the diagnosis is based on the presence of a specific pattern of behaviours. Diagnosis can be complicated by the presence of overlapping symptoms with other developmental disorders, as well as differences in symptom expression as a function of age, severity and degree of intellectual impairment. As a result, a definitive diagnosis is often obtained from multidisciplinary centres with a specialisation in autism. Diagnostic teams commonly include a developmental paediatrician, psychologist, speech and language therapist, psychiatrist, and occupational and physiotherapists. A comprehensive assessment for autism requires gathering information from the child's parents and other care providers as well as observing the child in structured situations (such as developmental testing) and unstructured situations (such as play). A number of instruments have been developed for the purpose of gathering diagnostically relevant information through observations or parental report, and are presented in Box 11.1. One or more of these instruments will most likely be used during the course of a comprehensive diagnostic evaluation.

In recent years there has been increasing recognition of the importance of early identification of autism. The diagnostic label can provide the 'port of entry' to specialised early intervention, which can lead to marked cognitive and behavioural improvements for many young children with autism.[17–19] Moreover, a definitive diagnosis can alleviate family stress and uncertainty by helping parents and siblings understand the child's puzzling behaviours and begin the process of adaptation. The average age of symptom onset reported by parents of children with autism is 18 months,[20] suggesting that identification at an early age should be possible.

A brief description of each of the three core characteristics of autism is presented in

---

Box 11.1:   Diagnostic assessment instruments for autism

Observational scales
Autism Behaviour Checklist (ABC)[9]
Autism Diagnostic Observation Schedule (ADOS)[10]
Behaviour Rating Instrument for Autistic and Atypical Children (BRIAAC)[11]
Childhood Autism Rating Scale (CARS)[12]
Diagnostic Checklist for Behaviour-Disturbed Children (Form E-2)[13]
Ritvo-Freeman Real Life Rating Scale (RLRS)[14]

Parental interviews
Autism Diagnostic Interview – Revised (ADI-R)[15]
Parent Interview for Autism (PIA)[16]

Table 11.1 Characteristics of autism at different levels of severity

Social behaviour	Language and communication	Repetitive activities
Mild impairment Shows clear social interest but limited reciprocity. Seeks social interactions but relationships may be hampered by limited understanding of the perspective and feelings of others	Speaks in complete sentences but language may be rigid or inflexible. Conversational skills may be limited by persistence on particular topics and poor understanding of non-verbal cues. May show comprehension problems and difficulty with abstract concepts	Shows some behavioural rigidity and inflexibility. May have circumscribed areas of interest and specific routines or rituals that interfere only minimally with daily activities
Moderate impairment Shows enjoyment in a limited number of social routines, especially those involving physical activities or satisfaction of needs. Shows little interest in interacting with peers, though may engage in parrallel play or chasing games	Verbalisations may contain a combination of functional speech, jargon and immediate and/or delayed echolalia. Initiation of communication is for the purpose of satisfaction of needs rather than for the purpose of social interaction	Resists changes in routines or interruption of activities. Shows repetitive play with toys and may have motor stereotypies, such as rocking or spinning
Severe impairment Shows limited social awareness and interest. Social interactions may be restricted to simple routines with familiar adults. Shows little social initiation and inconsistent responsiveness to others	Uses no functional speech. Non-verbal communication is limited and may include using others' hands as tools	Shows extreme resistance to changes in activities and routines. Stereotyped motor behaviours may be persistent and difficult to interrupt. May focus on sensory aspects of toys or other objects

Box 11.1, with particular attention to behaviours that may be helpful in early identification. Whereas all children with autism demonstrate a triad of symptoms in the areas of social relating, communication, and restricted activities and interests, the specific behavioural manifestations of these characteristics may vary greatly from child to child. Moreover, all characteristics may not be readily observed during a relatively short clinic visit,[21] highlighting the importance of parental report as an essential tool in the diagnostic process. This variability in symptom expression is illustrated in Table 11.1 and in the case example at the end of this section.

Social impairments

Deficits in social relating and reciprocity are considered by many researchers to represent the core characteristics of autism. Children with autism may appear to have little social interest in their parents or peers, and they have difficulty forming reciprocal peer relationships based on mutuality and sharing. One of the earliest social deficits to appear is in the area of motor imitation. Children with autism often have difficulty imitating the actions of others; they may not imitate the gestures used in early social imitation games, such as peek-a-boo or pat-a-cake, or those used to blow a kiss or wave goodbye. They may establish eye contact with others for only brief periods, and may fail to use eye contact communicatively, for the purpose of conveying affect or directing another person's attention to an object or event of interest (i.e. establishing joint attention). Children with autism often have difficulty identifying or sharing in the feelings of others, and their own forms of emotional expression may be limited or idiosyncratic. For instance, they may retain a bland facial expression, demonstrate rapid shifts from one emotional extreme to another, or begin laughing for no apparent reason. Often physical games, such as tickling, are the only way parents are able to elicit positive affect and pleasure from their very young children. In older individuals with autism, even those who function at average or near average intellectual levels, the ability to experience empathy and to understand that others can have thoughts and beliefs different from one's own, is often impaired.

Language and communication impairment

A wide range of language and communication difficulties have been described for individuals with autism. Delayed speech development or lack of speech are seen frequently in children with autism, and represent the most common early concerns of parents whose children receive a diagnosis of autism. The majority of parents of autistic children report delayed speech to be among their initial concerns. A disordered pattern of language acquisition may also be evident. One such pattern, found in about one-third of children with autism, is the loss of previously acquired meaningful language before the age of 30 months.[22]

In addition to delayed and disordered speech development, other communication deficits are also apparent at young ages. For example, babbling and jargon, when present, may be used to provide self-stimulation rather than for the purpose of communicating with others. Children with autism may also fail to develop early communicative gestures, such as pointing to objects of interest or showing objects to others. Lacking such gestures, these children may attempt to satisfy their needs or desires by using another person's hand as a tool, such as placing an adult's hand on a jar lid to request that the jar be opened. Other non-specific communicative behaviours, such as vague reaching or handing objects to an adult, are also commonly seen in young children with autism, and often are not accompanied by eye contact.

Only about 50% of individuals with autism develop the functional use of speech. Those children who do acquire speech may show a number of unusual language features; these include immediate and delayed echolalia, 'pronoun reversal', repetitive language, neologisms, and idiosyncratic use of words and phrases. Abnormal prosody (i.e. the pitch, stress, rate and rhythm of language) is another aspect of disordered language development in individuals with autism. The ability to use speech and gesture in a communicative and socially appropriate manner (i.e. the pragmatic aspect of language) is also impaired in individuals with autism. Examples of pragmatic deficits include pedantic speech, a one-sided rather than reciprocal conversational style, difficulty understanding the non-verbal communication of others and a tendency to persevere on particular conversational topics. In contrast, the structural aspects of language, such as syntax and grammar, may be relatively unimpaired.[23]

Impairment of imagination

The impairment of imagination varies in each individual child with autism; it impacts on the child's development and behaviour in numerous and diverse ways. It is often measured in terms of the child's level of symbolic play when compared with non-autistic children of comparable developmental levels. Typically children with autism engage in less pretend play and absorb their free time with more physical and repetitive type play, such things as opening and closing the doors on a toy car, tipping the car over and exploring the movements of the wheels, for example. These repetitive play actions are frequently linked with repetitive motor stereotypies, the most commonly reported being spinning, rocking themselves, flapping and twirling their hands and fingers, but also incorporating various materials like sticks, threads, pieces of material, etc. Unusual sensory responses that include both hyporeactivity and hyper-reactivity have been reported for all sensory modalities. For example, some children with autism may inspect small details of objects for prolonged periods or may repeatedly run their hands along certain surfaces. A lack of response to loud sounds and/or hypersensitivity to sounds are also commonly reported. In older children, the need for sameness may be manifested in an insistence on particular routines or rituals and extreme distress when these routines are interrupted or prevented. These behaviours are thought to serve the common purpose of attempting to impose some degree of invariance on to the environment.[24]

Implications for service delivery

- The role of the family practitioner and the primary healthcare team is primarily one of initial identification and appropriate referral.

- The diagnosis of autism should always be made in consultation with the team of specialist clinicians who examine the child's pattern of strengths and weaknesses and who are then responsible for managing the case and providing appropriate support to the family. *See* Table 11.2 for some suggestions for primary healthcare teams.

- The primary goals of treatment for children with autism are threefold: to promote the development of social, communicative and adaptive living skills; to decrease maladaptive behaviours such as rigidity and stereotypies; and to alleviate family stress.[25,26] The most efficacious treatments for autism at the present time are educational and behavioural in nature. Successful educational interventions employ visual structure and routines to enhance comprehension and increase the predictability of events; provide individualised programming that follows a developmental model and that focuses on the specific deficit areas of autism; use typically developing peers as agents of change; employ behavioural techniques to promote acquisition of new skills and behaviours, reduce disruptive or self-stimulatory behaviour, and enhance attention and motivation; and involve parents in the teaching process to foster generalisation of skills.

- Specific intervention for language and communication problems in children with autism is often provided through an incidental teaching approach. This approach emphasises the importance of teaching language use within the child's natural context, using activities that are functional and meaningful for the child, and focusing on the expansion of spontaneous, rather than prompted, communication.[27]

- Medication has also been used in older children as an adjunct to educational and behavioural intervention for the purpose of ameliorating severe behavioural problems. Haloperidol and fenfluramine have been successful in reducing symptomatology in some individuals with autism, but their associated side-effects limit their usage. Clomipramine and naltrexone are other medications that have received some preliminary support. The most common class of medication used for autism is anticonvulsant medication, because of the high incidence of seizure disorders in this population.[7]

- As indicated above, the most effective intervention for autism may well be participation in specialised, early intervention programmes. For this reason, children who demonstrate a constellation of deficits in social relating, verbal and non-verbal communication, and restricted activities and interests should be referred for further evaluation and treatment at as early an age as possible.

Table 11.2 Suggestions for primary healthcare teams

Don't	Do
• Expect to make a formal diagnosis of autism during a single visit	• Recognise the constellation of symptoms and refer to a multidisciplinary team of specialists for diagnosis
• Expect the behavioural manifestations of autism to be the same from one child to another	• Recognise that variability in symptom expression can occur as a function of age, intellectual functioning and language development
• Fail to consider the possibility of autism in a child who shows affectionate behaviour towards parents	• Ask parents about other aspects of social relating, such as social imitation, affective expression, peer interactions and empathy
• Wait to refer a two-year-old child who is exhibiting a pattern of deficits in social reciprocity, communication and play	• Refer the child for assessment and early intervention as soon as autism is suspected
• Disregard parental expression of frustration, confusion or distress	• Become familiar with community resources for supportive counselling and behaviour management, and make referrals as necessary

Summary

In summary, autism is a pervasive developmental disorder characterised by a triad of symptoms: deficits in social relating and reciprocity; disordered development of verbal and non-verbal communication; and restricted and repetitive interests that can include motor stereotypies, unusual sensory responses and a need for routines. There is substantial evidence for an underlying organic aetiology. Because of individual variability in symptom expression, the formal diagnosis of autism is best made by a multidisciplinary team of specialists. Early referral for assessment enables the family to begin to understand and cope with the child's often challenging behaviours, and enables the child to participate in specialised early intervention programmes.

References

1   Zahner GEP and Pauls DL (1987) Epidemiological surveys of infantile autism. In: DJ Cohen and AM Donnellan (eds) *Handbook of Autism and Pervasive Developmental Disorders*, pp. 199–207. VH Winston & Sons, Silver Spring, MD.

2   Bryson SE, Clark BS and Smith IM (1988) First report of a Canadian epidemiological study of autistic syndromes. *Journal of Child Psychology and Psychiatry* **29**: 433–45.

3   Gillberg IC and Gillberg C (1989) Asperger syndrome – some epidemiological considerations: a research note. *Journal of Child Psychology and Psychiatry* **30**: 631–8.

4 Cialdella Ph and Mamelle N (1989) An epidemiological study of infantile autism in a French department (Rhone): a research note. *Journal of Child Psychology and Psychiatry* **30**: 165–75.

5 Ritvo ER, Freeman BJ, Pingee C *et al.* (1989) The UCLA-University of Utah epidemiologic survey of autism: prevalence. *American Journal of Psychiatry* **146**: 194–9.

6 Folstein SE and Rutter ML (1988) Autism: family aggregation and genetic implications. *Journal of Autism and Developmental Disorders* **18**: 3–30.

7 Tuchman RF, Rapin I and Shinnar S (1991) Autistic and dysphasic children. II: Epilepsy. *Pediatrics* **88**: 1219–25.

8 Gillberg C (1990) Autism and pervasive developmental disorders. *Journal of Child Psychology and Psychiatry* **31**: 99–119.

9 Krug DA, Arick JR and Almond PJ (1980) Behavior checklist for identifying severely handicapped individuals with high levels of autistic behavior. *Journal of Child Psychology and Psychiatry* **21**: 221–9.

10 Lord C, Rutter M, Goode S, Heemsbergen J, Jordan H, Mawhood L and Schopler E (1989) Autism Diagnostic Observation Schedule: a standardized observation of communicative and social behavior. *Journal of Autism and Developmental Disorders* **19**: 185–212.

11 Ruttenberg BA, Kalish BI, Wenar C and Wolf E (1977) *The Behavior Rating Instrument for Autistic and Other Atypical Children.* Stoelting Co., Chicago.

12 Schopler E, Reichler RJ and Renner BR (1988) *The Childhood Autism Rating Scale.* Western Psychological Services, Los Angeles.

13 Rimland B (1971) The differentiation of childhood psychoses: an analysis of checklists for 2,218 psychotic children. *Journal of Autism and Childhood Schizophrenia* **1**: 161–74.

14 Freeman BJ, Ritvo ER, Yokota A and Ritvo A (1986) A scale for rating symptoms of patients with the syndrome of autism in real life settings. *Journal of the American Academy of Child Psychiatry* **25**: 130–6.

15 Lord C, Rutter M and Le Couteur A (1994) Autism Diagnostic Interview – Revised: a revised version of a diagnostic interview for caregivers of individuals with possible pervasive developmental disorders. *Journal of Autism and Developmental Disorders* **24**: 659–85.

16 Stone WL and Hogan KL (1993) A structured parent interview for identifying young children with autism. *Journal of Autism and Developmental Disorders* **23**: 639–52.

17 Lovaas OI (1987) Behavioral treatment and normal educational and intellectual functioning in young autistic children. *Journal of Consulting and Clinical Psychology* **55**: 3–9.

18 Rogers SJ and Lewis H (1989) An effective day treatment model for young children with pervasive developmental disorders. *Journal of the American Academy of Child and Adolescent Psychiatry* **28**: 207–14.

19 Strain PS, Hoyson M and Jamieson B (1985) Normally developing preschoolers as inter-

vention agents for autistic-like children: effects on class deportment and social interaction. *Journal of the Division for Early Childhood* **Spring**: 105–15.

20   Siegel B, Pliner C, Eschler J and Elliott GR (1988) How children with autism are diagnosed: difficulties in identification of children with multiple developmental delays. *Developmental and Behavioral Pediatrics* **9**: 199–204.

21   Stone WL, Hoffman EL, Lewis SL and Ousley OY (1994) Early recognition of autism: parental report vs. clinical observation. *Archives of Pediatrics & Adolescent Medicine* **148**: 174–9.

22   Kurita H (1985) Infantile autism with speech loss before the age of 30 months. *Journal of the American Academy of Child Psychiatry* **24**: 191–6.

23   Tager-Flusberg H (1989) A psycholinguistic perspective on language development in the autistic child. In: G Dawson (ed) *Autism: nature, diagnosis, and treatment*, pp. 92–115. Guilford, New York.

24   Rutter M and Schopler E (1987) Autism and pervasive developmental disorders: concepts and diagnostic issues. *Journal of Autism and Developmental Disorders* **17**: 159–86.

25   Lansing MD and Schopler E (1978) Individualized education: a public school model. In: M Rutter and E Schopler (eds) *Autism: a reappraisal of concepts and treatment*, pp. 439–52. Plenum, New York.

26   Rutter M (1985) The treatment of autistic children. *Journal of Child Psychology and Psychiatry* **26**: 193–214.

27   Carr EG (1985) Behavioral approaches to language and communication. In: E Schopler and GB Mesibov (eds) *Communication Problems in Autism*, pp. 37–57. Plenum, New York.

CHAPTER 12

Behavioural difficulties

Geoff Thorley

Case study

At 18 months of age, Mark was uttering only a few words and by 24 months of age he had an expressive vocabulary of approximately 50 words. This slow progress continued and speech and language therapy services became involved following a referral by the health visitor. In other respects Mark was progressing well developmentally, although behaviourally and temperamentally was quite a 'handful' according to his parents. Over several months his parents became concerned about Mark's aggressive behaviour. This was directed to family members and later, to other children when he started nursery school at three and a half years of age even though by then, his expressive speech was improving rapidly. Another concern was over Mark's poorly regulated behaviour characterised by overactivity and impulsiveness both of which had been present from the time he started to walk. By six years of age, he was displaying a number of difficulties at school including aggressive behaviour towards peers, non-compliance and a failure to progress academically. By this time, his expressive speech was in the normal range and he was assessed as having an average level of verbal intelligence although non-verbal intelligence was in the low-average range.

By eight years of age Mark's formal learning skills, including reading and arithmetic, were lagging behind those of his peers, he found it difficult to make and sustain friendships, was viewed as quite immature and was disruptive in the classroom. The problems persisted and by nine and a half years of age his teachers felt that he had major problems in sustaining attention. Because of these difficulties and continuing behavioural problems at home, a referral was made to the child and adolescent mental health service. Mark was diagnosed as having Attention Deficit Hyperactivity Disorder (ADHD), which was viewed as underpinning behavioural and emotional problems as well relationship difficulties and low self-esteem. An intervention programme was instituted involving stimulant medication, family therapy and cognitive behavioural approaches implemented by parents and school staff.

Mark's profile is illustrative of research findings that show that up to 50% of children with a wide variety of communication disorders present with or develop psychological problems. Baker and Cantwell for example,[1] found that 44% of children with speech and language disorders qualified for a psychiatric diagnosis and that this prevalence increased with age.[2] In a study of 1655 five-year-olds, Beitchman and colleagues[3-5] found a similar pattern. They found that whereas 12% of non-impaired children had psychiatric disorders, almost 50% of the 11% that had communication disorders also had a concurrent psychiatric disorder. As in the Baker and Cantwell cohort, a follow-up at 12 years of age revealed no reduction in the prevalence of psychiatric disorder. This poor outcome was despite improvements in the severity of the speech and language disorders as the children developed.

The association between speech and language disorders (SLD) and a range of mental health problems is an important finding which argues for early screening and intervention of SLD children for the presence of psychological problems and disorders. Quite often the temptation clinically is to focus on the communication difficulties and if mental health problems are identified, assume that they will resolve as a consequence of successfully addressing the communication difficulties. Unfortunately, delays in dealing with psychological problems can substantially increase the risk of poorer outcome long term. A disorder such as ADHD with core problems of overactivity, impulsiveness and inattentiveness can quickly become more serious as secondary problems develop, such as academic failure, conduct and emotional problems, relationship difficulties and low self-esteem.

The range of psychological problems and disorders associated with communication difficulties is varied but the research findings reveal certain important clusters of mental health impairments.

Key associations between communication difficulties and mental health problems

Impaired social interaction

Research by Leitao et al.[6] suggests that a wide variety of children with communication difficulties, including those who are speech impaired, language impaired or with mixed disorders, are at increased risk for impaired social skills and relationships. Illustrative of this finding is a study by Paul and Kellogg[7] involving 28 children with slow expressive language development at two years of age. On follow-up at six years of age they were rated as being more aloof, shy and less socially outgoing than normal controls. These impairments were also found to be positively associated with sentence length in spontaneous speech. Similar risks to social skills have been identified in late talkers. Paul et al.,[8] in a study of late talkers at 18 months of age, found that at follow-up at 36 months of age, the children were at significant risk for receptive communication and socialisation difficulties.

An interesting question is whether the relationship between communication problems and social impairments is a causal one. In other words, do speech and language problems *cause* social difficulties. In a study by Vallence and colleagues of children with language and learning disabilities it was evident that the children showed impairments in social discourse skills as well as social interactional skills.[9] Once discourse skills were controlled for in statistical analyses, it was evident that these skills failed to exert an independent effect, suggesting that social skills deficits represent the major risk factor. The authors speculate, however, that what might underpin the failure to acquire social skills may be the presence of social discourse difficulties initially.

It is likely, however, that social discourse difficulties may represent one of several sets of risk factors for later social impairments. Early communication difficulties are also associated with other impairments and these may singly, or in combination, represent risk factors for later social difficulties. A study by Frisk[10] showed that children with cognitive delay as measured by slow reaction times have poor outcome in terms of social adjustment. Interestingly, the range of problems is very similar to those shown by children with communication difficulties. Hence the risk to social adjustment faced by children with communication difficulties is not unique to communication difficulties and may represent a non-specific effect of a wide range of impairments related to cognitive functioning and early mental health problems. Some support is provided for this non-specific effect and association in the study by Paul et al.[8] of late talkers. They found that in late talkers identified at three years of age, social skills remained affected even when communication skills moved into the normal range on follow-up at age six.

In practical terms, therefore, it needs to be recognised that children with communication difficulties are at risk for social impairment even though the mechanism by which this comes about is unclear. The impairment seems relatively enduring even with improvements in communication skills over time.

Co-morbidity with psychiatric disorders

Disorders of opposition and defiance

A number of studies suggest that one of the strongest associations with communication disorders is the presence of behavioural problems with such associations being found from as early as two to two and a half years of age.[11] These associations seem to be relatively enduring in childhood as indicated in a study by Beitchman et al.[12] Children as young as five with speech and language disorders were found to have behavioural disturbance by 12 years of age. This finding held true even controlling for the severity of behavioural disturbance in early childhood. The authors note that receptive and pervasive speech and language impairment in early childhood was associated with the greatest risk at follow-up.

Attention Deficit Hyperactivity Disorder (ADHD)

This disorder is characterised by core problems of overactivity, impulsivity and inattentiveness but is complicated by the development of secondary problems such as conduct problems, emotional difficulties, educational failure, poor social relationships and low self-esteem. Ornoy et al.,[13] for example, found a high association of speech delay with ADHD in children under four years of age with a variety of developmental problems. Other studies provide evidence to suggest that the more severe the ADHD as in subtypes such as Hyperkinetic Disorder or situationally pervasive forms, the more likely it is that communication difficulties are present.[14] In addition to gross speech pathology, minor problems which may impair communication skills and the development of social relationships are often seen in children with ADHD. Sandler et al.,[15] for example, found high rates of overly talkative behaviour in children with ADHD.

Other psychiatric disorders

The range of psychiatric problems associated is quite extensive with the presence of Emotional Disorder being a significant mental health risk.[12] More severe forms of mental illness such as Early Onset Schizophrenia have been found to have a high co-morbid association with communication disorders.[16] A further association has been found with selective mutism. In a study by Steinhausen and Juzi[17] a third of 100 children with selective mutism were identified as having speech and language problems before the onset of selective mutism. Associations with Autistic Spectrum Disorders are also well-established.

Cognitive difficulties, educational delay and impact on formal learning

Children whose language difficulties persist after the age of five and a half years show a tendency to develop reading and oral language problems. Even if reading accuracy is age-appropriate, reading comprehension is delayed. Phonological language problems by themselves in early childhood appear not to have such adverse implications.[18] Beitchman et al.,[4] in a seven-year follow-up (5–12 years) of children with speech and language disorder, showed that pervasive speech/language impairment in early childhood was associated with increased risk of poor linguistic and academic outcome at follow-up. As in the Bishop and Adams study,[18] they noted that children with isolated articulatory problems had a more favourable outcome.

Other problems, such as problem-solving skills, are found to be more impaired in language-impaired children compared to normal controls even when matched on cognitive ability.[19] Wider cognitive problems are also associated with communication disorders particularly where there are combined expressive and comprehensive language difficulties. In addition there is some evidence that communication difficulties are associated with poor fine motor skills.[20,21]

It is important to appreciate that the associations between communication disorders and psychiatric disorders, psychological problems, educational delay, cognitive and motor difficulties are likely to be interactive. The presence of one associative problem may increase the severity or cause the presence of another. In addition, children with mental health problems such as ADHD behave in such a way that others, including carers and other children, develop negative attitudes towards them. This can have important clinical implications in the sense that it can become difficult to improve the commitment of some carers to address either mental health or communication problems.

Causal pathways

Why is there such a strong association between communication disorders and the range of other problems – psychological, social and educational? Research has revealed a number of possible processes that may bring about such associations.

Cerebral development

It has been suggested that links between communication disorders and psychiatric disorders such as autism and ADHD are suggestive of an underlying neurodevelopmental immaturity.[22] Some support for this is provided by Plante and colleagues[23,24] in studies of four family groups each containing a child who had a specific language impairment. A structural anomaly was found involving atypical perisylvian asymmetries which the authors suggest provides an indication of there having been a prenatal alteration of brain development. Taken further, this may indicate that disruption to normal brain development which affects language also affects other aspects of cognitive development. Our ability to learn language is innate, but not necessarily domain-specific. That is, language development may be based on a relatively plastic mix of neural systems that also serve other cognitive and perceptual functions. Any disruption to the development of brain structures may thus have widespread effects and not simply on communication skills alone.

Further support for this hypothesis is provided in studies of the outcome for very low birth weight (VLBW) infants for whom there is a high risk of cognitive and language difficulties.[25,26] This association holds true even when neurological impairments were controlled for.[27] In the Scottish Low Birthweight Study[28] involving over

600 infants at four and a half years of age, language development was found to be negatively associated with birth weight but interestingly the association did not hold for expressive language and the authors also found a high frequency of behavioural and attentional problems (47%) in the study cohort.

Genetic factors

There have long been indications of genetic factors being involved in the aetiology of communication disorders. Tallal *et al.*,[29] in the San Diego longitudinal study, revealed that 70% of language-impaired children had parents with learning or language problems. Beitchman *et al.*[5] also found a significantly higher prevalence rate of language-related problems in families of speech- and language-impaired children than in normal language controls. Of note is that girls with speech and language impairments had more affected relatives than boys, suggesting that girls with this type of family history are at a greater risk of developing speech or language related problems.

In recent years there have been considerable advances in quantitative and molecular genetics relating to the development of psychiatric disorders. Recent findings and reviews point to moderate to high heritability rates for a range of mental health disorders such as autism, ADHD and depression[30] but with indications that these genetic influences encompass a broader range of communicative disorders.[31] It may transpire that a number of mental health disorders have similar genes in common and that these genes may be implicated in communication skills. This would certainly help to explain the high rates of association between communication disorders and mental health problems and disorders.

Implications for assessment and treatment

The research findings argue strongly for developing an awareness of the risks to mental health of children who present with communication disorders. At one level, as Rapin[32] states it is to, 'minimize secondary behavioural consequences of inadequate communication'. It is not certain, however, that such consequences are indeed secondary features of communication disorders. A model of co-morbidity may well be more appropriate for many mental health problems. Research will undoubtedly help us to continue to clarify these relationships. Whatever the aetiological underpinnings, it is difficult to escape the conclusion that children with communication disorders are at a high risk of presenting with a range mental health problems.

This argues for mental health screening of children who are identified as having speech and language problems. Speech and language therapy services need to establish expertise to achieve this or alternatively develop formal links with child and adolescent mental health services. Once children are identified as having a mental health problem through such screening, early therapeutic intervention is called for. In practice, most of these children should be managed by paediatricians in their gatekeeper role (*see* Chapter 4). The hope is that this will attenuate later morbidity and perhaps enhance efforts for the remediation of communication problems. A child presenting, for example with ADHD, will find it difficult to focus on learning remedial strategies and the disorder will interfere with the acquisition of social interactional skills. In addition, carers and teaching staff will be tempted to focus on addressing behavioural irregularities rather than supporting the child in overcoming communication deficits.

It is likely that the expertise to configure services in this way is generally available within health service settings. Greater inter-agency collaboration is likely to be necessary for training and resource allocation to enable the mental health needs of children with communication disorders to be satisfactorily met.

References

1   Baker L and Cantwell D (1982) Psychiatric disorders in children with different types of communication disorders. *Journal of Communication Disorders* **15**: 159–70.

2   Baker L and Cantwell D (1987) A prospective follow-up of children with speech/language disorders. *Journal of the American Academy of Child and Adolescent Psychiatry* **26**: 546–53.

3   Beitchman J, Nair R, Clegg M, Ferguson B and Patel P (1986) Prevalence of psychiatric disorders in children with speech and language disorders. *Journal of the American Academy of Child and Adolescent Psychiatry* **26**: 546–53.

4   Beitchman JH, Brownlie EB, Inglis A, Wild J, Ferguson B, Schachter D, Lancee W, Wilson B and Mathews R (1996) Seven-year follow-up of speech/language impaired and control children: psychiatric outcome. *Journal of Child Psychology and Psychiatry* **37**(8): 961–70.

5   Beitchman JH, Hood J and Inglis A (1992) Familial transmission of speech and language impairment: a preliminary investigation. *Canadian Journal of Psychiatry* **37**(3): 151–6.

6   Leitao S, Hogben J and Fletcher J (1997) Phonological processing skills in speech and language impaired children. *European Journal of Disorders of Communication* **32**(2 Spec No): 91–111.

7   Paul R and Kellogg L (1997) Temperament in late talkers. *Journal of Child Psychology and Psychiatry* **38**(7): 803–11.

8   Paul R, Looney SS and Dahm PS (1991) Communication and socialization skills at ages 2 and 3 in 'late-talking' young children. *Journal of Speech and Hearing Research* **34**(4): 858–65.

9   Vallance DD, Cummings RL and Humphries T (1998) Mediators of the risk for problem behavior in children with language learning disabilities. *Journal of Learning Disabilities* **31**(2): 160–71.

10   Frisk M (1995) Mental and somatic health and social adjustment in ordinary school children during childhood and adolescence related to central nervous functions as expressed by a complex reaction time. *European Child and Adolescent Psychiatry* **4**(3): 197–208.

11   Carson DK, Klee T, Perry CK, Donaghy T and Muskina G (1997) Measures of language proficiency as predictors of behavioral difficulties, social and cognitive development in 2-year-old children. *Perceptual and Motor Skills* **84**(3 Pt 1): 923–30.

12   Beitchman JH, Wilson B, Brownlie EB, Walters H, Inglis A and Lancee W (1996) Long-term consistency in speech/language profiles: II. Behavioral, emotional, and social outcomes. *Journal of the American Academy of Child and Adolescent Psychiatry* **35**(6): 815–25.

13   Ornoy A, Uriel L and Tennenbaum A (1993) Inattention, hyperactivity and speech delay at 2–4 years of age as a predictor for ADD-ADHD syndrome. *Israel Journal of Psychiatry and Related Sciences* **30**(3): 155–63.

14   Tripp G and Luk SL (1997) The identification of pervasive hyperactivity: is clinic observation necessary? *Journal of Child Psychology and Psychiatry* **38**(2): 219–34.

15   Sandler AD, Hooper SR, Watson TE, Coleman WL, Footo M and Levine MD (1993) Talkative children: verbal fluency as a marker for problematic peer relationships in clinic-referred children with attention deficits. *Perceptual and Motor Skills* **76**(3 Pt 1): 943–51.

16   Baltaxe CA and Simmons JQ III (1995) Speech and language disorders in children and adolescents with schizophrenia. *Schizophrenia Bulletin* **21**(4): 677–92.

17   Steinhausen HC and Juzi C (1996) Elective mutism: an analysis of 100 cases. *Journal of American Academy of Child and Adolescent Psychiatry* **35**(5): 606–14.

18   Bishop DV and Adams C (1990) A prospective study of the relationship between specific language impairment, phonological disorders and reading retardation. *Journal of Child Psychology and Psychiatry* **31**(7): 1027–50.

19   Weismer SE (1991) Hypothesis-testing abilities of language-impaired children. *Journal of Speech Hearing Research* **34**(6): 1329–38.

20   Bishop DV (1990) Handedness, clumsiness and developmental language disorders. *Neuropsychologia* **28**(7): 681–90.

21   Owen SE and McKinlay IA (1997) Motor difficulties in children with developmental disorders of speech and language. *Child Care Health Development* **23**(4): 315–25.

22   Beitchman JH and Inglis A (1991) The continuum of linguistic dysfunction from pervasive developmental disorders to dyslexia. *Psychiatric Clinics of North America* **14**(1): 95–111.

23   Plante E (1991) MRI findings in the parents and siblings of specifically language-impaired boys. *Brain and Language* **41**(1): 67–80.

24   Plante E, Swisher L, Vance R, Rapcsak S, Thal D, Tobias S and Morrison D (1991)

Language and gesture in late talkers: a 1-year follow-up. *Journal of Speech and Hearing Research* **34**(3): 604–12.

25   Smith L, Ulvund SE and Lindemann R (1994) Very low birthweight infants (less than 1501 g) at double risk. *Journal of Development and Behavioural Pediatrics* **15**(1): 7–13.

26   Holdgrafer G (1995) Language abilities of neurologically normal and suspect preterm children now in preschool. *Perceptual and Motor Skills* **80**(3): 1251–62.

27   Hack M, Breslau N, Aram D, Weissman B, Klein N and Borawski-Clark E (1992) The effect of very low birth weight and social risk on neurocognitive abilities at school age. *Journal of Developmental and Behavioral Pediatrics* **13**(6): 412–20.

28   Anonymous (1992) The Scottish low birthweight study: II. Language attainment, cognitive status, and behavioural problems. *Archives of Disease in Childhood* **67**(6): 682–6.

29   Tallal P, Townsend J, Curtiss S and Wulfeck B (1991) Phenotypic profiles of language-impaired children based on genetic/family history. *Brain and Language* **41**(1): 81–95.

30   Eaves LJ, Silberg JL, Meyer JM *et al.* (1997) 2. Genetics and developmental psycho-pathology: the main effects of genes and environment on behavioural problems in the Virginia twin study of adolescent behavioural development. *Journal of Child Psychology and Psychiatry* **38**(8): 965–80.

31   Rutter M, Silberg J, O'Connor T and Simonoff E (1999) Genetics and Child Psychiatry: II Empirical Research Findings. *Journal of Child Psychology and Psychiatry* **40**(1): 19–55.

32   Rapin I (1996) Developmental language disorders: a clinical update *Journal of Child Psychology and Psychiatry* **37**: 643–56.

CHAPTER 13

Central Auditory Processing Disorders

James W Hall III

Over 40 years ago, Mylkebust[1] pointed out that hearing is a receptive sense ... and essential for normal language behaviour, and noted that the diagnostician of auditory problems in children has traditionally emphasised peripheral damage. It is desirable that he also include considerations of central damage. He also explained that central deafness (Central Auditory Processing Disorder) is a deficiency in transmitting auditory impulses to the higher brain centres while receptive aphasia (Language Disorder) is a deficiency in the interpretation of these impulses after they have been delivered. During this era, Bocca *et al.*[2] reported that surgically confirmed central auditory system pathology could be detected with sufficiently sensitive audiological procedures. These pioneering observations and studies have since been validated by many clinical investigations. There is now a variety of behavioural and electrophysiological techniques for the assessment of peripheral and central auditory system function, including Central Auditory Processing Disorders (CAPD). The term CAPD is used to describe a deficit in the perception or complete analysis of auditory information due to central auditory nervous system dysfunction, usually at the level of the cerebral cortex.[3,4] Central auditory processing takes place before language processing or comprehension.

Risk factors for auditory dysfunction

The assessment and management of auditory dysfunction, including CAPD, is described in Figure 13.1. For school-age children, comprehensive audiological assessment to rule out auditory dysfunction may be indicated by any of the following factors:

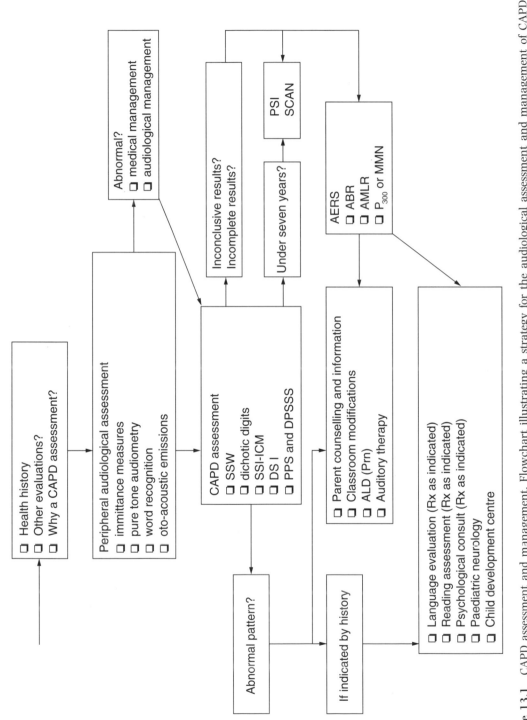

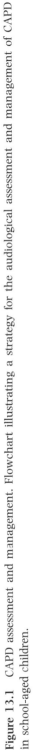

Figure 13.1 CAPD assessment and management. Flowchart illustrating a strategy for the audiological assessment and management of CAPD in school-aged children.

- parent or teacher concern about hearing or listening ability, such as difficulty following directions, distractibility in background noise, inattentiveness, short attention span, poor memory for auditory information and problems in spelling words that are dictated
- poor general academic performance despite normal hearing sensitivity, normal non-verbal intelligence, normal visual processing skills
- speech and language disorder
- reading disorder due to auditory-phonological deficits
- Attention Deficit Disorder (ADD) or Attention Deficit Hyperactivity Disorder (ADHD).

Assessment of auditory function

Peripheral auditory function

The first objective in the assessment of possible CAPD is to rule out a hearing loss caused by peripheral auditory dysfunction (*see also* Chapters 4 and 17). The peripheral auditory system is defined as the outer ear, the tympanic membrane and the middle ear, the inner ear (cochlea) and the eighth cranial (auditory) nerve. Audiology terms and procedures important in a discussion of CAPD assessment are defined in the Glossary. Pure tone audiometry is a measure of hearing sensitivity for pure tone stimuli (sinusoids) ranging in octave frequencies from 250 Hz up to 8000 Hz and, in CAPD assessment, also including 3000 Hz and 6000 Hz. Hearing test results, recorded as the threshold in decibels hearing level (dB HL) for these frequencies, are graphed on an audiogram. A young, perfectly normal person has hearing threshold levels of 0 dB HL across this frequency region. The clinically normal region on the audiogram, however, is from 0 to 20 dB HL.

Aural immittance measures are electrophysiological procedures that are often part of the basic audiometry test battery. Tympanometry, the most common of these, is a sensitive measure of tympanic membrane integrity and middle-ear function. Measurement of acoustic reflex activity, contractions of the middle-ear stapedial muscle to sound, is also clinically useful for estimating hearing sensitivity and differentiating among sites of auditory disorders within the middle ear, inner ear, eighth cranial nerve or auditory brainstem.[5] Aural immittance measures are particularly valuable with young or unco-operative children because they do not require a behavioural response, that is, close attention and a conscious response to sounds. The importance of middle-ear assessment is highlighted by recent investigations linking persistent conductive hearing loss due to chronic middle-ear disease to later auditory processing, language and reading deficits.[6]

Otoacoustic emissions (OAE), low intensity sounds detected within the external ear canal and produced by energy generated by outer hair cell movement within the inner ear in response to an acoustic stimulus, are an extremely sensitive measure of cochlear function.[7] There is now considerable research underway to document the effectiveness of OAE in the hearing screening of infants, and in other clinical applications in children and adults.

Speech audiometry is a measure of how well a person hears speech signals, such as words or sentences. Speech audiometry procedures are routinely used to estimate hearing sensitivity for words (the speech reception threshold which is reported in dB HL) or to roughly determine speech discrimination ability (word recognition scores which are reported in percent correct). Whenever possible, professionally produced (and commercially available) speech materials should be presented in prerecorded form, rather than spoken directly to the patient. There are a number of other, more sophisticated, speech audiometry test materials which are very useful in assessing central auditory processing abilities, as described below.

Central auditory function

The central auditory system consists of auditory regions within the brainstem and midbrain, the thalamus and the cerebral cortex, specifically Heschl's gyrus on the superior gyrus of the temporal lobe. Auditory evoked responses are electrophysiologic recordings of responses from within the auditory system that are activated by sounds.[8] The auditory brainstem response or ABR (also referred to as the brainstem auditory evoked response or BAER) is the most clinically applied auditory evoked response. The ABR is generated with very brief clicking sounds or tones and recorded with surface electrodes placed on the forehead and on the external ears. It is possible to present thousands of sound stimuli and to average reliable ABR waveforms in a matter of minutes. Extensive research has shown that the ABR wave components arise from the eighth cranial nerve and auditory regions in the brainstem. Analysis of the ABR waveform for high intensity stimuli provides information on cochlear and retrocochlear (eighth cranial nerve and brainstem) auditory function. Also, by systematically reducing the intensity level of the stimuli and analysing changes in the response, one can estimate a patient's hearing sensitivity level, at least for the high-frequency region. A major clinical advantage of ABR is that it can be reliably recorded from very young children, even newborn infants, and from children who are difficult to test by conventional audiometric techniques. ABR is not affected by patient state of arousal. In fact, because any patient movement produces muscle artefact that precludes valid recordings, children between the ages of six months and five years typically must be lightly sedated for ABR assessment. There is increasing interest in the application of cortical auditory evoked response techniques, including the P_{300} and the mismatch negativity (MMN) responses, for electrophysiological assessment of CAPD.[9–12] It is likely that the MMN will play an important role in the identification and confirmation of CAPD in select populations, such as infants or children who are difficult to test with behavioural techniques.

CAPD assessment is carried out with a battery of behavioural tests that have proven sensitivity to central auditory dysfunction (*see* Appendix to this chapter). If a peripheral hearing loss (unilateral or bilateral) is discovered, we initiate medical or audiological management and postpone further CAPD assessment. Typically, however, peripheral auditory function is normal and we proceed with the CAPD test battery. Behavioural CAPD tests are administered first. The overall goal is to measure reliable performance for each ear on a series of speech audiometry procedures, including a dichotic word test (dichotic digits and often the staggered spondaic word test), a dichotic sentence test (the dichotic sentence identification test or, for younger children with poor reading skills, the competing sentences test), a speech-in-competition test (the synthetic sentence identification test with an ipsilateral competing message) and reliable performance with binaural stimulation on one or more non-speech measures, such as the pitch pattern sequence and duration pattern tests. Auditory evoked responses are recorded if specifically requested by the referring person, or if we have any concerns about the reliability or questions about the interpretation of behavioural test performance. CAPD findings for children are analysed in comparison to age-corrected normative data. Minimal criteria for confirmation of CAPD are scores that are below the age-corrected normal region (below 2.5 standard deviations from the mean) for one or both ears for at least two different procedures in a child with normal peripheral auditory test findings.

Interpretation of CAPD tests is most straightforward when deficits are unilateral, which confirms that the patient understood the task and that the outcome was not due to a linguistic, cognitive or attention disorder. A pronounced unilateral abnormality, specifically a marked left ear deficit, is one of the most common patterns of CAPD test battery findings in our experience. Another rather definite CAPD test battery pattern is when reduced performance is apparent only on difficult (versus easier) portions of a test. This finding also implies an auditory versus linguistic, cognitive or strictly attentional explanation for the child's poor performance. Other important features of a clinically feasible CAPD test battery are: (i) resistance to the influence of even slight peripheral auditory dysfunction, (ii) the availability of adequate age-matched normative data, and (iii) professionally produced tape-recorded or compact disc-recorded test materials. Earlier concerns about the usefulness of CAPD assessment with rudimentary procedures lacking these criteria were justifiable.[13] Now, however, clinically feasible and commercially available procedures are available for young children, such as the Paediatric Speech Intelligibility (PSI) test,[14] as well as older children and adults.

Diagnosed or suspected ADD or ADHD is often cited as a reason for referral for CAPD.[15] Parents, and even professionals, seem to be unclear as to the definition of ADHD and its possible relation to language/learning disorders, as well as CAPD. Close examination of the diagnostic criteria for ADHD[16] fails to reveal a direct link between ADHD and CAPD. Although the attention-related criteria of ADHD sometimes involve communication activities (e.g. the child often does not seem to listen to what is being said, has difficulty following through on instructions from others), none of the criteria specifically addresses auditory skills or performance. Our experience clearly suggests that ADHD and CAPD are separate, although often co-existing, disorders.[17,18] There does appear, however, to be a relationship among certain CAPD measures and receptive language and reading skills.[19]

Implications for service delivery

Children with suspected communication difficulties need to be referred on to appropriate professionals either directly or via a paediatrician. However, even following such a referral and assessment by a multidisciplinary team, a diagnosis of CAPD is, as yet, relatively uncommon in the UK. Services for the assessment of CAPD are currently more advanced in their development in the USA than the UK.

US practice indicates that a diverse, individualised and multidisciplinary management strategy is usually necessary for children with confirmed CAPD,[4,20] the diagnosis usually being made at specialist hearing and balance centres. Following diagnosis and based on the pattern of CAPD results, and the suspicion or presence of a variety of medical, educational, emotional, and/or speech and language disorders, any of the following general referrals may be appropriate for subsequent intervention (*see also* Figure 13.1):

- a speech and language therapist for evaluation and/or therapy
- a neuropsychologist for evaluation
- a paediatric neurologist for neurodiagnosis and medical treatment as indicated
- a reading specialist for assessment and/or instruction utilising a multisensory non-phonetic approach appropriate for children with auditory processing and phonologic decoding deficits[21–23]
- otolaryngologist for medical or surgical treatment.

Audiological management may include:

- parent and teacher counselling and detailed information regarding characteristics and management of children with CAPD
- modification of teaching strategies at school and at home the use of earplugs during deskwork and homework to attenuate background sounds
- aural rehabilitation designed to develop auditory and listening skills with, for example, an intensive computer-based programme of auditory skill development, such as Fast ForWord or Earobics[23–25]
- the use of an assistive listening device (ALD) by teacher and child to enhance the signal-to-noise relationship in the classroom. The ALD consists of a directional microphone and transmitter worn by the speaker, and a receiver coupled either to some type of earphone which is worn by the listener (personal ALD), or to an array of loudspeakers placed at specific locations in a room (classroom ALD).

There is mounting evidence that this latter management strategy is beneficial in the classroom setting for certain students.[26–29]

Thorough audiological assessment of children with suspected or confirmed communication problems contributes to complete diagnosis and appropriate and effective management.

References

1 Mylkebust HR (1954) *Auditory Disorders in Children: a manual for differential diagnosis.* Grune & Stratton, New York.

2 Bocca E, Calearo C and Cassinari V (1954) A new method for testing hearing in temporal lobe tumors. *Acta Otolaryngologica* **44**: 219–21.

3 Jerger J, Johnson K, Jerger S, Coker N, Pirozzolo F and Gray L (1991) Central auditory processing disorder: a case study. *Journal of the American Academy of Audiology* **2**: 36–54.

4 Chermak GD and Musiek FE (1997) *Central Auditory Processing Disorders: new perspectives.* Singular Publishing Group, San Diego and London.

5 Hall JW III (1984) The acoustic reflex in central auditory dysfunction. In: ML Pinheiro and FE Musiek (eds) *Assessment of Central Auditory Dysfunction: foundations and clinical correlates*, pp. 103–30. Williams & Wilkins, Baltimore.

6 Gravel JS and Wallace IF (1996) Early otitis media, auditory abilities, and educational risk. *American Journal of Speech-Language Pathology* **4**: 89–94.

7 Hall JW III, Chase PA, Baer JE and Schwaber MK (1994) Clinical application of otoacoustic emissions: what do we know about factors influencing measurement and analysis? *Otolaryngology – Head and Neck Surgery* **110**: 22–38.

8 Hall JW III (1992) *Handbook of Auditory Evoked Responses.* Allyn & Bacon, Needham, MA.

9 Jirsa RE (1992) The clinical utility of the P_3 AERP in children with auditory processing disorders. *Journal of Speech and Hearing Research* **35**: 903–12.

10 Musiek FM, Baran JA and Pinheiro ML (1992) P300 results in patients with lesions of the auditory areas of the cerebrum. *Journal of the American Academy of Audiology* **3**: 5–15.

11 Kraus N and McGee TJ (1994) Mismatch negativity in the assessment of central auditory function. *American Journal of Audiology: A Journal of Clinical Practice* **3**: 39–51.

12 Kraus N, McGee TJ, Carrell TD, Zecker SG, Nicol TG and Koch DB (1996) Auditory neurophysiologic responses and discrimination deficits in children with learning problems. *Science* **273**: 971–3.

13 Kamhi AG and Beasley DA (1985) Central auditory processing disorder: is it a meaningful construct or a twentieth century unicorn? *Journal of Childhood Communication Disorders* **9**: 5–13.

14   Jerger S, Martin RC and Jerger J (1987) Specific auditory perceptual dysfunction in a
     learning disabled child. *Ear and Hearing* **8**: 78–86.

15   Gascon G, Johnson R and Burd L (1986) Central auditory processing and attention
     deficit disorder. *Journal of Childhood Neurology* **1**: 27–33.

16   American Psychiatric Association (1987) *Diagnostic and Statistical Manual of Mental
     Disorders (DSM-III-R-1987)* (3rd edn). APA, Washington DC.

17   Hall JW III and Mueller HG III (1997) *Audiologists' Desk Reference*, vol I. Singular
     Publishing Group, San Diego.

18   Chermak GD, Hall JW III and Musiek FE (1998) Differentiation of CAPD and ADHD.
     Journal of the American Academy of Audiology (in press).

19   Keith RW and Novak KK (1984) Relationships between tests of central auditory function
     and receptive language. *Seminars in Hearing* **5**: 243–50.

20   Chermak GD and Musiek FE (1992) Managing central auditory processing disorders in
     children and youth. *American Journal of Audiology* **1**: 61–5.

21   Lindamood P, Bell N and Lindamood P (1992) Issues in phonological awareness assess-
     ment. *Annals of Dyslexia* **42**: 242–59.

22   Shaywitz SE, Shaywitz A, Fletcher J and Shupack H (1986) Evaluation of school perfor-
     mance: dyslexia and attention deficit disorder. *Pediatrician* **13**: 96–107.

23   Wright BA, Lombardino LJ, King WM, Puranik CS, Leonard CM and Merzenich MM
     (1997) Deficits in auditory temporal and spectral resolution in language-impaired
     children. *Nature* **387**: 176–8.

24   Merzenich MM, Jenkins WM, Johnston P, Schreiner C, Miller SL and Tallal P (1996)
     Temporal processing deficits of language-learning impaired children ameliorated by
     training. *Science* **271**: 77–80.

25   Tallal P, Miller SL, Bedi G, Byrna G, Wang X, Nagarajan SS, Schreiner C, Jenkins WM
     and Merzenich MM (1996) Language comprehension in language-learning impaired
     children improved with acoustically modified speech. *Science* **271**: 81–4.

26   Blake R, Field B, Foster C, Platt F and Wertz P (1991) Effect of FM auditory trainers on
     attending behaviors of learning-disabled children. *Language, Speech, and Hearing Services
     in Schools* **22**: 111–14.

27   Flexer C and Savage H (1992) Using an ALD in speech-language assessment and
     training. *The Hearing Journal* **45**: 26–35.

28   Hawkins DB (1984) Comparisons of speech recognition in noise by mildly-to-moderately
     hearing-impaired children using hearing aids and FM systems. *Journal of Speech and
     Hearing Disorders* **49**: 409–18.

29   Mueller HG III and Hall JW III (1998) *Audiologists' Desk Reference*, vol II. Singular
     Publishing Group, San Diego.

30   Jerger J and Jerger S (1975) Clinical validity of central auditory tests. *Scandinavian Audiology* **4**: 147–63.

31   Pinheiro ML and Musiek FM (eds) (1984) *Assessment of Central Auditory Dysfunction*. Williams and Wilkins, Baltimore.

32   Hall JW III, Baer JE, Prentice C *et al.* (1993) Central auditory processing disorder: a case report. *Seminars in Hearing* **14**: 254–64.

Appendix Test battery used for assessment of peripheral auditory function and central auditory processing disorders (CAPD)

Procedure	Description	Reference
Peripheral auditory function		
Pure tone audiometry	Hearing thresholds for octave frequencies of 250 through 8000 Hz	17
Word recognition	Perception of single syllable words presented in quiet	17
Aural immittance measures	Tympanometric measurement of middle ear function and acoustic reflex thresholds for ipsilateral and contralateral signals	5,17
Otoacoustic emissions (OAE)	Electrophysiological measure of cochlear function	7
CAPD: behavioural audiometry		
Children 8 years and older		
Dichotic digits	Different pairs of numbers presented simultaneously to each ear	10
Staggered spondaic word test	Two-syllable words presented simultaneously to each ear	10,30,31
Dichotic sentence identification	Different non-meaningful sentences presented to each ear	32
Synthetic sentence identification with ipsilateral competing message (SSI-ICM)	Non-meaningful sentences presented to one ear with meaningful story in the same ear at different intensity levels	30,32
Competing sentences test	Sentences presented to each ear with attention to one ear	10
Pitch pattern sequence (PPS) test	Randomised sequence of three tones of two frequencies	10,31
Duration pattern sequence (DPS) test	Randomised sequence of three tones of two durations	4
Children less than 8 years		
Paediatric Speech Intelligibility	Single words and sentences presented with a competing message at varying levels of difficulty; performance adjusted for language age	3,14
PSI test		
SCAN	A screening procedure consisting of three subtests (filtered words, auditory figure-ground and competing words)	19
Goldman-Fristoe-Woodcock Test auditory discrimination	Auditory Discrimination assessed with picture-pointing task in quiet and in noise	

Appendix Continued

Procedure	Description	Reference
CAPD: auditory evoked responses		
Auditory brainstem response (ABR)	Electrophysiological measure of eighth cranial nerve and auditory brainstem	8
Auditory middle latency response (AMLR)	Electrophysiological measure of primary auditory cortex function	8
Auditory P$_{300}$ response	Electrophysiological measure of hippocampal and auditory cortex function	8
Mismatch negativity response (MMN)	Electrophysiological measure of auditory cortex function (does not require subject attention or participation)	11
All behavioural CAPD test materials are available on analog or digital tape or CD format from:	AUDiTEC of St Louis, 2515 S. Big Bend Blvd. St Louis, Missouri, USA 63143-2105 (Tel: 800-669-9065; Fax: 314-781-4946) Precision Acoustics, Vancouver, Washington, USA	VA Medical Centre CD 1.0 and 1.1. Available from: Richard Wilson. Audiology-126, VA Medical Centre, Mountain Home, TN 37684, USA

CHAPTER 14

Cerebral palsy

Helen Cockerill

Case study

At the age of 12 months Liam was referred by his GP to the speech and language therapy department of a specialist centre for cerebral palsy for advice on feeding. He had been diagnosed as having athetoid cerebral palsy by his local hospital paediatrician and was not yet able to sit independently. He had a history of feeding difficulties, poor weight gain and failure to develop chewing skills. Liam presented as sociable child, with apparently good understanding and an interest in age-appropriate toys. He could only produce undifferentiated vowel sounds and was not babbling. By the age of 15 months, when presented with two objects he could make clear choices by reaching and eye-pointing. Because of the high risk of speechlessness, an augmentative system of communication was introduced. A chart with symbols and photographs, representing the things Liam might want to communicate about, enabled him to ask for objects which were not physically present. This helped to fill the gap between what he wanted to communicate and what he was able to convey through non-verbal signals.

Liam initially received services from a multidisciplinary team (physiotherapy, occupational therapy, speech and language therapy, psychology, paediatric neurology) on an outpatient basis, accompanied by his parents, and then in a specialist nursery from the age of two and a half years.

By the age of seven Liam was a multimodal communicator: he had a small repertoire of spoken words or initial sounds, e.g. 'b' for ball; a range of non-verbal communication including pointing, eye-gaze and facial expressions; a number of manual signs; a 400-symbol communication chart; and he was learning to use a voice-output communication aid (VOCA). He could build sentences using symbols and could combine symbols to create words which were not on his chart, e.g. 'wind' + 'machine' + 'hair' for 'hairdryer'. He used an expanded keyboard to write on the computer. He moved around using a walking frame or bunny-hopping, taking his communication chart with him. Liam's family had requested direct work on his articulation for speech but this proved a frustrating experience and Liam refused to continue.

Liam then moved to another school for children with physical disabilities. Here a greater emphasis was placed on speech, within the context of an adapted conductive education curriculum, and Liam had limited access to technology for communication or education. He continued to need his chart to communicate about events outside the immediate situation and to convey abstract thoughts. After two years he moved again to a residential school where his parents felt he would have access to the technology required to achieve his educational and communicative potential.

Currently, at age 14, Liam is embarking on a range of GCSE courses. His speech has improved to the extent that he is intelligible to his family and friends. When communicating with less familiar people and for addressing groups of children (e.g. in assembly or class discussions) Liam uses a computer-based communication aid, mounted on his wheelchair, on which he types messages, facilitated by predictive typing software, or chooses pre-stored messages which are produced via a speech synthesiser.

Prevalence

There are no figures concerning the prevalence of speech and communication difficulties in children with cerebral palsy, but it is known to be high. Incidence of cerebral palsy is estimated at around 2.0–2.5 per 1000 live births. There is evidence suggesting diminished incidence in the 1960s, possibly due to improvement in neonatal care, with a subsequent rise during the 1970s and 1980s, probably reflecting increased survival of very low birth weight infants (for a review of incidence, aetiology, classification and clinical manifestations of cerebral palsy *see* Aicardi and Bax[1]).

Aetiology

Cerebral palsy has no single cause or consistent set of symptoms. It is defined as a disorder of posture and movement resulting from a non-progressive abnormality of the immature brain. Increasingly, research is pointing to problems during intra-uterine development and prematurity as being the most common aetiologies, rather than perinatal causes (such as anoxia at birth) as had been assumed hitherto.

Cerebral palsy is often classified according to the predominant pattern of motor impairment. Differences in classification between studies have made it difficult to establish the relative proportions of the types of cerebral palsy, and to link these to speech and language difficulties. However, certain patterns of features are often noted, and may indicate likely communication difficulties. Children with spastic hemiplegia (unilateral distribution) which accounts for approximately 30% of the cerebral palsy population, and spastic diplegia (lower limbs more affected than upper limbs), estimated at 40% of the population, may have epilepsy, mild to moderate learning difficulties, visual impairment or visuo-spatial problems. Speech is rarely affected, although a small minority may have severe bulbar difficulties. Language delays or disorders may reflect the degree of learning disability. These groups may also have specific literacy difficulties and so require technology to support written communication.

Children with spastic quadriplegia (affecting all four limbs, the trunk, oral and pharyngeal muscles), who account for around 8% of the population, are often totally dependent. They frequently have severe learning difficulties, seizures and sensory impairments, which in combination with bulbar problems lead to profound communication impairments. Dyskinetic cerebral palsy (approximately 10%) is characterised by fluctuating tone throughout the body, often with involuntary movements. Bulbar problems are very common, often evidenced by early feeding difficulties, leading to dysarthric speech. The majority of children have normal intelligence or mild learning difficulties. Epilepsy or visual problems are not common.

Children with ataxia (around 7–15%) have difficulties with balance, leading to a wide-based gait in those who walk, and intention tremor. Some degree of intellectual impairment may occur, but severe learning difficulties are rare. A small number of children will have dysarthric or dyspraxic speech, sometimes with abnormal voice quality, resulting in severe communication difficulties.

Extreme caution must be exercised in predicting which children are likely to have communication difficulties merely on the basis of a given diagnostic label. This is partly due to difficulties of diagnosis and classification in cerebral palsy (with a proportion being described as having a 'mixed' type), but also to the complex interplay of cognitive, motor and sensory factors in the development of speech and language.

Identification

Many infants with cerebral palsy will be known to medical services from the early months of life. This may be due to prematurity, medical problems in the neonatal period, early onset of seizure disorders, etc. Some babies will be referred to speech and language therapists because of feeding difficulties and failure to thrive, particularly if there are hospital-based services. These infants should be referred on to community services on discharge from hospital. However, for many children with cerebral palsy where there is no clear aetiology, the neonatal periods and early months of life may be uneventful. Parents frequently describe a gradual realisation that their babies are developing slowly in terms of motor milestones or showing atypical behaviours, such as using only one side of the body to reach or excessive drooling. Many families undergo periods of great anxiety if their observations are not investigated and they receive inappropriate assurances that there is no cause for concern. Experiences of the period leading up to diagnosis and the way in which parents are told about their child's condition can affect their relationship with medical and therapy services for years to come. It is not uncommon for parents to repeatedly retell those experiences with feelings of sadness and anger.

Referral

It can be a difficult task to identify which children will not develop speech, but children with early feeding problems and abnormal bulbar signs, such as excessive drooling or opening of the mouth, are likely to be at risk. Children with seizure disorders, sensory or cognitive impairments will show delayed or atypical communication development which may or may not relate to the degree of motor disability. Assessment of the complex factors contributing to the development of communication requires a co-ordinated, specialist team approach. Core members of the team will include a paediatrician or paediatric neurologist, physiotherapist, occupational therapist and psychologist in addition to a speech and language therapist (for a review of multidisciplinary services required by children with cerebral palsy *see* McCarthy and Finnie[2,3]). Most health districts have a preschool special needs therapy team who can provide community services, often on a domiciliary basis, to young children and their families. These are often based in child development centres and have established links with specialist clinics, such as dietetics, audiology and ophthalmology, or hospital-based services. Some children will have ongoing medical needs which require inpatient investigations or treatment, and community nursing services. For many families there will be a need for social work and respite care. In collecting information about a child's condition which will have relevance for the development of communication skills, and in implementing any intervention, liaison between professionals and with the family is essential.

The contexts in which communication takes place and the range of communication partners with whom the child interacts are of the utmost relevance when planning communication goals and means to attain them. As the child grows these will extend beyond the immediate family to nursery and school settings. There has been an increasing move towards integration of children with disabilities into mainstream schools, usually with individual support, although a substantial number of parents and professionals continue to feel that special schools offer the best option for some children. As children move into school the emphasis of communication intervention shifts to enabling the child to access the curriculum and convey information, in addition to expressing basic needs and interacting socially.

Implications for service delivery

As illustrated by the case study above, early intervention for children with cerebral palsy may focus on the development of feeding skills. Historically it was considered that oral-motor patterns for feeding lay the foundations for speech, but the link between eating and speaking is not clear. Currently a more holistic approach prevails in which consideration is given to maintaining safety (i.e. reducing the risk of aspiration), optimising nutrition and promoting health. The aims of intervention are the reduction of anxiety for parents and children and the development of communication within the context of family meals, in addition to stimulating efficient oral-motor skills.

Increasingly the importance of working in partnership with parents to set goals and create environments which foster communication has been recognised. The multidisciplinary team must consider how children with physical disabilities are making sense of their environment, particularly if the children have sensory impairments, and work with parents to develop strategies which facilitate comprehension. The use of specialist seating and standing frames and adapted toys can give a child access to play materials and promote early learning and communication.

Speech and language therapists are particularly involved in helping parents to identify and develop early communication signals. The motor and sensory impairments of children with cerebral palsy can give rise to limited or atypical movements, creating difficulties in the preverbal stages of communication development where parents are interpreting the actions of infants as having communicative intent, e.g. crying means hunger, looking at an object indicates interest, etc. It is through the consistent responses of parents that babies develop a sense of their own ability to influence the world around them and build up a repertoire of meaningful signals. For children with cerebral palsy, movement patterns can appear random and undirected, the ability to use eye-gaze may be inhibited by poor head control and reaching is often limited by postural control. The speed of movements and cognitive processing can result in mistiming of responses and consequent misinterpretation of intent. Any symbolic communication system, whether speech, manual signing, graphic symbols or electronic communication aids, must be based on unambiguous, consistent and intelligible signals between the child and communication partner to avoid frustration or the common problem of passivity on the part of the child and overdirectiveness of the parents. Assessment of a child's skills in this area, and the monitoring and shaping of the home and school environments to foster intentional communication can be a process which is carried out over several years, particularly for children with multiple disabilities.

For a minority of children it may be appropriate to work directly on speech. However, there is limited evidence that articulation drills carry over into speech. Such intervention is likely to be of no benefit to children with severe dysarthria who have very limited speech. Children who are using speech as their main mode of communication may benefit from articulation therapy as they get older and are able to think about both what they are saying, and how they are producing speech. Providing postural support through adaptive seating can facilitate improved head and neck alignment and more efficient breathing patterns which in turn can improve voice, speech production and phrasing. Many adults with severe physical disabilities are understandably angry about the time spent struggling to practise oral movements during their childhood, time and effort which could have been more profitably directed towards developing effective augmentative systems of communication including symbol charts and VOCAs.

Augmentative and alternative methods of communication (AAC)[4,5] should be introduced to children considered at risk of speechlessness at an early age. Waiting to see if speech develops can lead to frustration and reduced opportunities for language learning. A total communication approach is recommended, i.e. developing all possible modes of communication, including manual signs, graphic symbol and VOCAs. While limited fine motor skills may preclude the development of signing as the primary expressive system, such an unaided system of communication can be very effective with familiar communication partners and as a supplement to dysarthric speech. Successful introduction of graphic symbols systems such as Bliss, Picture Communication Symbols or Rebus will depend on skilled assessment of vision, learning and physical accessing (how the child will select the symbols, e.g. through pointing or eye-gaze), in addition to creating opportunities within the environment for communication through aided systems. It will take years to develop a system which reflects the child's changing communication needs and there are many practical difficulties to be surmounted in selecting vocabulary and producing chart systems.

The development of electronic VOCAs over the past 15 years has enabled many children who have limited speech to communicate complex ideas to peers and unfamiliar partners, to communicate over a distance via telephone or computer, and to access the school curriculum. Specialist teams, usually based in Communication Aid Centres or special schools, are necessary to make appropriate recommendations regarding equipment and training. Funding of such equipment, training and ongoing support remains a difficult issue. The variety of funding sources includes GP budgets, speech and language therapy departments, education, joint funding between health, education and social services, private funding by families or charities, or through court awards. Hi-tech equipment will only be useful if carefully matched to the needs and abilities of the child, and supported by the child's environment, which has implications for delivery of therapy and educational services to families of children with cerebral palsy.

Summary

- Cerebral palsy is a life-long condition with the needs and priorities of individuals changing over time, requiring medical involvement at different stages in the life span.
- A multidisciplinary approach is necessary for the assessment and management of communication difficulties in children with cerebral palsy.
- The prognosis for speech can be uncertain, therefore early referral for speech and

language therapy is recommended for children with feeding or other bulbar problems, rather than a wait-and-see approach. The early introduction of AAC systems, when a child is considered at risk of speechlessness, will not inhibit speech development.

- Motor impairment and associated disorders, such as visual impairment, learning disability, epilepsy, etc., will have a major impact on the development of communication skills between children and their parents.
- Communication skills are central to educational and social achievement and emotional development for children with cerebral palsy.
- A total communication approach where several modes of communication are involved, e.g. speech, signing, symbols and voice output communication aids may be necessary for effective and efficient communication.

References

1 Aicardi J and Bax M (1998) Cerebral palsy. In: J Aicardi (ed) *Diseases of the Nervous System in Childhood* (2nd edn). MacKeith Press, Cambridge.

2 McCarthy GT (1992) *Physical Disability in Childhood: an inter disciplinary approach to management*. Churchill Livingstone, Edinburgh.

3 Finnie NR (1997) *Handling the Young Child with Cerebral Palsy at Home*. Butterworth-Heineman, Oxford.

4 Millar S and Wilson A (1996) *Communication Without Speech*. CALL Centre (an accessible introduction to augmentative and alternative communication, available from the CALL Centre 0131 650 4269).

5 Glennen SL (1997) *Handbook of Augmentative and Alternative Communication*. Crocus Books, London.

CHAPTER 15

Nasal emission, cleft lip and palate

Timothy Milward

An unrepaired cleft palate causes nasal emission (also known as nasal escape) and hypernasality. Nasal emission refers to abnormal and inappropriate escape of air through the nose during speech due to inadequate closure of the soft palate against the posterior pharyngeal wall. The effect of nasal emission is to make speech muffled and indistinct, and, if severe enough, unintelligible. Hypernasality or hypernasal resonance refers to excess voice resonating in the nasal space due to inadequate velopharyngeal closure during speech.

In the UK these speech problems are dealt with by the various cleft lip and palate teams set up across the country. The usual composition of such a team is:

- Plastic surgeon (usually the team leader), who carries out corrective surgery.
- Orthodontist, who will correct any teeth malpositioning, some of which may affect speech by interfering with the placement of the tongue when articulating some sounds.
- ENT surgeon, who deals with any problems of hearing deficiency, particularly associated with glue ear.
- Specialist speech and language therapist, who assesses the speech, offers therapy when appropriate and advises on the need for surgical intervention.
- Oral and maxillofacial surgeon, who will carry out later corrective work to the bony facial skeleton.

Many teams also incorporate:

- restorative dentist
- community paediatrician
- child psychologist

- clinical geneticist
- clinical nurse specialist.

The majority of children with potential hypernasality and nasal emission are those born with a cleft palate who will have had it repaired between six and 12 months of age (depending on the team's protocol). Approximately 15% of these will need further surgery between the ages of four and six because of persisting hypernasality and nasal emission. A further group of children may be referred for their first appointment, up to the age of six, on account of late detection of hypernasality or nasal emission.

This group requiring late surgery are comprised of the following subgroups:

- nasal escape following cleft palate repair (in approximately 15% of repairs) (60%)
- submucous cleft palate (difficult to diagnose at birth) (5%)
- an anatomically normal soft palate but with nasal emission (20%)
- a soft palate with poor function due to neuromuscular problems (15%).

Children with a submucous cleft palate benefit from a repair of the split levator palati muscles by various techniques, whereas the other three groups are best treated with a pharyngoplasty after full investigation and a trial of speech and language therapy. Pharyngoplasty is an operation designed to narrow the velopharyngeal isthmus to assist closure of the velopharyngeal sphincter and thus correct the hypernasality or nasal emission. In our experience this operation improves the speech in about 90% of patients.

Prevalence

Cleft lip and palate occurs in 1 in 600 live births. Approximately 305 of these have a cleft lip only. Those with a cleft palate with or without a cleft lip occur in approximately 1 in 1000 live births.

Aetiology

In cleft lip, with or without cleft palate, the inherited element is strong. The male incidence is twice the female incidence. If a parent only or a sibling only is affected then there is a 4% incidence of a new baby being born with a cleft. If the parent and sibling are both affected then the incidence rises to 12%. In isolated cleft palate the inherited element is weak. The female incidence is twice that of the male incidence.

Though the majority of babies with cleft lip and palate are not syndromic there are a number of described complex syndromes in association with isolated cleft palate, e.g. Velo-Cardio-Facial syndrome. As time goes by the detection of syndromes associated with isolated cleft palate is increasing to the extent that it is good practice to carry out chromosomal analysis on all babies born with isolated cleft palate. The Pierre Robin sequence (a combination of a cleft palate and a small lower jaw) is not inherited in the vast majority of cases. It is thought to be a developmental abnormality relating to the fetal compression in the uterus, perhaps due to oligohydramnios compressing the chin against the chest restricting growth of the lower jaw and also forcing the tongue into the nasal cavity, preventing natural fusion of the palatal shelves leading to cleft palate. This theory is supported by the fact that in the majority of Pierre Robin children, the projection of the lower jaw becomes normal in due course.

Identification and referral

Before the development of speech, if any abnormal appearance of the palate or the uvula or any invisible but palpable notch in the back of the hard palate is detected, the general practitioner should refer the baby to the Cleft team for assessment. After speech development has started, speech problems, especially poor intelligibility or air leaking down the nose, should be reported to the GP who will consider referral to the community speech and language therapy team for assessment and clarification. He or she may well request a second opinion from the cleft team speech and language therapist who has special expertise in differentiating between the many speech problems and identifying those that are related to soft palate malfunction.

If in doubt, refer to your local cleft team. It is better not to tell parents that their child 'will grow out of it' before having it checked out with the team.

A recent government report by the Clinical Standards Advisory Group (CSAG) has made radical recommendations about how cleft palate teams should be organised in the country, recommending a major reduction in the number of teams into fewer but larger specialised units. This reorganisation will be occurring over the next few years.

Case study 1: Primary cleft of the palate

Debbie was born with a wide cleft of the hard and soft palate. The surgeon and speech and language therapist visited her and her parents in the maternity unit within 12 hours of being notified of her birth, according to local guidelines. The background to the cleft was explained, as well as the need for an operation and simple details about it. They were given a leaflet to support what was said to them. A firm date was fixed for the operation to repair the soft palate at six months of age. The speech and language therapist also gave them the helpline number to provide support for feeding. The team orthodontist was contacted to visit within 24 hours to discuss the fitting of a feeding plate because the cleft was so wide. In most cleft babies, however, feeding is satisfactory, though slow, using a squeezy bottle with or without an enlarged hole in the teat. The team speech and language therapist has a range of bottles and teats as babies differ to some degree in what suits them best. At one month of age Debbie and her parents met the team again in the fortnightly cleft clinic and the operation date was confirmed. At six months of age the repair was carried out. Debbie spent three nights in hospital with her mother sleeping in the same room. This is usually the maximum length of admission. Feeding by bottle was commenced on the evening of surgery.

Nowadays great stress is put on minimal trauma from the cleft palate surgery. There is no doubt that the more scarring there is from surgery the more chance of restriction of growth of the upper jaw. Debbie's surgery was a Von Langenbeck repair using lateral tension-relieving cuts on the outside edge of the hard palate as the cleft was so wide. In many patients, narrower clefts the repair can be done just incising the edges of the cleft itself with no other cuts. Great attention was also paid to freeing up the levator palati muscles and repositioning them at the back of the soft palate. This is thought to improve the function of the soft palate significantly.

Debbie then attended the cleft clinic regularly with assessment by the speech and language therapist at each visit until normal mature speech was established aged five. In parallel she was seen by the ENT surgeon who specialises in cleft children's ears as they have a greatly increased risk of glue ear. This is due to malformation of the Eustachian tube from an abnormal tensor palati muscle. She needed grommets in her eardrums to restore normal hearing. Normal hearing is very important as children with hearing difficulties have problems reproducing normal speech sounds.

Between 15 and 20% of cleft palate children develop some degree of hypernasality and nasal emission after cleft palate repair requiring some form of pharyngoplasty.

Case study 2: Submucous cleft palate

Harry was not noted to have any abnormalities at birth. However, when he started speaking his parents noted that his speech was odd, quite unlike his elder sister at the same age. They found him hard to understand. He also became frustrated trying to make himself understood. His GP suggested a 'wait-and-see' policy for a while but eventually referred him to the speech and language therapy department when he was aged four. The community speech and language therapist diagnosed a limited speech sound system due to nasal escape and hyper-nasal resonance and noted on examining his palate that he had a bifid uvula. Oral assess-ment revealed an invisible bony notch on the hard palate leading to a confident diagnosis of a submucous cleft palate. On the advice of the therapist Harry was referred to the cleft palate team.

Harry was assessed by the surgeon and specialist speech and language therapist. The diagnosis was confirmed and the need for surgery established following a detailed speech assessment. Surgery was designed to repair the cleft levator palati muscle which was hidden under intact soft palate mucosa. Following the repair the hypernasality and nasal emission were reduced. Harry underwent a course of speech therapy at his local clinic. Within 18 months normal speech was established.

Because of difficulty in getting a view of the uvula in a newborn baby these clefts are sometimes missed at birth by paediatricans. Consideration may need to be given to make feeling for a notch in the back of the hard palate part of the basic neonatal examination as it is a far more reliable test of submucous cleft than trying to visualise the uvula. When submucous cleft is diagnosed at birth, because 50% of these children do not develop related speech problems, the child is followed up in the cleft clinic to assess whether speech is affected rather than operating at birth. Surgery is typically only offered between three and four years if an abnormality that does not respond to speech and language therapy is identified.

Case history 3: Non-cleft palate nasal escape

Stephen's speech had been late in developing. He was aged four before he could say sentences. His speech never sounded normal. His parents first took him to the GP, who referred him to the speech and language therapy department. The community therapist felt the problem might be associated with enlarged tonsils and adenoids and he was referred on to the ENT surgeon. Aged four he had his tonsils and adenoids removed and grommets inserted because of reduced hearing acuity, but this produced no significant improvement in his speech. Further assessment by the community speech and language therapist suggested that there was nasal emission during speech and the specialist therapist from the cleft team was asked for a second opinion, following which he was referred to the whole team when he was five and a half years. Assessment of his speech showed sound system problems, marked nasal escape of air accompanying many consonants and hypernasality. His speech was very difficult to understand. Examination of his palate showed no obvious sign of submucous cleft palate or cleft palate.

The initial plan was:

1 A six-week course of intensive speech therapy.
2 Assessment of the palatal movements on lateral videofluoroscopy. This is a technique where a video is taken of a moving X-ray of the child's soft palate during speech. Analysis of the film with soundtrack can give a clear idea as to how normal the palate movements are.

Speech and language therapy treatment had no effect on the quality of Stephen's speech. The lateral videofluoroscopy showed that the soft palate had very poor muscular movement and had failed to reach the posterior pharyngeal wall and therefore close off the nose. At a further consultation with the parents this was explained to them and a pharyngoplasty operation advised with the aim of narrowing the velopharyngeal opening to help him achieve closure and eliminate nasal escape.

When Stephen was six he underwent surgery. A dynamic pharyngoplasty (Orticochea type) was carried out.[1] In this method the ends of the palatopharyngeus muscles in the side of the pharynx are joined to make a muscular sphincter around the velopharyngeal isthmus. The muscles were noted to be of poor quality and scarred by the previous tonsillectomy. There were reservations therefore about the likely outcome of surgery. Despite these reservations assessment of Stephen's speech showed steady improvement of quality and intelligibility. At a final consultation 14 months after the operation no further nasal emission was detected. The sound system problems resolved after further therapy at the local clinic.

Summary

- If any abnormality of the palate or the uvula is noted by the parents or by primary healthcare professionals this should be reported to the GP with a suggestion that the local cleft palate team might give an opinion on this.
- If, after the development of speech, problems are noted, particularly with the intelligibility of the speech, then this should be reported by the primary healthcare professionals to the GP. The local speech and language therapy department will offer advice on the actual diagnosis of the speech problem. They will have links with the local cleft palate speech and language therapist who specialises in speech disorders related to palatal dysfunction. The team therapist can then undertake more detailed assessment and suggest appropriate management.

Reference

1   James NK, Twist M, Turner M and Milward T (1996) An audit of velopharyngeal incompetence by the Orticochea pharyngoplasty. *British Journal of Plastic Surgery* **49**: 197–201.

Further reading

Wyatt R, Sell D and Russell J *et al.* (1996) Cleft palate speech dissected – a review of current knowledge and analysis. *British Journal of Plastic Surgery* **49**: 143–9.

CHAPTER 16

Dyslexia

Susie Hoddell

'Dyslexia' has often, over the years, been dismissed as a term used by pushy, middle-class parents to explain the difficulties their child is experiencing with reading and spelling at school. Even today some education authorities in the UK still refuse to recognise this problem. Dyslexia was first acknowledged towards the end of the last century, when it was felt to be the result of visual processing difficulties. It is only in the past 20 years that research has pointed to a specific reading and spelling difficulty resulting from an underlying language deficit. These difficulties may be compounded by other factors, such as general intellectual ability, visual problems and motivation, but are not felt to be as a direct result of them. The implications for a child with dyslexia are not confined to reading and spelling and therefore early identification and appropriate intervention are crucial in minimising the long-term effects on a child. Dyslexia is a developmental disorder and a dyslexic child will continue to experience difficulties, although these may change, through into adulthood. Dyslexia cannot be 'cured' and therefore any intervention is aimed at reducing long-term effects rather than providing a cure. The incidence of dyslexia is reported as being between 4% (British Dyslexia Association) and 20%.[1]

Case study

Ben was referred for assessment by his mother, who felt that although he was generally very creative and imaginative, and capable in areas such as drawing, construction tasks and computer games, he was struggling at school with reading and spelling. This was borne out by teachers' reports as well as comments that he was 'lazy' and 'not very clever'. Ben's mother was particularly concerned about his increasing lack of confidence.

Background

Ben had an uneventful birth and all his milestones were normal. He is generally a healthy child and has not suffered any serious illnesses or ear infections. He does, though, have hay fever and asthma and tends to become hyperactive if he eats a lot of chocolate. Ben also has had problems with bed-wetting, tantrums, sleeping and concentration. He is generally good-tempered and gets on well with adults, but has some difficulty socialising with other children. He uses his right hand for writing but for other fine motor activities he does not appear to have a preference. He is generally rather a clumsy child. His maternal aunt had spelling difficulties. Her speech was reported to be 'muddled' and she had difficulty with writing. Although Ben started saying words at an appropriate age, he was not understandable outside his family by the age of three, he mispronounced many sounds including /b,d,f,v,th,l and h/ and his mother was concerned about his speech and language development from when he was about two. His speech is now intelligible, but immaturities continue to be evident, e.g. /f/ for /th/. He needs instructions repeated and simplified before he is able to understand them and says he often forgets information. Sometimes it is hard to understand what he is talking about because his language is poorly organised and long-winded and he becomes frustrated when he cannot find the right words. He has had speech and language therapy for his speech difficulties, but no help with his language. He has had a considerable amount of specific support with his reading and spelling. Ben has been to three schools, the first change because of moving house, the second change because of the negative attitude of teachers.

Results of assessment

Verbal language

The assessment results show that at nearly eight years Ben's receptive and expressive language skills are delayed. By contrast his non-verbal skills were found to lie within the average range. Although this discrepancy between verbal and non-verbal skills is common in dyslexic children it is not a prerequisite for the diagnosis of dyslexia.

Ben finds it hard to process and retain verbal information and his vocabulary knowledge is restricted, which means that he often needs repetition and simplification of what is said to him. Although his speech is only slightly immature, he is sometimes hard to understand because he omits syllables in words, e.g. 'efent' for 'elephant', and is unsure of word boundaries, e.g. 'oneatime' for 'once upon a time'. He also experiences difficulty retrieving words quickly (word finding) and his language can appear dysfluent and repetitive as he tries to grope for words. His grammar is also immature, e.g. 'Oneatime there was a naughty bus and the man drive him then he left the man ... away then, then the bus goed away and left him behind then a big bus a bus camed then there was a train camed'.

To put Ben's language difficulties into context, a 'normal' eight-year-old's sound system should be free of errors and their basic knowledge of language should be complete with mature grammar. From eight years old the development of language takes place in the form of subtle refinements, e.g. with the increased understanding and use of vocabulary, idioms, riddles, figurative language, etc.

Literacy skills

Ben's literacy skills are also immature for an eight-year-old, but at a higher level than his verbal language skills, probably as a result of the support he has had with reading and spelling. He tends to read quickly, but inaccurately, and does not hesitate even when what he reads does not make sense. This means he often does not understand what he reads, which therefore reduces his motivation to read. Ben's restricted phonic skills are seen in both his reading and spelling errors, e.g. reading 'ceiling' as 'killing' and spelling 'story' as 'storee'. On one occasion when asked to write about something of his choice, he was very reluctant to do so, but in the end he wrote one sentence: 'I can Stop charlie playing at feetball', which highlights immature grammar and content as well as a limited awareness of punctuation. Although he completed all the reading and spelling tests, his anxiety was obvious and he needed constant breaks to help maintain his concentration. Ben's phonological awareness, particularly for rhyme, is weak and his sound/symbol knowledge is erratic. By eight years old one would expect a child to be able to appreciate rhyme and alliteration, to have a good sound/symbol knowledge, a wide sight vocabulary and the ability to decode unfamiliar words.

Conclusions

Although many children with dyslexia do not have such significant language difficulties as Ben, many of the language problems mentioned are typical of a child with dyslexia.

The anxiety that he appears to be experiencing is also typical of a dyslexic child. They often have to put in far more effort during the school day with little reward and sometimes, understandably, they become unmotivated. Hence all too often they are labelled as 'lazy', 'doesn't try' and 'lacks perseverance'. Ben's need for frequent breaks is also common with dyslexic children as they find it hard to listen, attend and maintain concentration, particularly if they have receptive language difficulties as well and do not always understand what is said to them. In a one-to-one situation it is usually easier to keep a child's attention. In a large classroom situation, where there are more distractions, it is not always possible to give them the breaks and reinforcement they need and poor listening and attention may be a significant problem.

Aetiology

There has been much research into the aetiology of dyslexia, the greater part of it falling into neurological and cognitive categories. There have been considerable advances in the neurobiology of dyslexia[2] and there is convincing evidence of heritability. Finucci *et al.*[3] found that 81% of children with dyslexia have a close family member with the same difficulty. This chapter will focus on cognitive causes, specifically the underlying language processing deficit.

The link between language and literacy

Dyslexia or specific learning difficulty, as it is sometimes referred to, relates to specific reading and spelling problems.[4] The link between speech and language development and dyslexia, may not be obvious. Indeed for many years, dyslexia was felt to be the result of visual processing difficulties, although the causal role of a visual impairment should not be dismissed entirely.[5] It also does not rule out the possibility that such difficulties may coexist and compound the reading problem.[6]

Research over the past 19 years[7,8] has shown that dyslexia is the result of an underlying linguistic deficit. Catts[9] even defines dyslexia, in some instances, as a 'developmental language disorder'. This is not to say that all dyslexic children will have a speech and/or language difficulty or that all children with a speech and language difficulty will be dyslexic, but there is no doubt that there is a strong connection.

For all areas of speech and language to develop (*see* Chapter 1), a child has to remember and discriminate between individual sounds and sequences of sounds. The child has to be able to store the precise composition of words and then retrieve words, organise them into the correct sequence and assemble, time and co-ordinate articulatory movements. Children with speech and language difficulties often have poor phonological awareness. This means that they lack awareness of words, syllables and sounds for talking and listening. When it comes to learning to read and spell, a child needs to learn that words can be broken up into sounds and that the sounds can be represented by letters. If a child is unsure of the sounds or sequence of sounds in a word, he or she will have difficulty in appreciating the correspondence between letters and sounds – the alphabetic principle – on which written English is based. Phonological awareness may be assessed by testing a child's ability to detect and generate rhyme and alliteration, and assessing their awareness of syllable number and phonemes (sounds) within a word. Any past or current history of speech and/or language may indicate the existence of reading and spelling difficulties. Leitao *et al.*[10] completed research on four groups of children: speech impaired (speech), speech and language impaired (mixed), language impaired (language) and normally developing children (normal). Their results showed that it was the 'mixed' children who are more at risk of developing literacy problems, followed by the 'language' children.

Historically, importance has been placed on the measured difference between reading ability and general intelligence. Stanovich[11] cites Siegel, who feels that reading disability should be defined solely on the basis of decoding deficits without reference to discrepancies in aptitude measures. Catts[9] states that if children have problems processing phonological information, they are at risk of reading difficulties regardless of their measured IQ. Torgenson[12] also states that low IQ is not a sufficient cause of poor reading.

Identifying characteristics of children with dyslexia

Dyslexia is a developmental disorder with different problems arising at different stages in a child's development. However, as dyslexics are a heterogeneous group it is impossible to refer to a rigid 'dyslexic profile'. There are, however, certain characteristics that tend to be typical of a dyslexic child and these are provided in Tables 16.1–16.3

Table 16.1   Characteristics that are typical of a dyslexic child in the infant school years (4–7 years)

Verbal characteristics	*Non-verbal characteristics*
Poor phonological awareness as characterised by difficulties in and generation of rhyme, alliteration and syllable number	May be later than some children in deciding on preferred hand for writing and may be ambidextrous
Cannot remember their address and telephone number	Clumsy
Difficulties with rote learning, such as times table, months of the year. For dyslexic children such things may appear to be meaningless chunks of verbal information	May be artistic and good mechanically, e.g. with Lego
Great difficulty with learning sound/symbol correspondences	Lack of interest in books
Delayed speech and or language development, e.g. difficulties following verbal instructions, difficulties expressing themselves verbally	Relying on pictures and/or context when reading, so may read words that are similar in meaning, but are spelt completely differently, e.g. 'lolly' for 'ice-cream'
Poor short-term auditory memory and discrimination	Slow development of reading and auditory spelling tending to get 'stuck' at the alphabetic stage according to Frith[13]*
Poor listening and attention	Beginning to lose confidence

*Frith refers to three stages of reading development: the first stage, *logographic*, where words are read as whole units, often using only partial visual clues, e.g. 'milk' for 'lorry', 'guess' for 'grass'. Children at this stage may also confuse words they have learnt in a particular situation, such as labels on school furniture or names above pegs, e.g. reading 'chair' for 'table' or 'Robert' for 'Tommy'. The second stage, *alphabetic*, where sound symbol correspondence is developed enabling a child to decode unknown words. Initially a child may overgeneralise their knowledge, e.g. reading 'city' as 'kitty', and they tend to take time to read words as they try and decode individual letters and letter strings, often out loud, e.g. 's-o-ck, sock'. The final stage, *orthographic*, is where spelling patterns and rules are finally internalised and words can be read automatically.

Table 16.2   Characteristics that are typical of a dyslexic child in the junior school years (7–11 years)

Verbal characteristics	Non-verbal characteristics
Hesitant, dysfluent speech because of word-finding difficulties	Poor handwriting
Restricted use and understanding of vocabulary, including confusing similar sounding words, e.g. 'exhibition' and 'expedition'	Slow and inaccurate copying from the board because they are unable to recognise common letter strings or words as a whole and therefore have to keep referring back to individual letters
Immature grammar	Can learn spelling for a spelling test but spelling not retained in long term
Difficulty saying multisyllabic words because they may have stored 'fuzzy' representations of words due to their difficulties in remembering and/or discriminating between sounds and sequences of sounds	Slow to express themselves in writing. The content may be restricted as they will tend to only use words that they think they know how to spell
Unsure of more abstract concepts of time and space including 'left' and 'right'	The same word may be spelt in various different ways in one piece of writing as they have not stored an automatic representation of the word
Difficulty following verbal information without the back-up of visual clues	Weak phonic knowledge, e.g. 'storee' for 'story' and incorrect sequence of letters, e.g. 'dwon' for 'down'
Generally disorganised as they may have difficulty verbally rehearsing what they have to do. This may also be linked with their poor concept of time	Inconsistent ability, i.e. will appear 'able' one day and have forgotten everything the next
Poor comprehension of what they read due to restricted fluency, inaccuracies and restricted vocabulary knowledge	Says school is 'boring' because they often do not understand the content of lessons
Reluctant to read out loud in class	Increasing lack of self-esteem, sometimes associated with behavioural difficulties
Limited use and understanding of punctuation	May become much more tired than peers as they have to try much harder to keep up during the school day

for infant, primary and secondary school-aged children. The problems that a child shows with reading and spelling may vary enormously, depending on the severity of their underlying difficulties and affective factors, such as motivation and personality type. This is *not* an exhaustive list and 'normal' children will show some of these characteristics.

Table 16.3   Characteristics that are typical of a dyslexic child in the secondary school years (11 years+)

Verbal characteristics	Non-verbal characteristics
Restricted understanding of jokes and figurative language. If their language development is delayed they will often take things literally and will be unable to appreciate double meanings	Difficulty with study skills, e.g. revision and note taking
Often significant difficulty learning a second language	Improvement with reading, but poor spelling continued
	Untidy presentation of work, including lots of crossing out
	Seldom reads for pleasure
	Ability deteriorates under pressure
	Increasing lack of motivation and antisocial behaviour. Muter[14] cites Maughn who has found a substantial link between early reading failure and later social adjustment and delinquent behaviour

Implications for service delivery

The present assertion that dyslexia is the result of an underlying linguistic deficit has proved extremely valuable in the early identification of children with dyslexia. Until this assumption was made, children were often not diagnosed until eight or nine years of age, when the discrepancy between their reading age and chronological age had become apparent. As children's phonological awareness begins to develop prior to learning to read,[15] it is possible to identify those children at risk of dyslexia in the preschool years.

There is growing evidence that early intervention is crucial for many reasons. Hornsby[16] states that the younger a dyslexic child is identified and specialist help given the more effective the help will be. Muter[14] suggests that children whose difficulties are recognised at five or six years will have less educational ground to make up than children identified later on in their schooling. Concern should be expressed if a five-year-old is not appreciating rhyme or if a six-year-old's single-word reading bears little graphic resemblance to the word to be read, e.g. 'school' for 'table', or who cannot read simple consonant, vowel, consonant, three-letter words, e.g. 'sun'.

Therefore if a young child appears to be at risk of being dyslexic, or is showing signs of being dyslexic, it is very important that they are identified and referred on to appropriate agencies for more detailed assessment of their strengths and weaknesses, a diagnosis and a description of need for the individual child concerned. In the first instance referral should be made to a paediatrician, who will then arrange for assessment by appropriate professionals, such as speech and language therapists, educational psychologists and specialist teachers of dyslexia.

Specific intervention is not discussed in any detail in this chapter, but several basic principles are mentioned.

- One of the most important considerations is that teachers and parents are aware of the difficulties the child is experiencing so that they do not look upon him or her as being 'lazy' and 'unmotivated'.
- It is important that a multisensory approach is used with dyslexic pupils. Usually their auditory channel is the weakest, i.e. they often find it hard to remember and understand what is said to them.
- If the auditory information is supported by visual material, e.g. relevant pictures or diagrams, the child finds it easier to understand and retain the information because more than one sensory channel is being utilised.
- To facilitate his or her learning of spelling, a dyslexic child will be asked to employ as many sensory channels as possible, e.g. to see a word (visual), to hear it being said (auditory), to write the word (kinaesthetic) and to say it themselves (kinaesthetic and auditory).
- Dyslexics need to be set achievable targets to provide them with the experience of success. Specific help should be targeted at their phonological awareness.
- To help them remember and retain information they need constant repetition and recall of information.
- As the children become older they will often need continued support to help with study skills and extra time allocated for them in public exams.

Summary

- The most recent research shows that dyslexia is the result of an underlying language deficit, particularly related to poor phonological awareness.
- A child with a family history of reading, spelling, speech and/or language difficulties or a history of speech and/or language difficulties themselves, is at risk of being dyslexic.
- The implications of dyslexia are more far-reaching than just difficulties with reading and spelling, e.g. behaviour, peer group relationships and self-esteem.
- Early identification and support are extremely important to help minimise the long-term effects of dyslexia.
- Other possible factors, such as motor impairment, hearing loss and visual difficulties, should be investigated.
- Children, teachers and parents need support to appreciate the long-term implications of dyslexia. There is no quick and easy cure.

References

1 Shaywitz SE (1996) Dyslexia. *Scientific American*. November: 78–84.

2 Duane D (1996) Neurobiological issues in dyslexia. In: M Snowling and ME Thomson (eds) *Dyslexia. Intergrating Theory and Practice*. Whurr, London.

3 Finucci JM *et al*. (1976) The genetics of specific reading disability. *Annals of Human Genetics* **40**: 1–23.

4 Stackhouse J, Nathan L and Goulandris N (1997) *Speech Processing Skills in Children with Specific Speech Difficulties: phase one of a longitudinal study*. DHCS, UCL.

5 Lovegrove P (1991) Is the question of the role of visual deficits as a cause of reading disability a closed one? *Cognitive Neuropsychology* **8**(6): 435–41.

6 Snowling M (1996) Developmental dyslexia: an introduction and theoretical overview. In: M Snowling and J Stackhouse (eds) *Dyslexia, Speech and Language: a practitioner's handbook*. Whurr, London.

7 Bradley L and Bryant P (1985) *Children's Reading Problems*. Blackwells, Oxford and New York.

8 Hatcher P, Hulme C and Ellis A (1994) Ameliorating early reading failure by intergrating the teaching of reading and phonological skills: the phonological linkage hypothesis. *Child Development* **65**: 41–57.

9 Catts HW (1996) Defining dyslexia as a developmental language disorder: an expanded view. *Topics in Language Disorders* **February**: 14–28.

10 Leitao S, Hogben J and Fletcher J (1997) Phonological processing skills in speech and language impaired children. *European Journal of Disorders of Communication* **32**(2): 91–113.

11 Stanovich K (1996) The theoretical and practical consequences of discrepancy definitions of dyslexia. In: M Snowling and ME Thomson (eds) *Dyslexia. Integrating Theory and Practice*. Whurr, London.

12 Torgenson JK (1989) Why IQ is relevant to the definition of learning disabilities. *Journal of Learning Disabilities* **22**: 484–6.

13 Frith U (1985) Beneath the surface of developmental dyslexia. In: K Patterson, JC Marshall and M Coltheart (eds) *Surface Dyslexia*. Routledge & Kegan Paul, London.

14 Muter V (1996) Predicting children's reading and spelling difficulties. In: M Snowling and J Stackhouse (eds) *Dyslexia, Speech and Language: a practitioner's handbook*. Whurr, London.

15 Goswami U and Bryant P (1990) *Phonological Skills and Learning to Read*. Lawrence Erlbaum, Hove.

16 Hornsby B (1996) *Overcoming Dyslexia: a straightforward guide for families and teachers*. Vermillion, London.

Further reading

Broomfield H and Combley M (1997) *Overcoming Dyslexia*. Whurr, London.

Edwards J (1994) *The Scars of Dyslexia*. Cassell, London.

Hales G (1994) *Dyslexia Matters*. Whurr, London.

CHAPTER 17

Hearing loss

Tony Narula

Classification is the key to understanding hearing loss. The causes of hearing loss are usually divided into congenital and acquired. Acquired conditions are separated out according to whether they were acquired during the prenatal, perinatal or postnatal period. In addition, the distinction between sensorineural and conductive hearing losses must be understood. In general, almost all congenital deafnesses are sensorineural and almost all conductive deafnesses are acquired (postnatally). However, it must be appreciated that the two may coexist in some cases, in which case the effects are additive (not always the case in biological systems, which tend to be non-linear).

The prevalence of severe sensorineural deafness (requiring early fitting of a hearing aid) is approximately 1 in 1000 live births. By contrast the prevalence of otitis media with effusion (OME) is about 20% in the at-risk age groups (18 months to five years). This means that any screening programmes aimed at identifying the former condition during this period are liable to be swamped by the latter. Accordingly the identification of congenital sensorineural deafness is best achieved as early as possible – both for the purposes of beginning treatment and for practical reasons.

Sensorineural

Congenital prenatal

Most children with congenital familial deafness can be identified with careful screening in the antenatal setting. Thus a child will be known to be at high risk long before birth and special attention can be paid to assessing the hearing function (*see below* for testing). In the developed world, approximately 60% of familial deafnesses are picked up in this way, the remainder are recessive or the positive family history is

---

Box 17.1:   Syndromes associated with congenital hearing loss

Recessive genetic disorders
Michel/Mondini/Scheibe syndromes are all recessive with maldevelopment of the labyrinth (inner ear)

Dominant genetic disorders
Waardenburg's syndrome (white forelock and heterochromia)
Usher's syndrome (with retinitis pigmentosa)
Refsum's syndrome
Alport's syndrome (with renal disorder)
Pendred's syndrome (with thyroid malfunction)

Chromosomal disorders
Trisomy 13
Trisomy 18
Cri-Du-Chat syndrome

---

only identified retrospectively, i.e. once the child has been diagnosed (perhaps much later in life). Boxes 17.1 and 17.2 list conditions associated with congenital hearing loss and with acquired losses respectively.

Box 17.2:   Conditions associated with acquired hearing loss

Acquired prenatally
Rubella
Congenital syphilis
Toxoplasma
Viral infections
Toxic damage from drugs, e.g. thalidomide

Acquired perinatally
Prematurity with haemorrhage into the cochlea
Perinatal hypoxia
Kernicterus (bilirubin deposition into the cochlear nuclei)

Acquired postnatally
Meningitis
Mumps
Measles

Conductive hearing loss

A variety of middle-ear disorders can cause conductive deafness in childhood. The most common of these is otitis media with effusion (OME), also known as secretory otitis media, etc. This will be discussed below.

Congenital conductive hearing loss

These are uncommon. Some of the syndromes above, e.g. the chromosomal abnormalities, also present with external and middle-ear deformities in addition to inner-ear problems. Pure middle-ear problems, such as otosclerosis and osteogenesis imperfecta, may also present in childhood with abnormalities of the ossicles. In addition isolated ossicular anomalies may occur, such as fusion of the incus and malleus or stapes abnormalities (which often occur with cranial nerve VII abnormalities). These are also rare.

Acquired conductive hearing loss

The most common form of mild to moderate hearing loss in childhood is due to OME. This condition is common up to the age of ten but the highest prevalence is from 18 months to five years. Most often it is a transient phenemenon and therefore not important in the development of communication disorders, but a proportion of children develop a chronic form of the disease (i.e. present greater than three months) which is particularly relevant in the younger child. The impact of multiple episodes of short-lived OME on development is much less certain.

The management of OME is controversial, with the timing of intervention the subject of great debate. In general, no child should be treated if the condition has persisted for less than three months: at least 50% will resolve spontaneously in this time. Thereafter it is generally agreed that drug treatment has no proven role and that surgical intervention should be considered. The most effective treatment is aspiration of the fluid and insertion of a ventilation tube ('grommet') under general anaesthetic. Additional surgery to remove the tonsils or adenoids is not of proven benefit and is not recommended by the US Department of Health and Human Services Clinical Practice Guideline (1994). If for any reason surgery is not considered to be appropriate, a hearing aid should be fitted.

Case study 1

Sean, aged three and a half, was referred by his GP. His mother reported hearing problems for most of his life and said that he had failed every hearing test from the age of eight months onwards. He had poor speech development and was thought to be 'ignorant'.

Examination confirmed glue ear (OME). He underwent urgent fitting of ventilation tubes and postoperatively his mother reported that he was 'much improved all round'. An audiogram at this stage showed normal hearing thresholds. A speech and language assessment carried out shortly afterwards confirmed that he had many immaturities in his speech sound system.

Over the next two years Sean required a further operation to replace his ventilation tubes but made good progress in speech and behaviour, entering primary school in the normal way.

Case study 2

Ben, aged three and a half years, was brought by his mother. He had a complex neonatal history, having suffered from birth asphyxia which had left him with epilepsy and mild cerebral palsy. His mother reported that he had very few words in his vocabulary and that she had been concerned about Ben's hearing for at least the preceding six months. Interestingly, Ben had passed an otoacoustic emissions (OAE) screen at birth which therefore confirmed normal hearing.

Examination and audiometric testing showed evidence of OME. Surgical treatment resulted in an immediate improvement in vocabulary and balance skills as well as improved interaction with other children. Unfortunately in this case, Ben's poor speech development had been misinterpreted as a feature of his cerebral palsy rather than of his newly acquired middle-ear problem. The OAE pass at birth further confused the picture because it could not exclude later acquired hearing loss of any cause.

Identification of deafness

Clearly the identification of hearing loss is commonly linked to the child's communication skills. It is important to be aware of signs in the child's communication development which may point to this sort of problem. Of course these signs may also be common with the wide range of other conditions which may contribute to poor speech and language development highlighted elsewhere in this book. This does not discount their importance but merely serves to highlight the need for careful and comprehensive assessment of children with apparent delays of this type. Some key verbal indicators are given in Chapter 3.

There are a wide range of assessments which contribute towards the differential diagnosis of hearing loss in the young child. As indicated below the techniques utilised are age-specific.

Birth onwards

Auditory brainstem response

This is an electrophysiological technique based on averaging the posterior fossa waveforms in response to mutiple repetitive stimuli. The test usually uses a 'click' noise which is based around 3–4 kHz. It requires a still child, to avoid movement artefact, and can be done under sedation or even under a general anaesthetic. This represents the current gold standard but the lack of detailed frequency mapping can be a trap for the unwary. It is also time-consuming and requires considerable expertise; it is therefore expensive.

Otoacoustic emissions

This relatively new technique (first described in 1978) relies on the fact that the cochlea is an active mechanism and that incoming sounds are therefore reflected back from the inner ear with more energy than was put in – also known as the cochlear echo. This non-invasive test is quick and relatively easy to use. In general, a hearing loss >40 dB means that the emissions will be absent. This technique is now being promoted for universal use in all maternity units because it is quick and sufficiently reliable. At present it has not been introduced into community-based testing.

At six to ten months

Distraction tests

These are done in the community – usually by health visitors – and can be performed in any child who can support the trunk unaided; they are not of value in children with severe visual disorders. This test provides frequency-specific information and can be used as the basis of fitting hearing aids.

At 18 months

Toy tests

These are required because older children will not sit still for long enough to carry out distraction tests. The tests use matched pairs of toys which the child must identify.

At three years

Conditioning audiometry

The slightly older child can be conditioned to perform a repetitive task such as dropping a brick into a box in response to an external noise (free field audiometry) or in response to headphone stimuli.

At five years

Headphone audiometry

This is carried out using a precise psychophysical paradigm as laid down by the British Society of Audiology. By using a probe based on the mastoid bone, it is possible to obtain estimates of sensorineural function (i.e. bone conduction thresholds) as well as standard air conduction. Once a child can perform bone conduction measurements it becomes possible to obtain details of any conductive deafness which is the difference between air and bone conduction thresholds (the so-called air–bone gap). Audiometry of this kind is much more difficult to perform than it might seem because of the need to prevent sounds being heard in the contra-lateral ear. Noise is introduced into the non-test ear (masking noise) and children are easily confused by this. Accordingly bone conduction measurements in children may not be performed separately for each ear. One must be aware that a unilateral dead ear may therefore be overlooked.

The advantage of tests that can be performed at age five is that they can be done in school thus increasing the chance that all children will be tested.

Any age

Tympanometry

This non-invasive test measures the middle-ear pressures. It is very quick and can be done by an automatic device; its great advantage is that it allows easy demonstration of fluid in the middle ear (OME). Because OME is such a common condition, tympanometry is a vital adjunct to almost any method of measuring hearing thresholds where the levels obtained appear to be suboptimal.

Hearing aids

Hearing aids are the mainstay of treatment for children whose hearing levels are 40 dB or worse. Considerable expertise is required in fitting hearing aids. This is initially based on frequency-specific information and must be supported by ongoing evaluation. Parents and professionals play an important role in monitoring the benefit provided by hearing aids, especially when very young children are involved.

Cochlear implants

The 1980s and early 1990s have seen a rapid development of new technologies to assist children (and adults) with profound deafness. The most significant of these has been the development of intra-cochlear implantation. This depends on the fact that in many cases of profound deafness the end-organ is damaged but the cochlear nerve fibres are still viable. Accordingly, a fine wire carrying electrodes can be inserted into the cochlea and used to stimulate the auditory fibres directly. As an invasive surgical procedure for a non-life-threatening condition, cochlear implentation in young children continues to be controversial, however, reported results are promising.

Rehabilitation

Whether children use hearing aids or cochlear implants, family support and ongoing rehabilitation are essential. Effective rehabilitation relies on the co-ordinated efforts of a multidisciplinary team comprising otologist, audiologist, teacher of the deaf, speech and language therapist, educational psychologist, etc.

A variety of communication approaches is used with deaf children; these include oralism, total communication and bilingualism. Oral approaches advocate development of spoken language primarily through residual hearing and lipreading. Total communication approaches combine the use of spoken language with manual signs and finger spelling. Bilingual approaches identify deaf children as a linguistic minority and seek to develop sign language as a first language via an accessible modality, i.e. vision, with spoken language taught as a second language. The selection of approaches should always be based on the abilities and needs of the individual child. Many deaf children will be capable of education in mainstream schools, provided they receive the appropriate support. In certain areas, placement options may include resourced units for the hearing impaired or special schools for the deaf.

Summary

- Hearing loss is classified according to whether it is congenital or acquired and whether it first manifests in the prenatal, perinatal or postnatal periods.
- The condition may be sensorineural or conductive in nature. Occasionally the two manifestations may co-occur. In such cases the impact may be additive.
- The identification of hearing loss is a key role for the primary care professional. It

is important that care be taken to select the most age-appropriate method of measuring hearing.
- A wide range of professionals is needed to maximise the child's potential. It is critical that the medical end of the diagnostic process dovetails into the available educational services.

Further reading

Beazley S and Moore M (1995) *Deaf Children, Their Families and Professionals*. David Fulton Publishers, London.

Gregory S, Knight P, McCracken W, Powers S and Watson L (1998) *Issues in Deaf Education*. David Fulton Publishers, London.

Letinhardt E (1984) *Clinical Aspects of Inner Ear Deafness*. Springer-Verlag, Berlin.

Lingam S and Harvey DR (1988) *Manual of Child Development*. Churchill Livingstone, Edinburgh.

McCormack B (ed) (1988) *Paediatric Audiology 0–5 years*. Taylor and Francis, London.

McCracken W and Sutherland H (1991) *Deaf Ability, Not Disability*. Multilingual Matters, Cleveland.

Maw AR (1995) *Glue Ear in Childhood*. Cambridge University Press, Cambridge.

O'Donoghue G, Bates G and Narula A (1992) *Clinical ENT – An Illustrated Textbook*. Oxford University Press, Oxford.

CHAPTER 18

Spina bifida

Steven R Couch

Case study

A seven-year-old girl with lumbar myelomeningocele and shunted hydrocephalus was referred to a developmental evaluation centre due to difficulties in school. Her teacher described her as bright, sociable, well-liked by her peers and an excellent conversationalist. Nevertheless, difficulties with learning made her a candidate for repeating the year in school. Upon examination she was able to converse quite well, as long as she discussed familiar topics. When the conversation was steered towards unfamiliar areas she had an unexpected amount of difficulty understanding the content. Upon psychological testing, she was found to have a verbal IQ of 75, a performance IQ of 62 and a full-scale IQ of 69. Language testing showed her pragmatic understanding to be about two years behind age level, despite age-appropriate grammatical structure. She was referred to special educational services for individualised instruction in academic subjects and integration into regular classroom settings during non-academic activities.

Spina bifida, or myelomeningocele, is frequently associated with a series of findings within the central nervous system which may have effects on language and cognition. The Chiari malformation of the posterior fossa is present in about 90% of persons with spina bifida, and contributes to the development of hydrocephalus, which itself contributes to problems with the development of cognitive skills.[1] In a series of children with postmortem neuropathological examination of the cerebral cortex, focal areas of polymicrogyria were seen in 40%, disordered cortical lamination in an additional 24% and subependymal heterotopies seen in 44%.[2] Overall, malformations of the cortex were seen in 92% of the examinations. However, the degree of cognitive or language impairment associated with these impairments is unknown.

The cognitive and language development of children with spina bifida has some correlation to the level of the lesion and the development and treatment of hydrocephalus. In a sample of children whose hydrocephalus was untreated, Badell-Ribera[3] showed that children with hydrocephalus had lower IQ scores than children without hydrocephalus, given the same level of spinal disability. Those without hydrocephalus showed no effect of spinal disability on IQ, but those with hydrocephalus showed lower IQ with higher spinal disability level. Tew[4] found significantly lower IQ scores in children who had ventricular shunts, which were those with severe hydrocephalus. These authors also found children with 'arrested' hydrocephalus to have average IQ scores, between those with hydrocephalus and a shunt and those without hydrocephalus. Soare[5] found children with hydrocephalus to have significantly lower IQ compared with their siblings and with other children who have spina bifida but without hydrocephalus. McClone[1] noted cognitive deficits more strongly associated with a history of a shunt infection, particularly ventriculitis, than with the hydrocephalus alone. A weak interaction of the presence of a shunt multiplied by the motor level has been suggested by Shaffer[6] and Friedrich.[7] In contrast, Luthy[8] found no different average IQ in a group of children with different functional spinal levels, but identical anatomic neurologic levels. In summary, lower IQ scores are associated with a history of brain infection, especially ventriculitis; to a somewhat lesser extent with hydrocephalus, particularly untreated or incompletely treated hydrocephalus; and to a still lesser extent with higher levels of the spinal lesion.

In general, the language abilities of children with spina bifida and hydrocephalus are stronger than their visual performance abilities.[9] Verbal memory, fluency and grammatical structure are all described as typical of children with normal language development.[9,10] However, several investigators noted a tendency toward less coherent and less cohesive narratives,[11] and more irrelevant utterances,[12] particularly as the complexity of the language task increases. Horn et al.[13] noticed that introducing increasing amounts of irrelevant stimuli produced increased distractibility, interfering with word comprehension, in those children with hydrocephalus as compared to normal children, suggesting attentional problems as a secondary contributor to language difficulties. The consequence of normal fluency and grammatical structure may lead physicians, teachers and parents to overestimate the ability of children with spina bifida to understand spoken communication.

There are also important interactions between IQ and language skills that are unique to this disorder. When comparing children with less than average intelligence with and without hydrocephalus, children with hydrocephalus have more difficulty with new learning, recall and reacquisition of learned material, but not 'memory for a short story'.[14] In groups with average intelligence, children with hydrocephalus differed only in poorer 'memory for words', which suggests greater difficulty with encoding. However, Byrne[15] suggested that differences between groups were largely a function of intelligence rather than language. Nevertheless, the research consensus seems to be that language and intelligence interact in unique ways for children with hydrocephalus.

A specific language syndrome called the 'cocktail party syndrome' has been described in persons with spina bifida and hydrocephalus.[16] The features include 'fluent, well articulated speech, excessive use of social phrases, over-familiarity of manner, introducing personal experience into the conversation in inappropriate and irrelevant contexts, and perseveration of responses'.[4] A person with this syndrome is often able to participate in an active interpersonal conversation as long as there is little content. The prevalence is estimated as between 28 and 40%, and is not invariably present. It is associated with hydrocephalus and with low intelligence, but has been reported in children with normal cognitive function. 'Cocktail party syndrome' is reported to decline with age.[17] People who come in contact with persons manifesting this syndrome commonly overestimate the level of language understanding present.[16]

Implications for service delivery

- Untreated or partially treated hydrocephalus should receive prompt medical attention.
- Physicians need to be alert to the possibility of subtle language dysfunction in children with spina bifida and hydrocephalus. The high degree of fluency and well-developed syntax of these children can easily obscure receptive language difficulties and intellectual deficits.
- Early, broad-band screening should detect these difficulties and facilitate appropriate referral.
- Attention problems should also be addressed via environmental and behavioural modifications and in some cases stimulant medication.[18]
- Educational services should include intervention techniques aimed at minimising, remediating and adapting to deficits. Specific, developmentally appropriate language instruction will aid remediation of language deficits.

Summary

- The cognitive and language development of children with spina bifida is associated with the type of lesion and with the stage at which it is treated.
- In general, language skills are in advance of visual skills.

References

1   McClone DG, Czyzewski D, Raimondi AJ and Sommers RC (1982) Central nervous system infections as a limiting factor in the intelligence of children with myelomeningocele. *Pediatrics* **70**: 338–42.

2   Gilbert JN, Jones KL, Rorke LB, Chernoff GF and James HE (1986) Central nervous system anomalies associated with meningomyelocele, hydrocephalus, and the Arnold-

Chiari malformation: reappraisal of theories regarding the pathogenesis of posterior neural tube closure defects. *Neurosurgery* **18**: 559–64.

3   Badell-Ribera A, Shulman K and Padock N (1966) The relationship of non-progressive hydrocephalus to intellectual functioning in children with spina bifida cystic. *Pediatrics* **37**: 787–93.

4   Tew B (1992) The effects of spina bifida upon learning and behavior. In: CM Bannister and B Tew (eds) *Current Concepts in Spina Bifida and Hydrocephalus*. MacKeith Press, Suffolk.

5   Soare PL and Raimondi AJ (1977) Intellectual and perceptual-motor characteristics of treated myelomeningocele children. *American Journal of Diseases of Childhood* **131**: 199–204.

6   Shaffer J, Friedrich WN, Shurtleff DB and Wolf L (1985) Cognitive and achievement status of children with myelomeningocele. *Journal of Pediatric Psychology* **10**: 325–36.

7   Friedrich WN, Lovejoy MC, Shaffer J, Shurtleff DB and Beilke RL (1991) Cognitive abilities and achievement status of children with myelomeningocele: a contemporary sample. *Journal of Pediatric Psychology* **16**: 426–8.

8   Luthy DA, Wardingsky T, Shurtleff DB, Hollenbach KA, Hicock DE, Nyberg DA and Benedetti TJ (1991) Cesarean section before the onset of labour and subsequent motor function in infants with meningomyelocele diagnosed antenally. *New England Journal of Medicine* **324**: 662–6.

9   Fletcher JM, Francis DJ, Thompson NM, Davidson KC and Miner ME (1992) Verbal and nonverbal skill discrepancies in hydrocephalic children. *Journal of Clinical and Experimental Neuropsychology* **14**: 593–609.

10 Dennis M and Barnes MA (1993) Oral discourse after early-onset hydrocephalus: linguistic ambiguity, figurative language, speech acts, and script-based inferences. *Journal of Pediatric Psychology* **18**: 639–52.

11 Dennis M, Jacennik B and Barnes MA (1994) The content of narrative discourse in children and adolescents after early-onset hydrocephalus and in normally developing age peers. *Brain and Language* **46**: 129–65.

12 Culatta B and Young C (1992) Linguistic performance as a function of abstract task demands in children with spina bifida. *Developmental Medicine and Child Neurology* **34**: 434–40.

13 Horn DG, Lorch EP, Lorch RF and Culata B (1985) Distractibility and vocabulary deficits in children with spina bifida and hydrocephalus. *Developmental Medicine and Child Neurology* **27**: 713–20.

14 Cull C and Wyke MA (1984) Memory function of children with spina bifida and shunted hydrocephalus. *Developmental Medicine and Child Neurology* **26**: 177–83.

15 Byrne K, Abbeduto L and Brooks P (1990) The language of children with spina-bifida and hydrocephalus – meeting task demands and mastering syntax. *Journal of Speech and Hearing Disorders* **55**(1): 118–23.

16   Tew B (1979) The 'cocktail party syndrome' in children with hydrocephalus and spina bifida. *British Journal of Disorders of Communication* **14**: 89–101.

17   Hurley A, Dorman C, Laatsch L, Bell S and D'Avignon J (1990) Cognitive functioning in patients with spina bifida, hydrocephalus, and the 'cocktail party' syndrome. *Developmental Neuropsychology* **6**: 151–72.

18   Mayes SD, Crites DL, Bixler EO, Humphrey FJ and Mattison RE (1994) Methylphenidate and ADHD: influence of age, IQ, and neurodevelopmental status. *Developmental Medicine and Child Neurology* **36**: 1099–107.

CHAPTER 19

Learning disability*

Linda Ashford

Case study 1

Charlie, a five-year, one-month-old boy, was referred to a developmental diagnostic and evaluation centre by his paediatrician with concerns regarding language abilities, unusual behaviour and educational difficulties in kindergarten. His family history included an older half sibling with a diagnosis of Attention Deficit Hyperactive Disorder (ADHD), normal intelligence and mild emotional instability and a younger brother with the diagnosis of autism and learning disability. The assessment team included a psychologist, a speech and language therapist, pathologist, a paediatrician and a social worker. Charlie's behaviour during testing was remarkable for mildly unusual social interaction skills, significantly disordered communication skills and distractibility. His social/environmental history suggested restricted experiences with fewer resources.

Charlie was administered the Wechsler Preschool and Primary Scale of Intelligence – Revised which yields standard scores in both verbal (verbal IQ) and non-verbal processing (performance IQ) abilities and a full-scale IQ score. Results indicated that Charlie's full-scale IQ score was in the borderline range (74) with his performance IQ score in the average range (95) and his verbal IQ score within the mild learning disability range (57). The discrepancy between his performance and verbal scores is statistically significant; a discrepancy this large is found in less than 1% of the children his age who were in the normative sample. Charlie's adaptive behaviour functioning, as measured by the Vineland Adaptive Behavior Scales, is significantly delayed (57). The language evaluation revealed significantly impaired communication abilities and a severe language disorder. Had Charlie's ability to function in kindergarten been based solely on his apparent communication problems, it would not have been revealed that his non-verbal cognitive skills were

*Following differences in terminology and clinical practice between the UK and the USA this chapter was initially entitled *Language problems associated with mental retardation.*

within the average range. This information allows for more appropriate educational placement.

Case study 2

Rowland is a two-year, five-month-old boy who was referred to a speech and language evaluation centre by his paediatrician due to excessive drooling and suspected delayed communication abilities. Significant receptive and expressive language delays were confirmed and speech and language therapy was initiated. After several months of little to no progress being made, the speech and language therapist referred Rowland to the developmental evaluation centre for an evaluation of his cognitive abilities. His evaluation team consisted of a paediatrician, developmental psychologist and a social worker. Results from the Bayley Scales of Infant Development II and the Vineland Adaptive Behavior Scales indicated that Rowland was significantly developmentally delayed in all areas of development. In addition, this finding proved helpful in understanding and explaining the lack of progress in his speech and language development and in accessing appropriate educational resources.

Case study 3

Ian is a four-year, one-month-old boy who was referred by his paediatrician to a child clinical psychologist due to parental concerns regarding Ian's behaviour and questions of emotional disturbance. Ian was described as encopretic with episodes of faecal smearing. Other concerns centred around behaviour rages, disturbed sleep patterns and destructive behaviour. Ian began play therapy sessions with the psychologist. After several sessions, where Ian was described as compliant and co-operative with few concerns regarding his ability to control his behaviour, the psychologist referred him to a developmental evaluation centre with concerns about his cognitive abilities. The evaluation team consisted of a paediatrician, a developmental psychologist, a speech and language therapist, and a social worker. Results indicated that Ian had a severe communication disorder with his verbal IQ being in the borderline range (77), his non-verbal IQ being in the high average range (113) and his overall IQ in the average range (92). The discrepancy between his verbal and non-verbal abilities (a difference of 36 points) is significant and found in less than 1% of the population. Many of Ian's behaviours can best be explained by a lack of understanding of his verbal world. It appeared that he had 'mis-learned' many words, using them inappropriately and suggesting that he was not very well connected with reality. For example, he referred to sleeping babies as 'dead', suggesting that he had overgeneralised the meaning of dead from still and quiet to sleeping. In addition, as an effort to 'communicate' in a standard question–answer format, Ian often answered many questions with what could be considered to be 'typical' answers. He answered many questions that adults asked him with colour names, letter names or number names, since these were frequently asked questions. However, when these answers are randomly provided in response to questions, many misconceptions about a child's intent can be construed. The evaluation of his cognitive abilities as well as his speech and language abilities allowed a clearer understanding of his impairment, clarified some confusing information and documented some important strengths in his intellectual make-up which are all important for meeting his complicated needs in service delivery.

Although theoretical controversy continues to abound regarding the relationship between language and thought, for the purposes of this discussion, it is believed that cognitive underpinnings are necessary precursors to language acquisition. While Piaget[1] argued strongly that cognitive structures and mental representation are necessary conditions for the later development of language, Bloom[2] suggests that one of the motivations for children to develop language is that they have ideas which they want to communicate to others. When a health professional becomes aware of a child with language acquisition concerns or problems, the challenge is to make the appropriate referral to determine the relationship between the individual child's cognitive development and current language status. A developmental assessment team including a speech and language therapist, a psychologist and a paediatrician is needed to make the appropriate diagnosis.

Determining whether a child has the cognitive infrastructures to support the development of language is not an easy task. Furthermore, children who present in paediatric practices with stories of delayed language and other developmental milestones, unusual or difficult behaviour and lags in the acquisition of typical self-care acts are wake-up calls, alerting the paediatrician to the possibility of global developmental delay. According to the American Association on Mental Retardation[3] mental retardation refers to 'significantly sub-average intellectual functioning which exists concurrently with related delays in two or more adaptive skill areas with onset occurring before 18 years of age'. Adaptive functioning refers to how well children cope with common life demands and how well they reach personal independence in comparison with similar-aged peers.

The aetiology of global developmental delay is broad and varied. In 30–40% of individuals who have received extensive evaluations, no known cause can be attributed to the diagnosis.[4] Some known causes of learning disability are:

- Hereditary (5%), which includes inborn errors of metabolism, single-gene abnormalities and chromosomal aberrations.
- Early alterations of embryonic development (30%), which includes chromosomal changes, prenatal damage due to toxins and other teratogenic agents.
- Pregnancy and perinatal problems (10%), which includes prematurity, fetal malnutrition, trauma and hypoxia.
- Medical conditions acquired in infancy and childhood (5%).
- Other influences (15–20%), which include environmental deprivation and disorders such as Autistic Spectrum Disorder.[4]

Although the prevalence rate of learning disability is only 1%, its occurrence is similar across all socioeconomic groups. When no known aetiology can be determined, the lower socioeconomic groups are over-represented. Potentially negative contributory factors (lead poisoning and prematurity) are believed to occur more frequently in lower socioeconomic groups. In addition, learning disability is found more frequently in males than females with a ratio of 1.5:1.[4]

To ascertain whether a child's developmental difficulties are best explained by a general learning disability, a comprehensive evaluation is necessary. In addition, the comprehensive evaluation presents a view of the whole child with emphases on cognitive strengths and weaknesses, learning style, temperament, behaviour, and language use and understanding. This evaluation should include the administration of a standardised measure of intelligence and a measure of adaptive behaviour functioning as well as measures of language development. The tests of intelligence and adaptive behaviour functioning are typically administered by a psychologist. Their task is to determine if the child's measured cognitive abilities are commensurate with or disparate from the child's measured communication abilities. Discrepancies can be of two types. When a child's score on the measure of cognitive ability is within the average range and the estimate of the child's language development is significantly discrepant from this score, the resulting diagnosis is one of communication delay or disorder. However, when cognitive and language abilities are believed to be approximately consistent and significantly delayed compared with chronological age, the resulting diagnosis is developmental delay or mental retardation. Some children may also score significantly below the average range on a test of intellectual abilities with language scores being yet more significantly delayed. These children would be diagnosed as having a primary diagnosis of learning disability or developmental delay and a secondary diagnosis of language delay.

Appropriate assessment tools when ruling out learning disability depend on the age of the child and the extent to which the child is able to communicate. Appendix 2 lists some of the tests of cognitive abilities, ages at which the tests are standardised and the types of items which are included. Some tests of general intellectual ability contain both verbal and non-verbal scales. Verbal scales typically assess verbal comprehension, factual information, vocabulary and verbal reasoning. Non-verbal scales typically assess visual reasoning, visual-motor integration skills, spatial relations, and visual analysis and design construction. Children with general developmental delay would be expected to perform equally poorly on both scales, while children with a communication disorder or delay would typically score more poorly on the verbal portion of the test. However, some children may not show this pattern due to multiple handicaps (motor and verbal) or concomitant receptive language delays which interfere with the child's ability to understand the instructions for non-verbal items. Test selection is a very important part of the assessment, as the psychologist must attempt to measure underlying cognitive structures rather than the extent of the communication disability.

DSM-IV[4] reports four categories of mental retardation which are based on the degree of severity and reflect the level of intellectual functioning or measured IQ

Table 19.1 Degrees of learning disability

Category	IQ level	General characteristics
Mild	50–55 to 75	Comprises 85% of those diagnosed learning disabled. Often are not distinguishable from typically developing children until school age. As adults may require no to minimum support in independent living
Moderate	35–40 to 50–55	Comprises 10% of those diagnosed learning disabled. Acquire communication skills during childhood. Benefit from training in all arenas. As adults can work in sheltered workshops or with support in work force. May require supervised living settings
Severe	20–25 to 35–40	Comprises 3–4% of those diagnosed learning disabled. May learn communication skills in late school years. May read some 'survival' words. Adults may learn simple tasks in highly supervised settings. Will need group home or family living support
Profound	IQ less than 20–25	Comprises 1–2% of those diagnosed learning disabled. Usually has identifiable neurological condition. Constant and individualised supervision needed

score. Table 19.1 provides the traditional system for categorising the degree of learning disability and includes the categories themselves, the cut-off scores and some common characteristics associated with each category.

Implications for service delivery

- Mild and sometimes moderate mental retardation is easy to underdetect. These children have some language facility and their motor milestones may be obtained on time. They typically lack obvious morphological or organic signs. Monitoring children's progress in nurseries and schools will support the identification of mild learning disabilities.
- Because the diagnosis of learning disability requires the administration of measures of intelligence and adaptive behaviour, routine child health clinics may not be in the best position to make what can be an emotionally difficult diagnosis. Rather the identification of a possible learning disability should lead to a referral to other professionals who are skilled in psychological assessment and in providing appropriate support to the child and the family (see discussion of curriculum-based assessment in Chapter 5). This helps the family maintain a positive, working relationship with their primary healthcare provider and ensures that the diagnosis is made in a careful thoughtful manner.

- The professional should refrain from making long-term pronouncements on the outcomes of patients with learning difficulties. There is tremendous variability in the condition, and the efficacy of intervention with children and adults with learning difficulties results in substantially more independence and skill attainment than has been the case in prior decades.
- The professional should expect that families will need time to adjust. One of the ways adjustment proceeds is by viewing development more incrementally. Families learn to be enthusiastic about relatively small gains in skills. Professionals sometimes misinterpret this as denial when, in fact, it is an effective coping mechanism and one which helps families teach their children more effectively by breaking large tasks down into small steps. Families should also be expected to maintain high expectations for the outcome of the children with learning disability as do parents of normally intelligent children.

Summary

- There is a wide range of possible causes for learning disabilities. Typically the aetiology is not known.
- Traditional classification systems label children according to their IQ from mild to profound.
- An alternative view and one widely accepted in the UK is that the assessment of a child's educational and social needs should not be confined to psychometric measurement. Rather it should reflect how the child communicates and learns in a range of social contexts.

References

1   Piaget J (1970) *Genetic Epistemology*. Columbia University Press, New York.

2   Bloom L (1973) *One Word at a Time: the use of single word utterances before syntax*. Mouton, The Hague.

3   American Association on Mental Retardation (1992) *Mental Retardation: definition, classification, and systems of supports* (9th edn). American Association of Mental Retardation, Washington DC.

4   American Psychiatric Association (1994) *Diagnostic and Statistical Manual of Mental Disorders (DSM-IV)* (4th edn). American Psychiatric Association, Washington DC.

CHAPTER 20

Convulsive disorders

Janet Lees

Case study

Chris had a history of early developmental delay in feeding, speech and motor development, but this did not give cause for greater concern. His first seizure was at the age of four years nine months: a left-sided partial seizure which began in his hand and arm, followed by secondary generalisation. This was followed by a transient left-sided weakness and an increased slurring of his speech. He seemed less communicative for a few days. He was treated with phenytoin. The next episode was when Chris was seven years old. Again a left-sided partial seizure which began with shaking in his left arm, spreading to his left leg, which lasted about 20 minutes. Again there was transient left-sided weakness and reported difficulties with communication: slurred speech and reduced communicative drive. He had his first EEG at seven years six months, which showed right mid-temporal and frontoparietal spikes.

The third and most severe episode began at the age of nine years with a deterioration in school performance, communication and motor difficulties: pausing in his speech, dropping things from his left hand. IQ assessment confirmed a low average ability. He continued to have motor difficulties throughout the next year: mild ataxia in his left arm, and episodes of dribbling, jerking and apparent deafness. He was treated with sodium valproate. At the age of ten years, a year after this episode began, it was clear that he had no verbal comprehension. Several treatments were tried: a ketogenic diet produced a possibly transient improvement, corticosteroids were not effective. He continued on phenytoin, which was thought to be most effective in the upper end of the therapeutic range.

Other investigations included a computerised tomography (CT) scan and brainstem-evoked auditory responses at 11 years which were normal, and a further electroencephalogram (EEG) which showed an increase in the abnormality in the right temporal region as well as a focal sharp and slow wave abnormality in the left temporoparietal region. He was admitted to a residential school for children with severe speech and language disorders at age 12 years, at which time his performance IQ on the WISC-R was 92. Hearing for speech was within the normal range.

He made good educational and language progress such that at 13 years seven months his scores for verbal comprehension and confrontational naming had returned to within the normal range for his age. His Schonell Spelling score was at an age equivalent of 11;6 years, his Neale Reading score was at an age equivalent of 11;9 years for accuracy and 11;2 years for comprehension. He returned to mainstream education at age 14 years, and obtained four passes at GCSE level at the appropriate time (age 16 years). An example of his expressive language scores recorded at aged 16 years:

> There was a old farmer who owned a stubborn donkey. He wanted to put his donkey into the stable. But it refused. The farmer thought he could frighten the donkey so he got his dog to bark. It refused. Then the farmer decided to get his cat to scratch the dog. The cat scratched the dog. The dog barked. The donkey jumped in the stable.
> (The Farmer Story, an example of a story-telling technique used to elicit spoken narrative, the full scripts of which are given in ref. 1.)

At 17 he went on to attend a course of further education in cabinet making and woodwork, a profession in which he won a five-year apprenticeship at 19 years. He continued to be a somewhat reticent young man, who worked diligently, gaining several commissions for his woodworking, and who, at aged 23 years was planning to move into his own flat.

It has been accepted for at least half a century that epilepsy in the young child can have an adverse effect on the child's speech and language development. The prevalence rate is unknown, although one specific disorder in which epilepsy and language disorder co-occur, the Landau–Kleffner syndrome (LKS), is generally considered to be rare. However, epilepsy is itself common in childhood with a prevalence of about 5 per 1000.[2] It is recognised that there is an increasing prevalence of epilepsy in children with learning difficulties. Corbett[3] gives figures of 6% for children with IQs in the range 50–70 and nearly 50% for those children with IQs below 20.

In respect of its association with speech and language difficulty few, if any, large-scale studies have been done. Robinson[4] reported that 21% of children in a school for children with severe long-term speech and language disorders had epilepsy, with a 'questionable history' of epilepsy in a further 11%. Of the relationship between the seizures and the language impairment he said that three were possible:

- the seizures may cause the language disorder
- the same genetic factors which predispose the child to developmental language disorder may also lead to epilepsy
- the seizures may indicate abnormal brain development or damage, which may also lead to language impairment.

Deonna[5] states that 'the association of language disorder with epilepsy is frequent in children, but there is usually no causal relationship'. He uses the term 'acquired epileptiform aphasia in children' to include the whole range of possible presentations, including LKS. As he says, 'a child with one single two-week episode of aphasia and a clinical epileptic syndrome otherwise typical of BCECS (Begnin Childhood Epilepsy with Centro-temporal Spikes) would be a milder case, and a child with an insidious and complete aphasia would be the other extreme, with all the intermediate possibilities'.

The phenomena of seizure disorders and communication difficulties will be categorised differently depending on the emphases of those involved with the child and family. A medical model classifies seizures into various types of epilepsy, which, in conjunction with other behavioural and developmental observations, are then stratified into a number of syndromes. For example, the co-occurence of bilateral symmetrical spasms (contractions of the trunk) and developmental regressions, including the loss of social smiling, interest in objects, voluntary grasp and visual tracking, in infants aged between four and seven months, resulting in developmental delay and autistic features, is the recognised clinical presentation of West syndrome.

Seizure disorder syndromes of childhood in which effects on speech and language have been reported include: Begnin Rolandic Epilepsy (BRE),[6] Continuous Spike and Wave in Slow Sleep (CSWSS),[7,8] Epileptic Gait Disorder (EGD),[9] Landau–Kleffner syndrome (LKS) (numerous papers, see ref. 10 for a review), Lennox–Gastaut syndrome (LGS),[11] West syndrome (WS).[12]

A linguistic model would describe the different speech and language disturbances which might arise when epilepsy affects speech and language development. They could be very generally described as receptive or expressive language difficulties. The most severe receptive deficit is verbal auditory agnosia, when all auditory-verbal comprehension is lost. More specific descriptions of expressive problems might relate to the linguistic level(s) which are affected: phonology, syntax, morphology, semantics, pragmatics. A practitioner might favour terminology which relates to a particular model of language impairment. Two commonly used classification systems are the Goodglass and Kaplan classification of aphasic syndromes in adults[13] and the Rapin and Allen classification of developmental language impairments.[14] However, recent work suggests that these are inadequate to describe the majority of acquired aphasias in children, of which these epilepsy-related speech and language disturbances are one subgroup.[15] In the literature a wide range of descriptions of speech and language behaviours are used, some general and others more specific, with the trend towards more objective and detailed linguistic descriptions developing since the early 1980s. More recently a few papers have begun to explore the use of a psycholinguistic framework in the speech and language therapy management of children with acquired aphasias.[16]

By contrast, a developmental model would indicate which domains of development have been affected. Cass *et al.*[17] have proposed such a model, in which the developmental domains of language, play, behaviour and non-verbal cognition are assessed in terms of the developmental level attained and the level of disorder present. They propose that this model can be used to objectively measure change in children who present with early developmental regression and epilepsy who are undergoing treatment, both anti-epileptic drugs and surgery.

The case history at the beginning of this chapter attempts to include medical, linguistic, developmental and social information to provide a comprehensive profile. On the whole these conditions have complex effects at all of these levels. Initially the child's loss or deterioration in speech and language might come to the attention of a range of different people:

- the child, who might respond with behavioural change
- the parents and family, who might not find it easy to convince professionals of their observations
- the class teacher or nursery officer, who might notice the child's changed or fluctuating behaviour
- the health visitor or general medical practitioner, to whom parents might go with initial concerns.

At the stage of such initial concern:

- the child needs security and reassurance, as well as appropriate support in situations of communication difficulty
- siblings and family members may also need these, and contact with a voluntary organisation or support group is recommended
- a teacher or nursery officer might need information about what can be expected from the child on a daily basis and how to support communication difficulties
- primary healthcare staff need to know what medical treatment is appropriate, and who to refer to for secondary or tertiary services as necessary.

Such children are currently best managed by a child-centred multidisciplinary team of which the family is an integral part. This team should be able at least to consult a paediatric neurologist with experience in epilepsy, a specialist speech and language therapist, and a neuropsychologist. These professionals should:

- be able to advise local primary services
- arrange and interpret results of specialist medical tests and psychological and linguistic assessments.

Aetiology

While most of these disorders affect more males than females, little is known about inheritance patterns or genetic factors underlying these conditions. Normal CT or magnetic resonance imaging (MRI) scans are the usual finding in LKS, BRE, CSWSS and EGD. Encephalitis has been suggested as a cause for LKS but no entirely convincing findings have been reported to date to support such a hypothesis. Focal arteritis in the temporal lobe(s) has also been suggested and one case of neurocystercosis reported (see ref. 8 for review of these aetiologies).

Current research has centred on the mechanism of subclinical seizure activity in relation to aphasia. Treatment, both pharmacological and surgical, aims to eradicate this activity. As Lees and Neville[1] have said:

The working hypothesis for the mechanisms causing language regression and recovery in the context of focal epilepsy is that subclinical seizure activity may be more important than overt seizures in the developing brain. Such discharges, often at a high rate in sleep, may prevent homologous language areas in the opposite (normal) side, or those close to the source of the epilepsy on the same side, from functioning. Thus by the removal of the epileptogenic zone, or disconnecting from the normal language areas, some recovery of these functions may occur.

Identification at different ages

Aicardi[8] states that 'In children, the factors of age, growth and development are of primary importance in determining not only whether or not epilepsy develops but also the clinical and electrical manifestations of seizures and the type of seizure disorders encountered'. Usually the younger the onset the poorer the prognosis, even within the same epileptic syndrome. Bishop[18] discussed this finding in respect of LKS specifically and noted it was the opposite to the usually reported finding in children with acquired aphasia of traumatic origin (although more recently even this long held assumption has begun to be questioned). Aicardi[8] divides childhood into four age periods in respect of onset of epilepsy. The first, the neonatal period, from birth to three months of age, is too early to cause speech and language regression, although it is noted that the severe prognosis for seizures during this period means that all aspects of subsequent development, including speech and language, are likely to be significantly compromised. From three months to three to four years of age occasional seizures may occur and some syndromes associated with communication difficulties may begin: WS and LGS being two examples. The third period is between three to four years and adolescence. Many of the syndromes mentioned earlier begin in this period as shown in Box 20.1.

In the last period, nine to ten years onwards, some of these syndromes begin to subside and even remit, while other types of seizures, especially those related to structural brain damage, may increase in frequency. However, even in those situations where so-called 'benign' epilepsies remit, it is important to establish whether the child has any residual speech and language problems which may be associated with social or educational needs, as in some reports of LKS. These may be high-level auditory-verbal processing problems or difficulties in the social use of language. A recent study of 20 children with Begnin Rolandic Epilepsy found that 13 had significant language problems.[6] This group of children has recently been followed up and forthcoming reports will confirm that these problems persisted in most of these children three years later.

Box 20.1:   Childhood epilepsy syndromes associated with speech and language difficulties and their usual age of onset

Begnin Rolandic Epilepsy (BRE)	4–10 years
Continuous Spike and Wave in Slow Sleep (CSWSS)	8 months to 12 years (mean age of 4;7 years)
Epileptic Gait Disorder (EGD)	Of the two children reported, one was 5;6 years at onset, in the other myoclonic jerks in the legs (predominantly left and occasionally right) from the age of 6 months
Landau–Kleffner syndrome (LKS)	2–14 years; most commonly 4–7 years
Lennox–Gastaut syndrome (LGS)	Usually before the age of 8 years, with a peak between 3–5 years; with 2–10 years as lower and upper limits
West syndrome (WS)	Peak onset 4–7 months; almost always before 1 year of age

Implications for service delivery

There are no controlled studies of intervention to improve speech and language in children with acquired epileptic aphasia including LKS. In the literature case reports and short time series, studies predominate in which details of speech and language skills vary considerably. Since the late 1970s a range of antiepileptic drugs, including steroids, have been reported as having good effects on the epilepsy or language or both. Yet no one series reports more than a handful of cases and objective measures of recovery are rarely reported. Similarly there are a few small series in which the results of neurosurgical intervention is reported. Of 14 children with LKS treated by Morrell et al.[19] by multiple subpial transection, half were said to have regained normal language after a presurgical aphasic period of at least two years.

Furthermore, there are no published efficacy studies of speech and language therapy for these children either. There is one longitudinal follow-up study from the UK of children who attended a residential school in the 1970s to 1980s[20] and one single case study of a younger child in a residential school.[21] A summary of these studies suggests that:

- many children with LKS previously left residential schools with little or no verbal language
- as signing communicators they often found a more natural home in the deaf community
- most were employed, married and seemed well settled[20]
- an integrated approach to language and learning which uses all modalities in an intensive programme is commended
- it includes the use of intensive auditory training, signing and cued articulation, visual sequencing, social skills training, and reading and writing in a comprehensive programme.[21]

There is clearly much more to be done in studying the management and outcome of these children. A controlled study using single case design with 20 children with epileptic aphasias, using the assessment schedule described by Cass et al.,[17] has recently been reported. The children were aged from 1;3 to 6;0 years at onset of the regression in their speech/language/communication skills and aged 3;4 to 9;3 years at treatment. All had abnormal EEGs, but not necessarily overt seizures, in which the abnormality had a left centrotemporal focus in 14 and a right centrotemporal focus in eight (i.e. two had bilateral EEG abnormalities). Twenty-three treatment episodes were monitored: prednisolone in 18 and other AEDs in five. Fifty-two percent of the group made a significant improvement on the target treatment. Further studies with a group of children who have had both resective surgery and mutiple subpial transection are currently underway.

Summary

Overall the clinician needs to be aware of the following:

- Take a detailed case history. Developmental regression may occur in association with epilepsy in childhood. The child's case history needs to be taken seriously. It is particularly important to respond to a history of lost or fluctuating skills in young children.
- Test hearing. Initial presentation of verbal auditory agnosia in LKS may be reported as deafness. While tests of peripheral hearing are important, non-compliance may mean that brainstem-evoked responses are necessary in some children.
- A referral to a paediatric neurologist is advised as early as possible. Primary medical investigations for suspected epilepsy and aphasia in childhood would be EEG, both while the child is awake and asleep.
- Speech and language assessment. Where comprehensive speech and language evaluation is not immediately possible then a recorded sample of the child's level of function should be made.
- Developmental/educational/behavioural assessment. Other aspects of the child's

development may be affected. Comprehensive assessment needs to be considered according to the child's specific pattern of difficulty.

- Caring for a child with such a rare and complex disorder can put a significant strain on any family. The maze of medical and educational options to be negotiated can be quite trying. A parent-run support group for the families of children with LKS now operates in the UK as a national charity: FOLKS. It has run two successful family days and provides an information pack.

- Follow-up. Long-term follow-up is advised in case there are further fluctuations or periods of regression and to monitor response to treatment, particularly antiepileptic drugs.

References

1   Lees J and Neville B (1996) Fit for neurosurgery? *Bulletin of the Royal College of Speech and Language Therapists* **535**: 9–10.

2   Cowan LD, Bodensteiner JB, Leviton A and Doherty L (1989) Prevalence of the epilepsies in children and adolescents. *Epilepsia* **30**: 94–106.

3   Corbett J (1985) Epilepsy as part of a handicapping condition. In: E Ross and E Reynolds (eds) *Paediatric Perspectives on Epilepsy*. John Wiley, Chichester.

4   Robinson RJ (1991) Causes and associations of severe and persistent specific speech and language disorders in children. *Developmental Medicine and Child Neurology* **33**: 943–62.

5   Deonna TW (1991) Acquired epileptiform aphasia in children (Landau–Kleffner syndrome). *Journal of Clinical Neurophysiology* **8**(3): 288–98.

6   Staden U, Isaacs E, Boyd SG, Brandl U and Neville BGR (1998) Language dysfunction in Rolandic epilepsy. *Neuropaediatrics* **29**(5): 242–8.

7   Tassinari CA, Bureau M, Dravet C, Dalla Bernardina B and Roger J (1992) Epilepsy with Continuous Spikes and Waves During Slow Sleep – otherwise described as Eses (Epilepsy with Electrical Status Epilepticus During Slow Sleep). In: J Roger, M Bureau, C Dravet, FE Dreifuss, A Perret and P Wolf (eds) *Epileptic Syndromes in Infancy, Childhood and Adolescence* (2e). John Libbey, London.

8   Aicardi J (1994) Syndrome of Acquired Aphasia with Seizure Disorder (Epileptic Aphasia, Landau–Kleffner syndrome, Verbal Auditory Agnosia with Convulsive Disorder) and Continuous Spike-Wave During Slow Sleep (Electrical Status Epilepticus of Slow Sleep). Chapter 12 of *Epilepsy In Children*. International Review of Child Neurology. Raven Press, New York.

9   Neville BGR and Boyd SG (1995) Selective Epileptic Gait Disorder. *Journal of Neurology, Neurosurgery and Psychiatry* **58**: 371–3.

10 Paquier P and Van Dongen HR (1993) Current trends in acquired childhood aphasia: an introduction. *Aphasiology* **7**(5): 421–40.

11 Beaumanoir A and Dravet C (1992) The Lennox–Gastaut syndrome. In: J Roger, M Bureau, C Dravet, FE Dreifuss, A Perret and P Wolf (eds) *Epileptic Syndromes in Infancy, Childhood and Adolescence* (2e). John Libbey, London.

12 Jeavons PM and Livet MO (1992) West syndrome: infantile spasms. In: J Roger, M Bureau, C Dravet, FE Dreifuss, A Perret and P Wolf (eds) *Epileptic Syndromes in Infancy, Childhood and Adolescence* (2e). John Libbey, London.

13 Goodglass H and Kaplan E (1972) *The Assessment of Aphasia and Related Disorders*. Lea and Febiger, Philadelphia.

14 Rapin I and Allen DA (1987) Developmental dysphasia and autism in preschool children: characteristics and subtypes. Proceedings of The First International Symposium on Speech and Language Disorders in Children. AFASIC, London.

15 Lees JA (1993) Differentiating language disorder subtypes in acquired childhood aphasia. *Aphasiology* **7**(5): 481–8.

16 Vance M (1997) Christopher Lumpship: developing phonological representations in a child with an auditory processing deficit. In: S Chiat, J Law and J Marshall (eds) *Language Disorders in Children and Adults*. Whurr, London.

17 Cass HD, Lees J, Burch V, Taylor DC and Neville BGR (1996) A model for the description and classification of neurodevelopmental impairment in epilepsy-related regressive disorders. Paper presented at the 22nd meeting of the BPNA, Southampton, January 1996.

18 Bishop DVM (1985) Age of onset and outcome in 'Acquired Aphasia with Convulsive Disorder' (Landau–Kleffner syndrome). *Developmental Medicine and Child Neurology* **27**: 705–12.

19 Morrell F, Whisler WW, Smith MC *et al.* (1995) Landau–Kleffner syndrome: treatment with subpial intracortical transection. *Brain* **118**: 1529–46.

20 Ripley K and Lea J (1984) Moor House School: a follow-up study of receptive aphasic ex-pupils. Moor House School Oxted, Surrey.

21 Vance M (1991) Educational and therapeutic approaches used with a child presenting with Acquired Aphasia with Convulsive Disorder (Landau–Kleffner syndrome). *Child Language Teaching and Therapy* **7**(1): 41–60.

Further reading

Neville BGR, Harkness W, Cross JH, Cass HD, Burch VC, Lees J and Taylor DC (1997) Surgical treatment of severe autistic regression in childhood epilepsy. *Pediatric Neurology* **16**(2): 137–40.

CHAPTER 21

Selective Mutism

Alice Sluckin

Case study 1

Mary, aged eight, was referred to the educational psychology service for not talking to her teacher or her peers. On starting school at five she had talked a little, but over the years in an open-plan classroom she had become increasingly silent. She came from a socially isolated, two-parent family and had a foreign-born mother. There was no evidence of delay in her mental or physical development. Mary was the younger of two sisters who were close in age.

Case study 2

Raj, aged six and a half, was referred to the educational psychology service by her headmistress. She was the youngest of three, the daughter of recent Indian immigrants. After three years at her school, which was predominantly Indian in composition, she had spoken only once, in anger, when another child snatched her pencil. Apart from that she communicated non-verbally, seemed to enjoy learning and joined in all activities, and at school she was not shy. She appeared a bright, happy child and was living in a child-centred family who were gradually rebuilding their lives in this country after having been expelled from Africa.

Case study 3

Trevor, aged six, was referred to the author by his headmistress at the suggestion of a speech and language therapist. 'He does not involve himself with any conversation with his teacher, or chatter with his peers.' Trevor had been at school for the best part of two years and was the eldest of three. He belonged to a close-knit, prosperous two-parent family with a good support network, and had been a very much wanted child, but late in coming. The only place where Trevor did not speak was at school, though he appeared well settled in every other respect.

Selective Mutism is an emotional disorder of childhood in which affected children speak fluently in some situations but remain consistently silent in others. The condition is known to commence early in life, and can be transitory, such as on starting school or being admitted to hospital, but in rare cases it may persist and last right through a child's school life. These children usually do not talk to their teachers, and in more serious cases they are also silent with their peers, though there may be non-verbal communication. Other combinations of non-speaking can also occur, affecting specific members of the child's family. Typically the child has no other identifiable problems and uses language age-appropriately at home or with close friends. Tramer,[1] a Swiss psychiatrist, coined the term 'Elective Mutism' to distinguish the condition from other forms of mutism, but as the child's silences are no longer thought of as deliberate acts, and are 'selective' in nature, the condition is now known as 'Selective Mutism', since reclassification in the Diagnostic and Statistical Manual of Mental Disorders.[2] However, both terms continue in use.

Prevalence

Selective Mutism is a rare condition and is found in fewer than 1–2% of patients referred to mental health establishments, although it may be that there are more such children who are never reported, as they are not troublesome. As communicating in class is now a requirement under the National Curriculum in the UK, more cases are likely to emerge. The average age of referral tends to be between six and eight years, but the onset is usually earlier, at preschool. According to the *Multiaxial Classification of Child and Adolescent Psychiatric Disorders*,[3] the condition is said to occur with approximately the same frequency in both sexes. However, there is now a consensus of opinion internationally that more girls than boys become selectively mute. The condition is also more prevalent among bilingual ethnic minority families, both in this country[4] and in Europe.[5]

Aetiology

The history and psychopathology of Selective Mutism has been fully dealt with in two textbooks, one American[6] and one British.[4] Kolvin and Fundudis,[7] in a controlled study of 24 cases in Newcastle, found the children to have delayed milestones, including speech problems. The most common pathology was that of an anxious child in an overprotective family. Although apathetic and withdrawn, some of the children described in the literature were also said to be manipulative and oppositional at home. Kolvin and Fundudis suggested the presence of genetic factors, and parental discord and social isolation were thought to be contributory factors. In a more recent investigation into 100 children with Elective Mutism, Steinhausen and Juzi,[5] Swiss psychiatrists, found, after studying a combined Swiss-German sample, that these children as a group had a history of complications during pregnancy, delivery and the neonatal period. Children with a history of parental migration proved more vulnerable. They concluded that hazards in early life may be a major factor, leading to social withdrawal and later refusal to speak in unfamiliar circumstances. Black and Uhde[8] evaluated 30 selectively mute children by means of parent and teacher rating scales and structured diagnostic interviews. They found that the children exhibited high levels of social anxiety and low levels of other psychiatric symptoms. A family history of social phobia was present in 70% of the families. These findings suggested that Selective Mutism may be 'a symptom of social anxiety rather than a distinct diagnostic label'. Dummit et al.[9] came to the same conclusion.

Thus, at least in the USA, Selective Mutism is increasingly seen as a manifestation of social anxiety, occurring to temperamentally predisposed children in vulnerable families. Hence it is not surprising that pharmacological treatment has been recommended 'in cases where symptoms are of long standing, causing significant impairment, and where other forms of treatment have failed'.[8] This shift of emphasis towards a more biological explanation was welcomed by the American parents' support group, Selective Mutism Foundation Inc., founded in 1993, who have for some time claimed that 'due to mischaracterisation of these children as controlling, manipulative, oppositional and angry, the strong association with anxiety has been neglected'.

Identification

The essential feature of Selective Mutism is, according to the DSM-IV,[2] the persistent failure to speak in specific social situations (e.g. at school, with peers and/or the teacher), despite being able to speak in other, more familiar situations. For the diagnosis to be made:

- the condition has to be sufficiently severe to interfere with the child's education and social and cognitive development
- the duration of the disturbance is at least one month beyond the first month at school
- the failure to speak must not be due to a lack of knowledge of the language
- the condition cannot be better explained by a communication disorder (e.g. stuttering) or any other known abnormality.[10]

If the non-speaking occurs in the school situation, the first place to start investigating the condition may be the classroom, once the problem has been discussed with the parents. Close observation with the help of sampling checks over a period of time can be useful, to identify the precise nature of the child's communication strategies, verbal as well as non-verbal. It is equally important to ascertain how the teacher responds, as such a child can easily be ignored and can become 'a fugitive from participation'. Associated behaviours may include no eye contact, no facial expression in extreme cases, immobility or nervous twitching or fidgeting when expected to perform in a social situation, refusal to participate in PE, to eat at school or use the lavatory.

In a recent paper by Dow *et al.*,[11] who run a Selective Mutism clinic in Bethesda, USA, some of the difficulties with regard to assessment are outlined. They conclude that 'selectively mute children deserve a comprehensive evaluation to identify primary and comorbid problems that might require treatment'. In short, it is necessary to look at the whole child and his or her family so that medical, neurological and psychosocial problems can be explored. An area that needs thinking about is the possibility, however remote, of physical or sexual abuse. Has the child perhaps been punished for not talking at school? If at all possible, an audiotape, or preferably a videotape, should be obtained of the child speaking at home in order to assess the quality of voice, the child's response to being talked to, sentence construction, etc. Meeting the child on his or her own home ground and getting to know other members of the family is likely to add much valuable information. In some cases the child is willing to speak to strangers at home. The therapist might then be able to join the family 'incognito' and become part of the child's 'speaking network'. Hearing the child will expedite assessment and treatment.

Parental assessment

Although parents invariably claim that their children have normal speech at home, this must not be taken at face value, as they may not be in a position to assess a possible difficulty. A full developmental history, such as the age at which the child began to talk, and circumstances surrounding onset of the non-speaking, is required. It is necessary to ascertain precisely who of the immediate family, children and adults, the child speaks to, and where. Is there consistency? Is there a history of past or present physical or mental illness or of non-speaking in either of the parents or any other member of the family? Were there any traumas, such as a family break-up, separation or deaths, which may have had a profound effect on the child and the family? What are the parents' expectations with regard to the grades? It is possible that an overambitious attitude can increase the child's anxiety. With a bilingual child from an ethnic minority background it is important to be clear about cultural norms: such a child may consider it impolite to make eye contact with a stranger; also the child may have difficulties understanding some of the subtleties of the English language, and on entering school may regress to the toddler stage, when remaining silent in such a situation is not unusual. More importantly, the family's attitude to having undergone a change of culture needs to be explored.

Referral

Referral by the school is usually to the educational psychology service, once parental permission has been obtained. Less entrenched cases are often resolved at this point, as the educational psychologist is in a position to pinpoint minor difficulties, which may inhibit the child either in the home or at school. Referral via the health service to child psychiatry and/or clinical psychology is more likely to take place if the child has additional emotional problems in the home and school setting and the parents are anxious for help. Unless this is the case, motivation for co-operating with psychiatric treatment may be lacking. Another NHS treatment resource is speech and language therapy, which is often 'the first port of call'. As indicated above many of these children do have related speech and language difficulties and such a referral may be appropriate to ensure that the assessment of the child's communication development is comprehensive.

Implications for service delivery

Psychological assessment

A full assessment by a clinical or educational psychologist can be very helpful, even though the child may remain mute during the test. One must keep in mind that some selectively mute children have a hidden learning problem, and may also have other special educational needs. From the results of the test it will emerge whether the child fully understands what is being said, and inferences can be made of his or her emotional state. Much can be learned from the child's attitude to other children and his or her schoolwork and drawings. If the findings and history suggest gross pathology, a referral to child psychiatry will then be made.

Helping the child, helping the school

Although some selectively mute children recover spontaneously, the problem should not be ignored as parents become increasingly worried and teachers more and more frustrated, and sometimes angry. It does not take long before the child is labelled a 'non-speaker' by his or her peers and is then virtually prevented from speaking in class. It is therefore not altogether surprising that in some cases of long-standing mutism a school transfer is beneficial, as it allows the child to 'get off the hook'. However, a word of warning: this is not a panacea, and must never be done without very careful preparations.

In the past, treatment was clinic-based, often of long duration and mainly directed towards improving family relationships in the hope that this would free the child's communication potential. While it is important to keep this aspect of the problem in mind, the most effective way of helping can be through a programme in which teachers and parents participate jointly. Such a programme aims to reduce the child's anxiety over speaking by a behavioural technique known as 'stimulus fading'. This involves moving the child by manageable small steps from the situation and person where there is speech, to another, where previously there had been none. The child's co-operation is gained by rewarding each step.[12] A useful additional tool may be making use of a tape recorder. The child is encouraged to read from his or her reading book into the tape recorder at home, and this is then played back to the teacher. This method encourages the child to keep up with reading, and his or her voice is also subsequently heard where there is normally 'no speech' – a step in the right direction. The case study below gives an example of a combined home–school programme.

Case study 4

Davida had been referred for not speaking at school at the age of eight. The family were described as isolated and the mother an immigrant from southern Europe. Davida was initially seen at home. From the home observation it emerged that Davida was grossly over-indulged by her mother. Davida was at first reluctant to respond to a stranger, but the family were surprised how quickly she made friends and began to chat. Verbal communication was established through drawing and painting and play with puppets. Davida particularly took to a battery-operated toy in the shape of an apple which, through a built-in microphone, ejected a worm when spoken to. After several sessions at home it was agreed that they would show the apple and the worm to the other children in her class. During a school visit jointly with the mother, all the children in chorus made the worm emerge from the apple. Then Davida and her mother jointly 'spoke' to the worm, and finally Davida worked the mechanism alone. The children were pleasantly surprised to hear Davida's voice for the first time, and praised her. From then on, encouraged by a sympathetic teacher, Davida started to speak in class. Her programme incorporated anxiety-reducing techniques such as stimulus fading, through-person fading and situation fading.

Such a combined home–school programme is only feasible if there is parental co-operation. In cases where the onus of remediation falls mainly on the school, use can be made of a structured treatment plan devised by Johnson and Glassberg,[13] a speech and language therapist and educational psychologist. They recommend to the school that such a child be given a key worker as a personal relationship and a very consistent approach over a period is of the utmost importance. Another great stand-by for teachers will be a recently published booklet by an Essex psychologist entitled 'Helping the Child with Elective Mutism – guidelines for schools'.[14] Teachers undertaking such programmes must show empathy and patience, as progress can be painfully slow. To quote Mark Twain, 'A habit cannot be tossed out of the window, it must be coaxed down the stairs a step at a time'.

Summary

- Selective Mutism is now a less puzzling condition than when it was first described, and treatment outcome appears more promising. Sluckin et al.[15] retrospectively followed up 25 children, who at one time had been selectively mute, by means of questionnaires administered via their present schools. Those given programmes involving stimulus-fading showed greater improvement on follow-up than those given standard school-based remedial programmes.
- A poor prognostic indicator is incidence of past or present mental illness in the family.
- There is evidence that intervention early in life is more likely to succeed, as it is known that the behaviour becomes entrenched in time.
- These children present as an 'at-risk' group, as they may become progressively more isolated and socially 'deskilled'. As Mich[14] points out: 'the impact of the difficulty does pervade many aspects of functioning at school, and should therefore be subject to planned intervention'.

References

1   Tramer M (1934) Electiver Mutismus bli Kindern. *Zeitschrift fur Kinderpsychiatrie* **1**: 30–35.

2   American Psychiatric Association (1994) *Diagnostic and Statistical Manual of Mental Disorder (DSM IV)*. American Psychiatric Association, Washington DC.

3   World Health Organization (1995) *Multiaxial Classification of Child and Adolescent Psychiatric Disorders*. Division of Mental Health, WHO, Geneva.

4   Cline A and Baldwin S (1994) *Selective Mutism in Children*. Whurr, London.

5   Steinhausen HC and Juzi C (1996) Elective Mutism: an analysis of 100 cases. *Journal of the American Academy of Child and Adolescent Psychiatry* **35**(5): 606–14.

6   Kratochwill T (1981) *Selective Mutism: implications for research and treatment*. Lawrence Erlbaum Associates, New Jersey.

7   Kolvin I and Fundudis T (1981) Electively mute children: psychological development and background factors. *Journal of Child Psychology and Psychiatry* **22**(3): 219–32.

8   Black B and Uhde T (1995) The psychiatric characteristics of children with Selective Mutism: a pilot study. *Journal of the American Academy of Child and Adolescent Psychiatry* **34**(7): 847–56.

9   Dummit ESI, Klein RG, Tancer NK *et al.* (1997) Systematic assessment of 50 children with Selective Mutism. *Journal of the American Acadamy of Child Adolescent Psychiatry* **36**(5): 653–60.

10   Tancer NK and Klein RG (1992) Elective Mutism, a review prepared for the DSM-IV sourcebook. Columbia University College of Physicians and Surgeons, NYS Psychiatric Institute, 722 West 168th Street, Box #78, New York 10032, USA.

11   Dow SP *et al.* (1995) Practical guidelines for the assessment and treatment of Selective Mutism. *Journal of the American Academy of Child and Adolescent Psychiatry* **34**(7): 836–46.

12   Sluckin A (1977) Children who do not talk at school. *Child: Care, Health and Development* **3**: 69–79.

13   Johnson M and Glassberg H (1998) *Breaking down the barriers created by selectively mute children.* A structured treatment plan written for speech and language therapists and teachers, sponsored and distributed by the Speech and Language Therapy Department, Kent & Canterbury Hospital, Ethelbert Road, Canterbury, Kent CT1 3NG.

14   Mich A (1998) Selective Mutism. The implications of current research for the practice of educational psychologists. In: *Educational Psychology in Practice.* **14**(1): 52–9, supplemented by 'Helping the Child with Elective Mutism – guidelines for schools', obtainable from Psychology and Assessment Services, A Block, County Hall, Chelmsford, Essex CM1 1LD.

15   Sluckin A, Foreman N and Herbert M (1991) Behavioural treatment programmes and selectivity of speaking at follow-up, in a sample of 25 selective mutes. *Australian Psychologist* **25**(2): 132–7.

CHAPTER 22

The effect of poverty

Theodora Phea Pinnock and Mark L Wolraich

Poverty refers to a host of related variables that adversely effect children's development: limited parental education, single-parent families, problematic parenting styles, low occupational status, overcrowded living conditions and troubled neighbourhoods. Societal forces act in consort to produce a 'caste-like minority group',[1] with a limited potential for changing status or employment resulting in what can amount to enforced ghettoization.[2] As a consequence, children from impoverished backgrounds have been termed 'culturally deprived, culturally alienated, culturally divergent, socioeconomically deprived, economically deprived, economically impoverished, poverty stricken, underprivileged, chronically poor, educationally disadvantaged, educationally disoriented, and experientially poor'.

The effects of poverty on development can be categorised into five components: physical, psychological, emotional, sociological and educational. Physical aspects can be subdivided into prenatal, perinatal and postnatal categories. The prenatal and perinatal aspects consist of a lack of adequate prenatal care,[3] increased infant morbidity and mortality,[4] risk of low birth weight[5] and maternal substance abuse.[6,7] The postnatal aspects consist of accidental death,[8] malnutrition,[9] chronic illness,[10] lead exposure[11] and developmental delay.[12] Some of the sociological, emotional and psychological factors include increased mental illness and behavioural problems,[10,13] poor school performance,[14] delinquency,[15] increased teenage pregnancy,[16] increased school dropout[17] and increased risk of suicide.[18]

The effects of poverty on language development, in particular, have been carefully explored and assessed because language is one of the most important determinants of a child's social, emotional and academic competence. Indeed, the cornerstone of the Head Start programmes in the USA and other early intervention programmes for at-risk children was the enrichment of language skills. It is therefore important to understand the impact of poverty on language development and the impact of language development on the overall function and outcome of children raised in poverty. This chapter reviews the effects of poverty on language development, subsequent outcomes, interventions and research initiatives, and some possible solutions.

Issues in the study of poverty and language development

There have been numerous and controversial conclusions about the language skills of disadvantaged children. One primary question is whether the tools used to measure language are culturally biased. Current literature suggests that both standardised intelligence and language tests may not be adequate measures for at-risk populations. Many tests were standardised on exclusively middle-class Caucasians whose culture differs substantially from that of many minority groups.[19] Thus, it may be that performance differences between minority and majority groups simply reflect cultural variation rather than ecologically meaningful strengths or weaknesses. A second and related issue is that tests are often applied and interpreted in a substantially different manner than the authors intended. Given that tests may provide invalid results to which invalid interpretations are applied, many investigators such as Cazden,[20] Shuy[21] and Menyuk[22] called for decisive changes in the content and format of testing with minority children. Recommendations included use of spontaneous speech samples and careful viewing of language function as an alter-native to standardised measures of the language of culturally disadvantaged children.

Concerns about how best to measure and account for language variability across cultures leads to another controversy surrounding lower IQ and language scores in impoverished children: is their language 'deficient' or simply 'different'.[3] Several researchers proposed that lower scores represented deficits associated with adverse, early environments which in turn decreased overall intellectual and language functioning.[23] Hess and Shipman[24] examined the speech of mothers to their toddlers and proposed the following explanation: punitive mother–child interactions, decreased verbal communications at home, and the noisy and chaotic home environment causes poor language development in impoverished children.

In contrast, the proponents of the 'different' hypothesis assert that disadvantaged children's language, although different in form, is not substandard when compared to middle-class peers. For example, Stewart[25] noted that 'Negro' dialect contained all the necessary elements of morphological constructs and meanings. Similarly Labov[26] noted that the language of inner city children was 'non-standard' and also had certain phonological differences such as omission of the consonant sounds 'r' and 'l' (i.e. tool = too), simplification of consonant clusters (i.e. past = pass) and weakening of final consonants (i.e. mend = men). Yet, this non-standard language possessed the same vocabulary basis, the same capacity to convey concepts or abstractions and the same amount of logic as standard middle-class English.

Baratz and Shuy[27] theorised that although impoverished children's language varied in structural characteristics, such as decreased use of possessives (i.e. John's house = John house), decreased past tense usage (i.e. she jumped = she jump) and different negative usage (i.e. he doesn't have any toys = he don't have no toys), it contained all the necessary logical structures. Anastasiow and Hanes[28] demonstrated that disadvantaged children would reconstruct the sentence that they were asked to repeat to conform to their own dialect, for example: 'he was tied up' = 'he got tied'. This ability to modify language efficiently certainly cast doubt on a deficiency model and supported the difference model.

Although the 'deficient' versus 'difference' argument has been the main framework of both theory and intervention, combinations of the two: 'different and deficient' may provide a strong explanation for the language and learning difficulties observed in some impoverished children. For example, parents who used more directive, non-reciprocal, verbal interactions with their children, instead of conversational, reciprocal, child-responsive interactions, are more likely to have children with impoverished language even using culture-specific standards. Teachers may also inadvertently contribute to language difficulties in minority children. Labov[26] pointed out that teachers often correct children's non-standard utterances with middle-class standard English. These 'corrected' utterances are not thought to hold any relevance or experiential reference for children who also tend to perceive them as confusing, demeaning and alienating.

Correlates of impoverished language

Whether or not language is impoverished, deficient or different, language skills have a profound influence on children's futures. Sameroff et al.[12] found that low socioeconomic status accounted for 35% of variance in verbal IQ scores and that scores decreased in proportion with the accumulated number of environmental risks. Escalona[29] noted that at 40 months of age, the IQ scores of impoverished, former low birth weight infants dropped from 99.8 at 15 months to 79.9 at 40 months, implying that the adverse environmental effects were obvious at two years or greater. Because of the strong relationship between IQ and school achievement, it is not surprising to find that disadvantaged children have lower reading competency scores and that these scores correlate closely with poor oral language skills.[30-33]

The consequences of poor school achievement also take a toll in social competence and sociodevelopmental outcomes of impoverished children. Quay[34] showed that juvenile delinquent adolescents had lower verbal IQ scores than performance IQ scores. Haynes and Bensch[35] showed that large discrepancies between verbal and performance IQ were associated with increased delinquent activity. Language difficulties underly this association: Karniski et al.[36] showed that juvenile delinquent males had poorer receptive and expressive skills than same age peers and that their poor language function made them at risk for delinquency. Similarly, poverty in conjuction with lower IQ and school achievement are associated with earlier teenage pregnancy.[37]

Intervention

In the USA, Head Start is among the early intervention programmes developed to address the effects of poverty on children. It is the largest federally funded early intervention system, and was initiated in 1965 to provide intervention for youngsters whose families were at or below the defined poverty line. The purpose of early intervention programmes is to provide supplementary education before children enter the formal education system.[38]

Research by the Consortium for Longitudinal Studies[39] studied 13 experimental intervention programmes for disadvantaged children. Initially, these programmes found that earlier IQ gains seemed to dissipate as school progressed. However, in following up students after school, it became apparent that other long-term gains were made. Children in intervention programmes were less likely to be retained in a grade (25% in intervention group versus 31% in non-intervention control group) and less likely to be referred to special education (5.3% of intervention group versus 29.4% of control group). Other studies, such as the Ypsilanti–Perry project had similar findings: after two years of early intervention (between the ages of three and five years) participants were less likely to drop out of high school at age 16. They also delayed child-bearing, had higher incomes and occupational status, decreased deliquency and less criminal behaviour, naturally resulting in considerable cost benefits.[40]

Ramey and Ramey[38] listed six principles which they believed to determine the degree and extensiveness of effects of early intervention. These principles are as follows:

- *The principle of timing.* Interventions that start earlier and continue longer give greater benefits to the participants than do those that start later and do not last as long. Programmes such as the Carolina Abecedarian Project went from infancy to kindergarten and had a strong emphasis on language development. Such programmes seemed to show larger para academic gains.
- *The principle of intensity.* Programmes that are more intensive, as defined by the number of hours per day, days per week and weeks per year, exhibit larger positive effects than do interventions that are less intensive. In a study, Ramey showed that the intensity of interventions had a linear relationship to the child's intellectual and behavioural development, reducing mild mental retardation.[41]
- *Principle of direct versus intermediary provision of learning experiences.* Children undergoing interventions that directly affect their daily learning experiences yield more positive and lasting results than do those that rely primarily on indirect routes to change competencies (e.g. home-based visitations or parent training only, health and nutritional services).
- *The principle of breadth.* Interventions that provide more comprehensive services and use various ways to enhance children's development have stronger effects,

compared with interventions that are narrower in their focus. That is, interventions that combine direct and indirect routes to improve children's learning and later school adjustment produce the most robust effects.

- *The principle of individual differences.* Some children show larger benefits from participation in educational interventions than do other children. These individual differences appear to relate to children's initial risk condition and the degree to which the programme matches the children's learning style.
- *The principle of environmental maintenance of development.* The initial positive effects of early interventions will lessen if there are no adequate environmental supports to maintain children's positive attitudes and behaviour and to encourage continued learning relevant to the children's lives. In a study by Horacek *et al.*,[42] children who had been in intervention programmes for the first eight years of their lives performed better in their maths and reading achievement scores than the group with intervention for the first five years or intervention from kindergarten to eight years of age. The principle of environmental maintenance also endorses the importance of family involvement in maintaining language and cognitive gains. Ramey and Ramey[40] advocated that interventions that included family and community would produce the most robust and long-lasting gains.

Implications for service delivery

In light of changes in health service delivery in both the UK and the USA, solutions for optimising language and general development in poor children must be incorporated into any new system of health care delivery. These include:

- Identifying children at risk for school failure by seeking and maintaining information on families' risk factors. Questionnaires can help doctors identify parents at increased risk for abusing their children (due to parents' history of abuse as a child and current domestic violence), those who are depressed or who have other mental health problems (*see* Chapters 3 and 9), those without high school educations, who are single parents, families with more than three children in the home, and those with frequent household moves.
- In the presence of risk factors, the primary healthcare team should refer children to secondary healthcare services for assessment of need and where appropriate access to early intervention. They may also need to explain carefully to parents the benefits of taking advantage of available services. Doctors may need to enlist the assistance of other healthcare and social workers who can help parents overcome practical and other obstacles to children's participation.
- Although participation in programmes is far superior to the intervention family doctors can provide in their surgeries, doctors can still have profound and helpful impact on family functioning. Since many impoverished children fail to attend well-child clinics, GPs should take advantage of opportunites arising when

children visit the clinic for other more obviously medical reasons to find out about all aspects of the child's development. Because risk factors have a cumulative effect and can change over time and because development itself is changing (e.g. the child with normal language development at 18 months may have significant delays by 30 months), physicians need to repeatedly check the development of at-risk children.

- Using the waiting room areas of hospital clinics or offices to present video, audio-taped computerised messages and pictorial brochures as ways to present material on language and development. This solution stems from the fact that the caregivers of poor children have a high rate of illiteracy.

- Offering parent training classes through community health centres and the GP's surgery and keeping an updated list of local services. Several such programmes not only train parents in effective parenting techniques but also build literacy skills.

- Use volunteer or part-time storytellers to present stories to children. This solution would help present visible models to caregivers, can transcend literacy skills and can be reinforced when physicians offer anticipatory guidance during well-visits.

- Intervening when problematic parenting is observed. GPs may wish to illustrate for parents alternative methods of talking to and interacting with children, such as asking them questions, pointing out attributes of objects (e.g. 'Did you see those big, red blocks?'), commenting on children's interests and activities, etc. Similarly, impoverished families often talk more to crying infants than to happy ones. This limits infants' opportunities to attend to their parents' faces and listen to their language. Healthcare professionals could demonstrate for parents how and when to talk with infants in order to build language skills. Where this is impractical, for example because of pressures of time, it may be appropriate to refer to speech and language therapy or other services specialising in promoting parent–child interaction.

- Paediatricians and medical professionals must offer leadership in establishing integrated networks of developmental and language services which link community, educational, medical, philantrophic and governmental resources to optimise outcomes for disadvantaged children and their families.[43] These might include advocating for changes in public school curricula in order to embrace the diversity of children in poverty, lobbying for increased funding for early intervention programmes, job training, parent training, etc.

Summary

The influences of poverty on children and their language has generated a large body of literature and some changes in national public policy over the last few years. Scientists and researchers have explored reasons and implications of such effects. In particular, attempts to explain the true effects of poverty on language have sparked considerable controversies and debates. These debates were intensified by the questions of standards of approach, assessment measures and observed results. The outcomes of impoverished children without intervention help formulate and produce many intervention strategies. Despite some positive outcomes, there remains a great need for better research. More importantly, it becomes a moral obligation for paediatricians and allied medical profesionals to effectively and extensively maximise the outcomes of disadvantaged youngsters.

References

1   Ogbu JU (1978) *Minority Education and Caste: The American system in cross-cultural perspective*. Academic Press, New York.

2   Drake St C (1968) The ghettoization of Negro life. In: LA Farman, JL Kornbluh and JA Miller (eds) *Negroes and Jobs*. University of Michigan Press, Ann Arbor, MI.

3   Esterman A, MacHarper T, Rohrsheim R and Roder D (1988) *South Australian Health Statistics Chartbook*. South Australian Health Commissioner, Epidemiology Branch, 71.

4   Mare RD (1982) Socioeconomic effects on child mortality in the United States. *American Journal of Public Health* **72**: 539–47.

5   Paneth N, Wallenstein S, Kielygd L *et al.* (1982) Social class indicators and mortality in low birth weight infants. *American Journal of Epidemiology* **116**: 364–75.

6   Chasnoff I, Burns K, Burns W and Schnoll S (1986) Prenatal drug exposure: effects on neonatal and infant growth and development. *Neurobehavioral Toxicology and Teratology* **8**(4): 357–62.

7   Chasnoff I (1992) Cocaine/polydrug use in pregnancy: two year follow-up. *Pediatrics* **89**: 284–9.

8   Wise PH, Kotelchuck M, Wilson ML *et al.* (1985) Racial and socioeconomic disparities in childhood mortality in Boston. *New England Journal of Medicine* **313**: 360–6.

9   Galler JR, Ramsey FC, Morley DS and Archer E (1990) The long-term side effects of early kwashiorkor compared with marasmus. IV: performance on national high school entrance examination. *Pediatric Research* **28**: 235–9.

10 Wood DL, Valdez RB, Hayashi T and Shen A (1990) Health of homeless children and housed, poor children. *Pediatrics* **86**: 858–66.

11 McMichael AJ, Baghurst PA, Wigg NR, Vimpani GV and Roberts RJ (1988) Port Pirie cohort study: environmental exposure to lead and children's abilities at the age of four years. *New England Journal of Medicine* **319**: 468–75.

12 Sameroff AJ, Seifer R, Barocas R *et al.* (1987) Intelligence quotient score of 4-year-old children: social-environmental risk factors. *Pediatrics* **79**: 343–49.

13 Offord DR, Boyle MH and Jones BR (1987) Psychiatric disorder and poor school performance among welfare children in Ontario. *Canadian Journal of Psychiatry* **32**: 518–25.

14   Dumaret A (1985) Scholastic performance and behaviour of sibs raised in contrasting environments. *Journal of Child Psychology and Psychiatry* **26**: 553–80.

15   Kapsis R (1978) Residential succession and delinquency. *Criminology* **15**: 459–86.

16   McDaniel G (1986) Teenage pregnancies in the United States more than double the rate in Canada. *Medical Post*.

17   Kominski R (1990) Estimating the national high school dropout rate. *Demography* **27**: 303–11.

18   Lewis SA, Johnson J, Cohen P, Garcia M and Velez CN (1988) Attempted suicide in youth: its relationship to school achievement, educational goals, and socioeconomic status. *Journal of Abnormal Child Psychology* **16**: 450–71.

19   Smitherman G (1977) *Talking and Testifying the Language of Black America*. Houghton-Mifflin, Boston.

20   Cazden CB (1972) *Child Language and Education*. Holt, Rinehart and Winston, New York.

21   Shuy R and Staton J (1982) Assessing oral language ability in children. In: L Feagan and DC Farran (eds) *The Language of Children Reared in Poverty*. Academic Press, New York.

22   Menyuk P (1986) Language development in a social context. *Journal of Pediatrics* **109**: 217–24.

23   Hunt J (1961) *Experience and Intelligence*. Ronald Press, New York.

24   Hess R and Shipman V (1965) Early experiences and the socialization of cognitive modes in children. *Child Development* **36**: 867–86.

25   Stewart W (1970) Toward a history of American Negro dialect. In: F Williams (ed) *Language and Poverty: perspectives on a theme*. Markham, Chicago, IL.

26   Labov W (1972) *The Language in the Inner City: studies in the Black English vernacular*. University Pennsylvania Press, Philadelphia.

27   Baratz J and Shuy R (1969) *Teaching Children to Read*. Center for Applied Linguistics, Washington.

28   Anastasiow NJ and Hanes ML (1976) *Language Patterns of Poverty Children*. Charles C Thomas, Springfield.

29   Escalona SK (1982) Babies at double hazard: early development of infants at biologic and social risk. *Pediatrics* **70**: 670–6.

30   Coleman JS (1972) The evaluation of equality of educational opportunity. In: F Mosteller and DP Moyniham (eds) *On Equality of Educational Opportunity*. Random House, New York.

31   Garman D (1981) Language development and first-grade reading achievement. *Reading World* **21**: 40–9.

32   Hyman JS and McNamara B (1980) The use of teacher training to modify oral language behavior in five ethnic groups. *Reading Improvement* **17**: 208–16.

33 Miller-Jones C (1984) Untangling the correlational relationship between language and reading acquisition. *Remedial and Special Education* **5**(3): 50–9.

34 Quay HC (1987) Intelligence. In: HC Quay (ed) *Handbook of Juvenile Delinquency*. John Wiley, New York.

35 Haynes JP and Bensch M (1981) The P-Greater than V sign on the WISC-R and recidivism in delinquents. *Journal of Consulting and Clinical Psychology* **49**(3): 480–1.

36 Karniski WM, Levine MD, Clark S, Palfrey JS and Meltzer LJ (1982) A study of neurodevelopmental findings in early adolescent delinquents. *Journal of Adolescent Health Care* **3**: 151–9.

37 Blaxter M (1989) Health services as a defense against the consequences of poverty in industrialized societies. *Social Science and Medicine* **17**: 1139–48.

38 Ramey SL and Ramey CT (1992) Early educational intervention with disadvantaged children – to what effect. *Applied and Preventive Psychology* **1**: 131–40.

39 Lazar I, Darlington RB, Royce JM, Snipper AS and Murray HW (1980) Preschool programs and later school competence of children from low income families. *Science* **208**: 202–4.

40 Ramey CT and Ramey SL (1990) Intensive educational intervention for children of poverty. *Intelligence* **14**: 1–9.

41 Ramey CT (1992) High-risk children and IQ – altering intergenerational patterns. *Intelligence* **16**(20): 239–56.

42 Horacek HJ, Ramey CT, Campbell FA, Hoffman KP and Fletcher RH (1987) Predicting school failure and assessing early interventions with high-risk children. *Journal of the American Academy of Child Psychiatry* **26**(5): 758–63.

43 Pierce D (1990) We help poor kids – and still get paid. *Medical Economics* **6**: 53–6.

CHAPTER 23

Traumatic brain injury

Doris J Wossum

Case study 1

Rosie was 16 months of age when she was involved in a road traffic accident. She suffered a closed head injury secondary to rapid deceleration injuries, as well as a left occipital skull fracture, and had numerous episodes of seizures in the days following the accident. She was ventilation-dependent for approximately two weeks post-injury. Rosie remained comatose until day 25, when she began responding to oral stimulation. Upon discharge to an inpatient rehabilitation hospital two months post-injury, Rosie was G-tube fed and was not speaking. While her premorbid developmental milestones were within normal limits, at the time of her admission to the rehabilitation hospital her language skills were estimated to be at a five- to seven-month level, with babbling and vocal play.

By discharge 9 months post-injury, she consistently localised to sound and would stop crying when someone talked to her. She attended to music or singing, and associated spoken words with familiar objects. It was estimated that at age 25 months her receptive language skills were at a six- to 11-month level. Her expressive skills were also improving. She played speech games such as pat-a-cake and peek-a-boo, and demonstrated communicative intent by gesturing. Babbling had increased with Rosie making a variety of consonant–vowel combinations produced spontaneously in strings. Gross motor control and co-ordination were at approximately a six-month level and she used a paediatric wheelchair. Fine motor and perceptual developmental age was around nine to 11 months.

At age two years five months – 13 months post-injury – Rosie's cognitive development, as measured by The Bayley Scales of Infant Development – Mental Scale was at the 16–17-month level. Motor skills, as measured by the Bayley Motor Scale were at the eight- to nine-month level. Personal and social sufficiency skills were significantly delayed and between the 10- and 14-month level.

By age three years three months, Rosie was still wheelchair dependent, with cognitive development at approximately the 19-month level and expressive language skills clustering at the 20-month level. She demonstrated a rather restricted repertoire of single words and did not readily imitate speech or gesture. Receptive language was a relative weakness, with skills clustering at the 14-month level.

Case study 2

Bruce was a popular high school student, with a B to C average. At age 17, he received a closed head injury while playing American football. With his helmet on, he struck his head against the thigh of another player during a tackle. Bruce walked to the sidelines and then collapsed. In the emergency room he was noted to have a dilated right pupil and was comatose. Computerised tomography (CT) scan indicated subarachnoid and subdural bleeding with mid-brain contusion and swelling. He subsequently developed numerous low-density lesions that were thought to be infarctions in the parietal-temporal area on the right. Right lateral ventricle enlargement was evident secondary to loss of brain tissue due to infarction. Bruce remained comatose for 53 days. At six months post-injury he was discharged from acute care to an inpatient rehabilitation hospital. A left homonymous hemionopsis was diagnosed. Left-sided hemiparesia was evident, and Bruce required a cane for navigating.

Sequential language testing had estimated receptive vocabulary skills at six years eight months; four months post-injury. Progress was evident at nine months post-injury, when Bruce had an age equivalency of 13 years eight months in this area. Neuropsychological testing eight months post-injury indicated behavioural and personality changes, compared to premorbid functioning, including irritability and lack of initiative and motivation. Bruce displayed a child-like, jolly overexuberance. Social isolation was a problem; his former high school friends no longer sought him out for companionship due to behavioural and cognitive changes.

IQ testing at his eight-month post-injury evaluation resulted in a full-scale IQ of 86, a verbal scale IQ of 99 and a performance IQ of 74. His lower score on the performance scale reflected impaired ability in non-verbal reasoning and difficulty with processing and integrating new information in a problem-solving situation. Severe memory and new learning deficits, especially for verbal material, were revealed. Sustained concentration was an area of difficulty, though immediate attention and concentration were unimpaired.

At age 21 years, Bruce moved from a special education service to a sheltered work environment. Repeat neuropsychological testing indicated a full-scale IQ score of 90, with a verbal scale IQ score of 96 and a performance scale IQ score of 85. Bruce performed better on verbal reasoning tasks than on measures of long-term memory and acquired knowledge. Memory testing indicated deficits in long-term retention of information, though memory was significantly better when Bruce had been given a repetition of the target when initially learning the information.

Formal testing as well as informal observation found Bruce to be a functional, effective communicator who could adequately convey as well as understand information. He demonstrated polite use of language as well as a sense of humour. However, functional communication skills, including written language, were assessed to be at the ten-year four-month level. Social skills were estimated to be at the same level. Receptive language skills were again assessed to be at the 13-year eight-month level, indicating little progress in this area since Bruce's nine-month post-injury evaluation.

The question of plasticity

The long-held notion that head-injured children are spared serious complications in cognitive and language functioning due to the plasticity of the developing brain has been abandoned in the light of mounting empirical evidence to the contrary. Indeed, there is growing evidence that young children are more susceptible to deficits compared to older children and adults. The effect of paediatric head injury on language development is influenced by many factors, including age at the time of injury; the severity of the injury; premorbid intellectual level, education and personality; post-injury treatment and support systems; and behavioural and emotional reactions to the injury by the patient.[1] The interaction of age with injury and the resulting long-term outcome has been a topic of special interest over the years. Yet controversies remain despite much clinical and research data. The belief that plasticity of the young brain protected children from adverse outcome following head injury stems from several factors. First, because the survival rate is higher in children and because children have better overall physical/motor outcome than do adults, researchers assumed that cognitive and language outcomes were also better in children.[1] Second, much of the early research on brain plasticity was with animal, rather than human, models and thus did not address the effect of injury on higher-level functions such as language. In addition, the subtle acquired language deficits seen in head-injured children differ qualitatively from deficits seen in congenital language disorders. Therefore, there has been an absence of agreed terminology to describe these unique symptoms, and as a result of this, these deficits have not been well-documented and or researched.[2]

Other evidence that bolstered a belief in early plasticity comes from clinical observations during the acute recovery phase. Functional language, even if there has been an initial post-injury period of mutism or dysphasia, usually recovers quickly in the paediatric head-injured population. In addition, there is often a rapid resolution of focal motor and sensory deficits resulting in children's ability to resume activities of daily living.[3] Nevertheless, recent research indicates that following closed head injury there is actually an increased risk of cognitive and language impairment in children under ten, relative to adolescents. The younger the child the greater the risk.[4] While the plasticity of the developing brain may increase the chances of recovery of cognitive functioning (especially language functioning) when a focal lesion occurs, the diffuse brain damage that often results with closed head injury leads to increased deficits in younger children.

Features of language in patients with head injury

In severe cases, subcortical damage can result in motor speech disorders. Children may retain the ability to communicate to some degree through non-speech channels, but have difficulty with spoken language. Other studies have shown dysarthria to be more common after injury in adolescence than in younger children.[1]

Head injury predominantly affects acquisition of new skills. In addition, some researchers have theorised that skills in rapid development at the time of injury may be the most affected, leaving well-consolidated skills less affected.[3] Thus, written language may be more likely to be affected in children than adolescents. Studies have shown increased expressive language deficits in children receiving injury before 31 months; perhaps because this is the developmental stage of rapid expressive language acquisition.[5]

While 'serviceable speech' often resumes after closed head injury, recent studies of language functioning after paediatric head injury demonstrate the presence of 'subclinical' deficits. In other words, functional language may appear intact, but impaired language processing is apparent upon standardised assessment by trained professionals and when increased academic and social demands are placed on the child. Expressive language deficits occur more often than receptive deficits. If receptive deficits are present in addition to expressive, the overall prognosis for language recovery is worse.[6] Specific problems often include word-finding difficulties, which may affect spontaneous interaction, decreased speech initiation and impaired confrontational naming. Studies also illustrated subtle deficits in higher-level language processing and verbally mediated thinking following head injury. These problems may manifest in a difficulty understanding ambiguous words, metaphorical speech, inference making and concepts such as antonyms and synonyms.[6]

Language functioning interacts with other post-head injury sequences such as organisational deficits and difficulty in the rapid processing of information. For example, students may have difficulty organising their thoughts over several sentences.[6] While reception of single words or phrases may be intact, rapid information processing required to understand and to integrate complex language may be difficult for the head-injured student. Reading comprehension deficits are also frequently seen.

The ability to carry on smooth, fluid conversation may be impaired[6] because of disruption in efficient mental processing. Attention and concentration can affect the child or adolescent's ability to sustain participation in a conversation. Facility in both quickly processing oral information and in formulating a response are difficult after a head injury. The ability to shift quickly from one idea to another, or to shift attention from one speaker to another can also prove difficult for a head-injured child. Furthermore, neuropsychological deficits may also produce difficulty in perceiving and understanding social cues and non-verbal communication involved in conversation. Thus, even subtle deficits may lead to conversation that is often ineffectual, disorganised, tangential or socially inappropriate. Because of these factors, those giving discipline and instruction to children must also take into consideration subtle deficits in language reception that may affect how rapidly they integrate what they are being told to do, and how well they understand what is told them.

Implications for service delivery

Ongoing education about the long-term effects of head injury is important for parents, teachers and others who will be working with her or him. It is important that children with previous head injuries receive comprehensive language and neuropsychological evaluation to document deficits that may affect their academic and social development. In addition, care providers need to be aware of subtle 'subclinical' deficits that may be present despite what appears to be functional language. Since there is a wide range of outcome from paediatric head injury, there is no standard treatment. Therefore, school and treatment recommendations must be individualised for each child.

References

1   Ylvisaker M and Feeney TJ (1994) Communication and behavior: collaboration between speech-language pathologists and behavioral psychologists. *Topics in Language Disorder* **15**: 37–54.

2   Jordan FM (1990) Speech and language disorders following childhood closed head injury. In: BE Murdoch (ed) *Acquired Speech and Language Disorders: a neuroanatomical and functional neurological approach*. Chapman & Hall, London.

3   Ewing-Cobbs L, Fletcher JM, Landry SH and Levin AS (1985) Language disorders after pediatric head injury. In: JK Darby (ed) *Speech and Language Evaluation in Neurology: childhood disorders*, pp. 97–112. Taylor and Francis, London.

4   Capruso DX and Levin HS (1992) Cognitive impairment following closed head injury. *Neurologic Clinics* **10**: 879.

5   Dennis M (1992) Word-finding in children and adolescents with a history of brain injury. *Topics in Language Disorders* **13**: 68–82.

6   Ylvisaker M (1986) Language and communication disorders following pediatric head injury. *Journal of Head Trauma Rehabilitation* **1**: 48–56.

APPENDIX 1

Speech and language assessment tools

Common measurement tools

Language

Title and author	Age range	Description
Bankson N (1990) *Bankson Language Test* (Second edition). Winslow Press, Bicester	3–7 years	Syntactic, semantic and pragmatic development
Boehm AE (1986) *Boehm Test of Basic Concepts: revised.* Psychological Corporation, San Antonio, TX	4–7 years	Basic concepts
Boehm AE (1986) *Boehm Test of Basic Concepts: pre-school version revised.* Psychological Corporation, San Antonio, TX	3–5 years	Basic concept development
Bracken BA (1984) *Bracken Basic Concept Scale (BBCS).* Psychological Corporation, San Antonio, TX	2 years, 6 months– 8 years	Concept development
Dunn L, Whetton C and Pintile D (1997) *British Picture Vocabulary Scales II (BPVS).* 2nd edn. NFER-Nelson, Windsor	3–16 years	Receptive vocabulary. Provides a standard score, age equivalence and percentile rank

Title and author	Age range	Description
Gathercole SE and Baddeley AD (1996) *Children's Test of Non-word Repetition*. Psychological Corporation, San Antonio, TX	4–8 years	Short-term memory
Wiig EH, Secord WA and Semel EM (1988) *Clinical Evaluation of Language Fundamentals* (Revised edition/ UK adaptation). The Psychological Corporation, San Antonio, TX	5–16 years	A comprehensive measure of receptive and expressive skills
Wiig EH, Secord WA and Semel EM (1992) *Clinical Evaluation of Language Fundamentals: pre-school*. Psychological Corporation, San Antonio, TX	3–9 years	Comprehension and expressive use of early content words, basic and linguistic concepts, and word and sentence structure
Masidlover M and Knowles W (1982) *Derbyshire Language Scheme*. Derbyshire County Council, Derby	1–5 years	Non-standardised. Comprehension in terms of ICWs and elicited spoken language
Kirk SA, McCarthy JJ and Kirk WD (1968) *Illinois Test of Psycholinguistic Abilities (ITPA)* (Revised edition). University of Illinois Press, Urbana, IL	2–10 years	Auditory and visual association, sequential memory skills, grammar and sound blending
Locke A (1985) *Living Language*. NFER-Nelson, Windsor	0–16 years	Receptive and expressive measurement of first words and phrases
Lee L (1971) *NorthWestern Syntax Screening Test*. Northwestern University Press, Evanston, IL	3–8 years	Receptive and expressive syntax

Title and author	Age range	Description
Dunn LM (1981) *Peabody Picture Vocabulary Test Revised (PPVT-R).* American Guidance Service, Circle Pines, MN	2 years, 6 months–adult	Receptive vocabulary. Provides a standard score, age- equivalent and percentile rank
Dewart H and Summers S (1997) *Pragmatic Profile of Early Communication Skills: preschool/school aged.* NFER-Nelson, Windsor	9 months–school age	Parent- and/or school-based interviews. A descriptive and qualitative assessment of the way children use language. Non-standardised
Zimmerman IL, Steiner V and Exatt Pond R (1998) *Pre-school Language Scale – 3UK (PLS-3UK): pre-school language scale.* Psychological Corporation, San Antonio, TX (UK adaptation by Boucher J and Lewis V)	2 weeks–6 years, 11 months	Receptive and expressive language. Standardised subscales plus a supplementary measure
Keirnan C and Reid B (1987) *Pre-verbal Communication Schedule.* NFER-Nelson, Windsor	Children and adults	Observation and testing. Pre-verbal and early verbal communication skills. Non-standardised
Bzoch KR and League R (1991) *Receptive-Expressive Emergent Language Scale (REEL-2).* 2nd edn. PRO-ED, Austin, TX	0–3 years	From an interview of the caregiver. Receptive and expressive skills. Results are expressed by age equivalence
Renfrew C (1988) *Renfrew Language Scales: word finding vocabulary.* Winslow Press, Bicester	3–9 years	Naming
Renfrew C (1989) *Action Picture Test.* Winslow Press, Bicester	3–8 years	Elicited sample analysed for MLU, content and grammar

Title and author	Age range	Description
Renfrew C (1991) *The Bus Story*. Winslow Press, Bicester	3–8 years	Narrative analysed for content and grammar
Reynell J (1985) *Reynell Language Development Scales (RDLS)*. 2nd revised edn. NFER-Nelson, Windsor	1–5 years	Receptive and expressive language. Standardised
Edwards S, Fletcher P, Garman M, Hughes A, Letts C and Sintia I (1997) *Reynell Scales III*. University of Reading, Reading	15 months–7 years	Receptive and expressive language. Standardised
Armstrong S and Ainley M (1988) *South Tyneside Assessment of Syntactic Structures*. STASS Publications, Tyne and Wear	3–5 years	Elicited spoken language sample analysed at phrase and clause level. Comparison with normative data, *see* Crystal D, Garman M and Fletcher P (LARSP)
Bishop DV (1986) *Test for Reception of Grammar (TROG)*. 2nd edn. The Age and Cognitive Performance Research Centre, University of Manchester	4–11 years	Standardised assessment of understanding of grammar
German DJ (1990) *Test of Adolescent/Adult Word Finding (TAWF)*. DLM, Allen, TX	12–19 years, 11 months	Assesses word-finding skills, including nouns and verbs, sentence completion, and category naming
Carrow E (1973) *Test of Auditory Comprehension of Language*. Learning Concepts, Austin, TX	3–7 years	Understanding of grammatical structures

Title and author	Age range	Description
Carrow E (1985) *Test of Auditory Comprehension of Language (TACL)* (Revised). DLM/Teaching Resources, Allen, TX	3–10 years	Comprehension of word classes and relations, grammatical morphemes and elaborated sentences
Wiig EH and Secord WA (1988) *Test of Language Competence (TLC).* Psychological Corporation, San Antonio, TX	5–18 years, 11 months	Recognition of ambiguous sentences, inferencing and explaining
Newcommer PL and Hammil DD (1988) *Test of Language Development 2: primary and intermediate.* Pro-Ed, Austin, TX	4–8 years, 11 months	Receptive and expressive language – 9 subtests
Wiig EH and Secord WA (1992) *Test of Word Knowledge.* Psychological Corporation, San Antonio, TX	5–8 years	Receptive/expressive vocabulary, word definition, opposites, synonyms, multiple meanings, figurative usage, conjunctions and transition words
Fisher JP and Glenister JM (1992) *The 100 Pictures Naming Test.* Australian Council for Educational Research Ltd through Winslow Press, Bicester		Naming skills
DiSimoni F (1978) *Token Test for Children* (Revised). Riverside Publishing, Chicago, IL	4–12 years	Comprehension of oral commands

Title and author	Age range	Description
Rinaldi W (1996) *Understanding Ambiguities: an assessment of pragmatic meaning.* NFER-Nelson, Windsor	8–13 years	Comprehension of ambiguous language

Speech

Title and author	Description
Wepman JM (1973) *The Auditory Discrimination Test.* Language Research Associates, Chicago, IL	Discrimination between speech sounds at word level
Grunwell P (1985) *The Phonological Assessment of Child Speech (PACS).* NFER-Nelson, Windsor	Phonological development
Connery V (1992) *The Nuffield Dyspraxia Assessment.* The Nuffield Hearing and Speech Centre, London	Imitative oral and verbal skills and motor sequencing
Armstrong S and Ainley M (1988) *South Tyneside Assessment of Phonology (STAP).* STASS Publications, Tyne and Wear	Phonology
Dean EC, Howell J, Hill A and Waters D (1966) *The Metaphon Resource Pack.* NFER-Nelson, Windsor	Use of phonological contrasts

Play

Title	Age range	Description
Lowe M and Costello A (1988) *The Symbolic Play Test.* 2nd edn. NFER-Nelson, Windsor	Up to 36 months	Relational and symbolic play
Lewis V and Boucher J (1998) *Test of Pretend Play (TOPP).* Psychological Corporation, San Antonio, TX	–	Pretend and imaginative play

APPENDIX 2

Tests of intelligence

Age of child	Test	Modality tested
0–42 months	*Bayley Scales of Infant Development II* (Bayley, 1993)	Verbal, non-verbal, sensory-motor. Global score only
3 years–7 years, 3 months	*Wechsler Preschool and Primary Scale of Intelligence* (revised) (Wechsler, 1989)	Produces separate verbal and non-verbal scores along with a global score
2 years, 6 months–12 years, 5 months	*Kaufman Assessment Battery for Children (K-ABC)* (Kaufman and Kaufman, 1983)	Produces separate verbal and non-verbal scores and a global score
2 years–23 years	*Stanford-Binet Intelligence Scale* (Fourth edition) (Thorndike, Hagen and Sattler, 1986)	Produces separate verbal and non-verbal scores and a global score
2 years, 6 months–8 years, 6 months	*McCarthy Scales of Children's Abilities* (McCarthy, 1972)	Produces separate verbal and non-verbal scores and a global score
6 years–17 years	*Wechsler Intelligence Scale for Children* (Third edition) (Wechsler, 1991)	Produces separate verbal and non-verbal scores and a global score
18 months–72 months	*Merrill-Palmer Scale of Mental Tests* (Stutsman, 1948)	Produces separate verbal and non-verbal scores and a global score
2 years–adult	*Leiter International Performance Scale* (revised) (Leiter, 1997)	Non-verbal score

Age of child	Test	Modality tested
3 years–8 years	*Pictorial Test of Intelligence* (French, 1964)	Non-verbal score
3 years–17 years	*Hiskey-Nebraska Test of Learning Aptitude* (Hiskey, 1966)	Non-verbal score

References

Bayley N (1993) *Bayley Scales of Infant Development* (Second edition). Psychological Corporation, San Antonio, TX.

French JL (1964) *Pictorial Test of Intelligence*. Riverside Publishing, Chicago, IL.

Hiskey M (1966) *Hiskey-Nebraska Test of Learning Aptitude*. Union College Press, Lincoln, NE.

Kaufman AS and Kaufman NL (1983) *Kaufman Assessment Battery for Children*. American Guidance Service, Circle Pines, MN.

Leiter R (1997) *Leiter International Performance Scale* (revised). Stoelton Co., Chicago, IL.

McCarthy D (1972) *McCarthy Scales of Children's Abilities*. Psychological Corporation, New York.

Stutsman R (1948) *Merrill-Palmer Scale of Mental Tests*. Stoelton Co., Chicago, IL.

Thorndike RL, Hagen EP and Sattler JM (1986) *Stanford-Binet Intelligence Scale* (Fourth edition). Riverside Publishing, Chicago, IL.

Wechsler D (1989) *Wechsler Preschool and Primary Scale of Intelligence* (revised). Psychological Corporation, San Antonio, TX.

Wechsler D (1991) *Wechsler Intelligence Scale for Children* (Third edition). Psychological Corporation, New York.

APPENDIX 3

Useful addresses and contacts

AUTISM SPECTRUM DISORDER
The National Autistic Society
276 Willesden Lane
London NW2 5RB
Tel: 0181 451 1114

The Scottish Society for Autistic Children
24d Barony Street
Edinburgh EH3 6NY
Tel: 0131 557 0474

CEREBRAL PALSY
Scope
Library and Information Department
12 Park Crescent
London W1N 4EQ
Tel: 0171 636 5020

Scottish Council for Spastics
Advice and Information Centre
ETAS Centre
11 Ellersley Road
Edinburgh EH12 6HY
Tel: 0131 313 5510

Scottish Centre for Children with Motor Impairments
1 Craighalbert Way
Cumbernauld G68 0LS
Tel: 01236 456100

The Aidis Trust
1 Albany Park
Cabot Lane
Poole
Dorset BH17 7BX
Tel: 01202 695244

The Bobath Centre for Children with Cerebral Palsy London
Tel: 0181 444 3355

The Foundation for Conductive Education Birmingham
Tel: 0121 456 5533

COMMUNICATION DISABILITY
Communications Forum
1 Royal Street
London SE1 7LL
Tel: 0171 261 1959

Royal College of Speech and Language Therapists
7, Bath Place
Rivington Street
London EC2A 3SU
Tel: 0171 613 3854

CRANIO-FACIAL ABNORMALITIES
Cleft Lip and Palate Association
1 Eastwood Gardens
Newcastle Upon Tyne NE3 3DQ
Tel: 0191 285 9396

DYSLEXIA
The Dyslexia Association
98 London Road
Reading
Berkshire RG1 5AU
Tel: 01734 668271

The Dyslexia Institute
133 Greaham Road
Staines
Middlesex TW18 2AJ
Tel: 01784 463851

DYSPRAXIA
The Dyspraxia Trust
PO Box 30
Hitchin
Hertfordshire SG5 1UU
Tel: 01462 454986

EPILEPSY
The National Society for Epilepsy
The Chalfont Centre for Epilepsy
Chalfont St Peter
Gerrards Cross
Buckinghamshire SL9 0RJ
Tel: 01494 873991

British Epilepsy Association
Anstey House
40 Hanover Square
Leeds LS3 1BE
Tel: 01532 439393
Helpline 0345 089599

Epilepsy Association of Scotland
48 Govan Road
Glasgow G51 1JL
Tel: 0141 427 4911

HEARING IMPAIRMENT
The National Deaf Children's Society
24 Wakefield Road
Leeds LS26 0SF
Tel: 0113 282 3458
Freephone parents only 1–5pm 0800 252380

LEARNING DISABILITY
Down's Syndrome Association
155 Mitcham Road
London SW17 9PG
Tel: 0181 682 4001

Scottish Down's Syndrome Association
158/160 Balgreen Road
Edinburgh EH11 3AU

Mencap
123 Golden Lane
London EC1Y 0RT
Tel: 0171 454 0454

Enable
6th Floor
7 Buchanan Street
Glasgow G1 3HL
Tel: 0141 226 4541

The Independent Panel for Special Education Advice
22 Warren Hill Road
Woodbridge
Suffolk IP12 4DU
Tel: 01394 382814

SPEECH AND LANGUAGE
AFASIC
347 Central Markets
Smithfield
London EC1A 9NH
Tel: 0171 236 3632/6487

ICAN
4 Dyers Buildings
Holborn
London EC1N 2QP
Tel: 0870 010 4066

SPINA BIFIDA
The Association for Spina Bifida and Hydrocephalus
42 Park Road
Peterborough
Cambridgeshire PE1 2UQ
Tel: 01733 555988

STAMMERING
The Association of Stammerers
15 Old Ford Road
London E2 9PJ
Tel: 0181 983 1003
Helpline 0181 981 8818

Further reference

Contact a Family (1991) *Directory of Specific Conditions and Rare Syndromes*. Contact a Family, London.

Glossary

The following are some terms used both in this book and by professionals.

Acoustic reflex
Contraction of the stapedial muscle within the middle ear in response to moderate to high intensity levels of sound. There are three components of the acoustic reflex arc. The afferent component includes the inner ear and the eighth cranial (auditory) nerve; the brainstem component includes nuclei and pathways in the pons; the efferent component is the seventh cranial (facial) nerve.

Aetiology
Causes of illness or disorder.

Age equivalent
Comes from the use of standardised tests and refers to the average age at which children receive a given score. Thus, a five-year-old receives a score equivalent to that of a three-year-old. The concept is widely used by therapists but we have to be careful in interpreting what it means. A five-year-old and a ten-year-old with an age-equivalent score of a three-year-old are unlikely to use language in the same way.

Aided systems of communication
Those requiring additional resources such as photographs, computers, etc. These augmentative types of communicaiton may be high or low tech. There is a contrast with unaided systems, e.g. signs, body posture, gesture, etc.

Alternative and Augmentative Communication (AAC)
The different systems that can be introduced to augment or enhance the child's communication skills. These may be manual, sign systems, technological aids or communication boards. These supplement the child's skills and are not intended to replace them.

Articulation
The process of using the tongue, lips, jaw and vocal folds to produce speech sounds. It refers to the child's ability to move the articulators in the mouth as opposed to the ability to plan an utterance in the brain.

Articulators
The moving parts in the mouth: tongue, lips, soft palate and the sphincter linking the oral and nasal cavities.

Assistive listening device (ALD)
An electronic device for improving speech and understanding in noisy listening settings, such as classrooms. A personal ALD consists of a microphone, an FM transmitter, an FM receiver and some type of earphone. The speaker, e.g. teacher, wears the microphone and transmitter, while the listener, e.g. student, wears the receiver and earphones. Amplifying ALDs are used by children with peripheral hearing losses. A no-gain (no-amplification) device is sometimes prescribed for children with CAPD to facilitate their ability to communicate in the classroom setting. With a classroom ALD, the speaker's voice is transmitted to high-fidelity loud speakers, rather than individual earphones.

Audiogram
A graph for displaying the results of a simple hearing test. The patient's hearing threshold levels in deciBels (dB) are plotted for six to eight audiometric test frequencies (octave frequencies from 250 to 8000 Hz).

Auditory brainstem response (ABR or BAER)
A non-invasive electrophysiologic measure of auditory system function. Sound stimulation, e.g. very brief clicking sounds, are presented to a patient via earphones. Small electrical potentials generated in response to the sounds by the eighth (auditory) nerve and auditory centres in the brainstem are detected by electrodes placed on the scalp and on the earlobes. ABR recording requires computerised auditory evoked response instrumentation. The ABR is commonly used as a hearing screening technique and to estimate hearing sensitivity or detect neurologic auditory dysfunction in infants and children.

Auditory evoked responses
Electrical potentials generated by regions of the auditory nervous system by sound stimulation (usually clicks or tones). Auditory evoked responses in clinical use include the auditory brainstem response (ABR), electrocochleography (ECochG) and auditory middle latency response (AMLR).

Auditory discrimination
The process of distinguishing differences among sounds.

Auditory memory
The process of encoding, storing and recalling what has been heard.

Auditory middle latency response (AMLR)
A non-invasive electrophysiologic measure of auditory system function. Sound stimulation, e.g. clicking sounds or tones, are presented to a patient via earphones. Electrical potentials generated in response to the sounds by the auditory thalamus and cortex are detected by electrodes placed on the scalp and on the earlobes. AMLR recording requires computerised auditory evoked response instrumentation.

Central auditory nervous system
Auditory nuclei and pathways in the brainstem (pons and midbrain), the thalamus and the cerebrum.

Central auditory processing disorders (CAPD)
A diagnosis given following non-invasive electrophysiologic measure of auditory system function. Sound stimulation, e.g. very brief clicking sounds, are presented to a patient via earphones. Small electrical potentials generated in response to the sounds by the eighth (auditory) nerve and auditory centres in the brainstem are detected by electrodes placed on the scalp and on the earlobes. ABR recording requires computerised auditory evoked response instrumentation. The ABR is commonly used as a hearing screening technique, and to estimate hearing sensitivity or to detect neurologic auditory dysfunction in infants and children.

Children Act (1989)
UK legislation drawing together all the existing legislation designed to protect the rights of the child. It emphasises the role played by the family and stresses the need to work through the family in all but the most exceptional of cases. The role of children in care and the need for the recognition of the needs of children with developmental and medical difficulties are highlighted. It stresses the need for interagency collaboration particularly between social, health and educational agencies.

Circumlocution
A 'roundabout' way of speaking when a person cannot recall a specific word for an object, action or event, e.g. shovel – that digging thing.

Code of Practice
Department for Education guidance published in 1994 for children with special educational needs to which schools, health authorities and social services have a statutory duty to 'have regard'.

Cognitive processsses
Mental processes conceived with thinking and understanding.

Cognitive referencing
The comparison of a student's score on a measure of language ability to the score obtained on a measure of cognitive ability (IQ).

Communication

The process of transferring messages from a speaker to a listener, or from a writer to a reader by means of a standard code, e.g. speech, signing language, etc.

Communication Aid Centres

Established by health or education authorities, or can be independently funded. They typically offer multi-agency assessment. Some focus on communication for learning, e.g. computers and the relevant softwear, and others carry out a complete assessment of a person's educational, social, leisure, etc. communication needs.

Comprehension

Verbal: The child's ability to comprehend the spoken word. Therapists always assess verbal comprehension to ensure that this is not at the root of the child's difficulties. Such assessments are often very structured in order to cut out extraneous clues which might help the child answer the questions.

Non-verbal: All the other ways in which children use the context to understand what someone is saying. Typically, this would be pointing and eye-pointing to requested objects, facial expressions, gestures, etc. It is very important to establish to what extent children are using such clues.

Conductive hearing loss

A temporary and often fluctuating hearing loss associated with infection or blockage in the middle ear, i.e. immediately inside the ear drum.

Content of language

We speak of the form, content and use of language. Content refers to the child's intended meaning. Does the child have a range of such meanings – requesting, denying, etc – at his disposal? If not, this may be a focus of intervention.

Developmental delay

This means that development in one or more areas is following the normal developmental pattern but at a slower rate than would be expected for his/her chronological age. Usually contrasted with a **disorder**, a term which suggests that the development is not following a normal developmental pattern.

Dichotic digits test

A test of central auditory nervous system function in which sets of two different numbers are presented to each ear simultaneously (two numbers to one ear and two numbers to the other ear). The patient repeats at least 20 sets of numbers, and the percentage of correct responses is calculated for each ear, and compared to age-corrected normative data. The term 'dichotic' refers to the simultaneous presentation of different sounds to the two ears.

Dichotic sentence identification (DSI)
A test of central auditory nervous system function in which two different nonsense sentences are presented to each ear simultaneously. The patient has a list of the sentences, each numbered, and identifies the two sentences heard from the list by number. Then the percentage of correct responses is calculated for each ear and compared to age-corrected normative data. The term 'dichotic' refers to the simultaneous presentation of different sounds to the two ears.

Didactic intervention approaches
Where the child is given a model by the adult who makes a direct attempt to elicit the production of the modelled item by the child.

Differential diagnosis
The process by which the doctor or therapist ascertains the nature of the child's problems by excluding other conditions.

Dysfluency
A condition where speech is produced with hesitations or repetitions that interrupt the usual flow of speech. Some dysfluency is normal within preschool speech and language development.

Dyspraxia
A diagnostic term intended for use with children who have difficulties planning what they intend to say. The effect is highly unintelligible speech. The children can often produce sounds in isolation but they become increasingly difficult to understand as they try to put the sounds into words and then into sentences.

Echolalia
Restatement or echoing of the previous speaker's utterance.

Expressive language
Language produced by the speaker: spoken words, phrases, sentences, paragraphs and stories. In contrast to receptive language.

Fluency
The ease and smoothness with which speech or language is produced.

Form of language
We speak of the form, content and use of language. Form refers to the outward aspects of language, the sounds, syntax and way in which words are modified to change their meanings, e.g. plural or verb endings.

Generalisation
The extent to which behaviours learned in one context can be transferred to another context or to other behaviours or stimuli, i.e. the use of trained behaviour in untrained situations.

Grammar
Often seen as meaning the same as syntax, the study of the rules for forming words and linking words to form sentences.

Graphic symbols
Representations of objects, events, feelings, etc. in stylised picture form.

Hearing level (HL)
A decibel (dB) scale used in audiometry. For example, 0 dB HL is the intensity level for tones or speech that is just audible to young, normal hearing persons. Any child who does not respond to sounds at intensity levels of 20 dB HL or greater has a hearing loss.

Hybrid intervention approaches
A combination of didactic and naturalistic approaches, such as milieu therapy.

Immittance (aural) measurement
Electrophysiologic audiologic technique for measuring the impedance to or admittance of energy flow through the eardrum and middle ear. Immittance measurement provides diagnostic information on the peripheral auditory system in children and adults. One commonly used immittance measurement is tympanometry.

Inclusive education
An approach to education that allows all students with disabilities to attend their home schools and become members of a regular class while receiving individual adaptations and support.

Integration
A term first introduced into law in 1981 to refer to the need for children with special needs to be kept within their classroom to mix with their peers. Often easier to talk about than carry out. The children's needs should be carefully considered in each case.

Kinaesthetic method
Using muscle movements, such as writing a letter in sand, to support auditory and visual stimuli to help dyslexics with reading and spelling.

Language
The set of symbols (usually words or signs) which are organised by convention to communicate ideas.

Comprehension: It is always important to be aware how a child makes use of what they understand of the non-linguistic context to help them understand what others are saying.

Delay: A term used to suggest that the child's language level is equivalent to that of a younger child and is usually contrasted with disorder. Recent research work suggests that the majority of children with language impairments fit into this category. It is probably most widely used up to the early school years. Thereafter, the child's experience is likely to mean that they will have very little in common with a child whose tested language levels are similar.

Disorder: Contrasted with delay (*see above*) and suggests that there is something abnormal about the child's language development above and beyond the delay. Such conditions become much more apparent as the child gets older.

Impairment: A generic term referring to all clinical levels of language difficulty. It suggests that there is something structurally different about the way the child responds to language which distinguishes him/her from 'normal' language learners.

Learning disability (LD): A developmental language disorder associated with learning disabilities, generally discovered after the child has failed to achieve academic expectations for age and intelligence.

Production: The child's capacity to express him/herself. Conventionally, this refers to speech but it can equally apply to the child's use of augmentative systems.

Processing: The process of hearing, discriminating, assigning significance to and interpreting spoken words, phrases, clauses, sentences and discourse.

Units: Children with pronounced speech and language impairments are sometimes placed within language units that provide specialist teaching and therapy. Units are usually set within mainstream schools and may be referred to as language classes or resource bases.

Learning difficulty/learning disability
Generalised reduction in cognitive abilities which usually impacts on language development (UK usage).

Linguistic comprehension
The ability to understand using only the language cues and language knowledge.

Mainstream school
Schools which have not been set up to provide specifically for children with special needs. They are usually contrasted with 'special schools'.

Mean length of utterance (MLU)
The average sentence length conventionally determined from a sample of utterances.

Metacognitive
The deliberate, conscious awareness of processes involved in thinking, creating, reasoning, problem solving and decision making.

Metalinguistics
A speaker's ability to think about the units and rules of language.

Mismatch negativity (MMN) response
An auditory evoked response generated by high levels of the central auditory nervous system (probably the hippocampus and auditory cortex) in response to sound stimulation, and detected non-invasively by electrodes on the scalp and ears. Two important clinical advantages of the MMN are that it can be stimulated by complex speech stimuli, and can be recorded from even very young children.

Modelling
Where the child is asked to listen while the adult produces an example (model) of a target.

Naturalistic intervention approaches
Where the adult responds to the child's focus of attention rather than imposing a different context specifically for intervention.

Neurodevelopmental
Descriptive term for the maturing neurological systems of the child, for example, motor skills and perception.

Norm-referenced measure
A score from a test that has been standardised on a population.

Otoacoustic emissions (OAE)
Sounds produced by outer hair cells in the cochlea (the inner ear) and detected by a microphone placed in a probe within the ear canal. OAE are recorded non-invasively, usually in response to acoustic stimuli, e.g. clicks or tones. Two types of OAE most often used clinically are transient evoked OAE (TEOAE) and distortion product OAE (DPOAE).

Parenthetical remarks *see* **Circumlocution**

Paediatric speech intelligibility (PSI) test
A test of central auditory nervous system function designed for use in the preschool paediatric population. A unique feature of the PSI is that the child's language age is taken into account in scoring the results.

Peripheral auditory system
The outer, middle and inner ear (cochlea), and eighth (auditory) cranial nerve.

Pharyngoplasty
An operation in which the size of the gap between the mouth and the nose (velopharyngeal isthmus) is narrowed surgically. There are a number of different techniques. In the dynamic pharyngoplasty (Orticochea or Hynes), little muscles from the side of the pharynx are wrapped round the back of the pharynx. This narrows the isthmus but, once healed, it is able to relax and contract, thus opening the isthmus wider for normal breathing and narrowing it for speech. In another type of pharyngoplasty a broad strip of mucosa from the posterior wall of the pharynx is brought across the velopharyngeal isthmus and sewn to the back of the soft palate narrowing it considerably. There is no muscle in it, so it is called a static pharyngoplasty.

Phonology
The rules which allow children to perceive and produce the differences between sounds in a highly regular manner. These rules are usually acquired in the first three or four years of life although the speed at which they can mark these differences varies considerably.

Phonological processing
The relationship between speech sound production (articulation) and higher level language processing abilities involving pragmatic, semantic and syntactic levels of language organisation.

Picture communication symbols
One of a number of commercially available systems.

Pitch pattern sequence (PPS) test
A test of central auditory nervous system function involving the identification of the pitch (high or low) of a sequence of three tones. The patient's correct percentage score in the identification of at least 40 sets of tone patterns is calculated, and compared to age-corrected normative data.

Pragmatics
The set of rules used by a language community or culture for communicating messages in natural contexts. The ability to use language in context as both a speaker and a listener: what is said and the way that it is perceived.

Pre-linguistic skills
Skills which are foundational for language development, including babbling, taking turns in simple play, eye contact, visual and auditory attention.

Probes
A series of questions or cues used to explore a child's ability to elaborate following an initial response. Probes may be used to explore comprehension, thought processes or learning potential.

Prompting
Where the child is encouraged to imitate or produce specific targets by means of questions or commands by the adult.

Prosody
The melody of speech determined by patterns in stress and intonation.

Pure tone audiometry
A simple hearing test using a calibrated audiometer in which the patient hears tones at octave frequencies of 250 Hz up to 8000 Hz. Tones are presented one at a time, first to one ear and then to the other via standardised earphones. At each test frequency, the instensity level of the tone is systematically decreased and then increased until the patient's threshold is determined. Hearing thresholds are then plotted in dB on an audiogram. Pure tone audiometry is conducted in a sound-treated room.

P300 response
An auditory evoked response generated by regions of the central auditory nervous system (probably the hippocampus and auditory cortex) in response to sound stimulation (tones), and detected non-invasively by electrodes on the scalp and ears. The P300 response, first described in 1965, has been studied in CAPD and extensively in adults with neurologic or psychiatric disorders.

Raw score
Used when counting the number of correct responses on a standardised test. It is contrasted with the standard score which refers to the child's score compared to what would be expected for the child's age.

Rebus
One of a number of commercially available symbol systems.

Receptive language
The understanding of spoken or read words, phrases, sentences, paragraphs or stories. In contrast to expressive language. Also referred to as 'verbal comprehension'.

Reinforcement
Where a correct performance by the child is rewarded by praise or a tangible reward.

SCAN
A well-designed test for screening school-age children for CAPD. Results on three subtests (filtered words, dichotic words, words in noise) are compared to age-corrected normative data. The SCAN is not a diagnostic audiologic procedure.

Semantics
The set of rules that govern the meaning of words, word combinations and grammatical structures in language.

Semantic pragmatic disorder
A specific diagnostic label used for a group of children who have great difficulty in holding a conversation. They may talk at length but they find interaction very challenging, often because they find it difficult to understand what their conversational partner has said or what he/she really means by what he/she has said. Now taken to be an autism spectrum disorder.

Semantic word errors
The use of inappropriate words due to a problem in understanding the semantic relationships or functional attributes of the word, e.g. my dress is too tall [long].

Sentence completion task
A task in which the child is expected to fill in the last word of a sentence that has been constructed, so that there are few possible correct response options.

Speech
The meaningful articulation of sounds.
Speech audiometry: Measurement of a person's threshold for words (described in dB), or a person's ability to identify correctly words or sentences (described in percentage correct). Speech audiometry is usually conducted for each ear separately via earphones using commercially available tape-recorded materials. *See* **Staggered spondaic word (SSW) test.**
Speech and language delay: A broad descriptive term for speech and language abilities which are considered to be below that expected for a child's chronological age, while still following the expected developmental sequence. Often qualified as mild, moderate or severe.
Speech and language disorder: A broad descriptive term for speech and language abilities which are considered to be developing in a manner distinct from the usual developmental sequence. May be further qualified by noting those aspects of speech and language most affected: semantics, pragmatics, phonology, syntax.
Speech and language impairment: A general term for a speech and language problem, whether this is diagnosed as a delay or a disorder.

Spontaneous language sample
A sample of spontaneous language usage in natural context that has been transcribed for analysis.

Staggered spondaic word (SSW) test
A dichotic test of central auditory nervous system function in which sets of two different words are presented to each ear simultaneously (one word to one ear and another to the other ear). The patient repeats at least 40 sets of words, and the percentage of correct responses is calculated for each ear and compared to age-corrected normative data.

Standardised tests
Tests developed on a representative sample of subjects. It is then possible to compare a given child's response to the test in question with that original sample. This allows us to calculate a number of ways of describing that child: standard score, age equivalent, percentile rank, etc.

Standard score
The single most important score derived from a standardised test, this allows you to express the child's performance in terms of where it comes relative to the group of children on whom the test was originally developed. The average on such tests is normally taken as 100 and the child's performance may be expressed as a function of the number of 'standard deviations' from the average (usually 15 points) or as a single score.

Statement of Special Educational Needs
A legal document to which parents and professionals contribute. This describes the child's special educational needs and the resources and provision required to meet those needs.

Syntax
The rules for combining words into phrases and sentences concerning grammatical structures.

Synthetic sentence identification (SSI)
A central auditory test in which the patient identifies nonsense sentences presented at the same time as a competing message, e.g. a story about Davy Crockett. The patient has a list of 10 sentences, each numbered, and identifies the sentences heard from the list by number. Then the percentage of correct responses is calculated for each ear and compared to age-corrected normative data. Difficulty of the SSI is manipulated by increasing the intensity level of the competition (the story) relative to the signal (the sentences).

Tangentiality
A response that is similar to the topic but is not the same.

Treatment
An explicit application of therapeutic/educational techniques intended to modify an individual's performance in a designated area associated with communication, i.e. expressive language, attention, etc.

Tympanometry
A measure of middle ear compliance (flexibility) as a function of change in air pressure in the ear canal. Tympanometry is a very sensitive technique for assessment of the middle ear. Patterns of abnormalities in tympanogram shape are associated with different middle ear disorders. Tympanometry is not a test of hearing, e.g. a child with a severe or profound sensory hearing loss may have a normal tympanogram.

Use of language
We speak of the form, content and use of language. Use of language is comparable to the term pragmatics (*see above*) and refers to the child's ability to use language in context.

Velopharyngeal incompetence (VPI)/velopharyngeal dysfunction (VPD)
A condition where, despite the conscious efforts of the speaker, air escapes through the nose when normally it should not. This causes muffled, indistinct or unintelligible speech.

VOCA
Voice output communication aid.

Index

assessment 110
developmental surveillance 49–51
impairment 19–20, 22
  diagnostic criteria 25
  differential diagnosis 26
  prediction 40
  traumatic brain injury 294
specific language impairment 156, 157
expressive language learners 23
expressive-receptive language disorder 25–6
extremely low birth weight (ELBW) children 82

family context 80–1
family history 83
Fast ForWord 212
fast mapping 12
fathers
  alcoholism 179
  with communication difficulties 40
  smoking during fetal development 40
feeding
  assessment 97
  difficulties
    cerebral palsy 222–3
    developmental surveillance 49
fenfluramine 193
Fetal Alchol Syndrome 81
fetal growth retardation 82
fluency
  assessment 114–15
  model of communication 7
  problems 20, 22–3, 114
    see also stammering
  spina bifida 252
Fluharty Preschool Speech and Language
  Screening Test 65
focal arteritis in temporal lobe(s) 266
focused simulation intervention 147
folic acid 81
food sensitivity 83, 85
formal assessment 94–5
  case study 99
  considerations 95–6
  linguistic skills 106–8, 109–10, 111, 113,
    115
  multicultural context 127
  underpinning abilities 100, 101, 102, 104,
    105
Fragile X syndrome
  autism, association with 188

case study 70–1
  macrocephaly 83
free field audiometry 248
fricative consonants 18
fundi, examination 84

gender factors 81
  and assessment 96
  Attention Deficit Disorder 180, 181
  autism 188
  behavioural difficulties 202
  cleft lip and palate 228, 229
  convulsive disorders 266
  learning disability 260
  Selective Mutism 274
general practitioners (GPs)
  impoverished children 285–6
  role 72, 73
genetic factors
  Attention Deficit Disorder 179
  autism 188
  behavioural difficulties 202
  cleft lip and palate 228
  consanguinity 125
  convulsive disorders 266
  development of communication 14–15
  dyslexia 235–6
  hearing loss 243–4
  investigation 86
  learning disability 259
  Selective Mutism 274
gestures
  autism 191
  developmental surveillance 50
glue ear *see* otitis media with effusion
gluten sensitivity 83, 85
glycosaminoglycans 85
Goldman–Fristoe–Woodcock Test 216
grammatical forms 51
  understanding
    assessment 107
    specific language impairment 157
  use
    assessment 111
    autism 192
    spina bifida 252
grommets 245
growth 83

Haemophilus b (Hib) vaccination 75